THE HIDDEN ZOO INSIDE YOU

An illustrated guide to pesky organisms and pandemics

Hand-written and drawn by

DR. ALLEN JONES, M.D.

GRANVILLE ISLAND PUBLISHING

Publisher's Cataloging-in-Publication data

Names: Jones, Allen Sohrab, author.
Title: The hidden zoo inside you : an illustrated guide to pesky organisms and pandemics / handwritten and drawn by Allen Jones, M.D.
Description: Includes bibliographical references and index. | Vancouver, BC, Canada: Granville Island Publishing, 2024.
Identifiers: ISBN: 9781989467664 (paperback) | 9781989467725 (hardcover) | 9781989467671 (ebook)
Subjects: LCSH Microbiology—Comic books, strips, etc.. | Microorganisms—Comic books, strips, etc. | Infectious diseases—Comic books, strips, etc. | Graphic novels. | BISAC COMICS & GRAPHIC NOVELS / Nonfiction / Science & Nature | HEALTH & FITNESS / Diseases & Conditions / Contagious (incl. Pandemics) | SCIENCE / Life Sciences / Virology
Classification: LCC QR57 .J66 2024 | DDC 579—dc23

Editor: Ed Zegarra
Proofreader: Antoinette Mazumdar
Book designer: Omar Gallegos

Granville Island Publishing Ltd.

604-688-0320 / 1-877-688-0320
info@granvilleislandpublishing.com
www.granvilleislandpublishing.com

DISCLAIMER: THIS IS INFORMATION ONLY. THIS IS NOT MEDICAL ADVICE. TALK TO YOUR DOCTOR REGARDING ANY HEALTH CONCERNS.

In memory of

Dr. Albert Otis Bush (1948-2010)
  Professor of Parasitolgy
  Department of Zoology
  Brandon University
  Brandon, Manitoba, Canada

What you taught me was:

  This is not intended to be easy.
  There is no curve.
  If you all fail, that is your problem.

  Do the work. Do it quietly.
  Do it without complaint.

  Create a safe space for people to
      ask questions.

  There is majesty in all living things.

- I am SOMPOO. I am your guide. You will learn a ton of stuff. Oh, and I like hyphens.

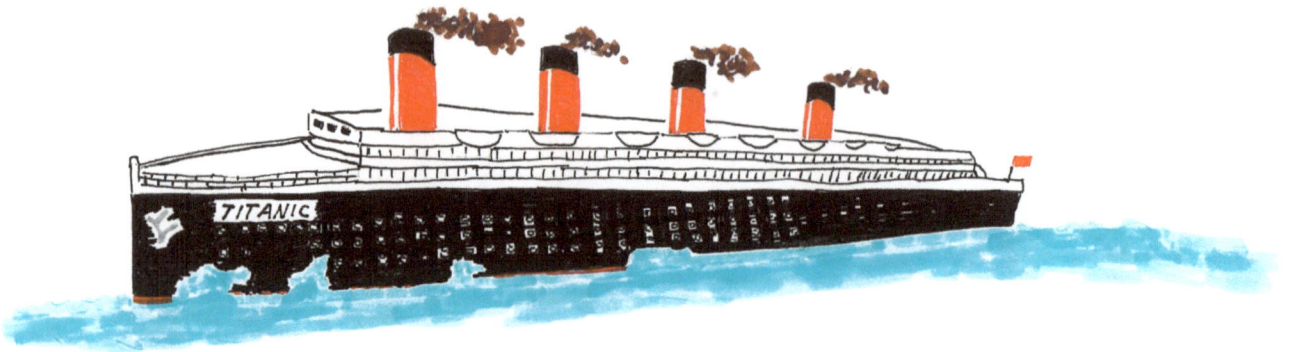

- If you were asked, "Why did the Titanic sink?", what background information would you need?

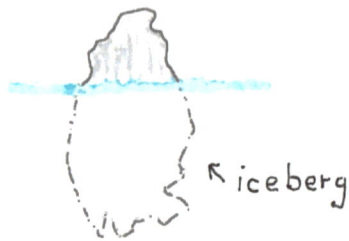

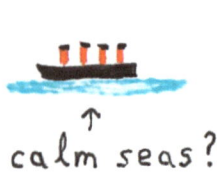

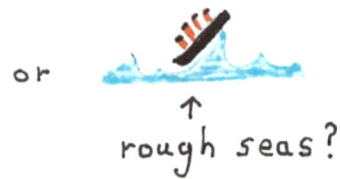

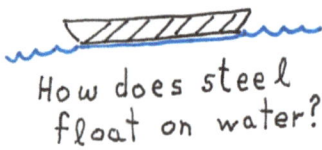

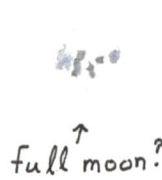

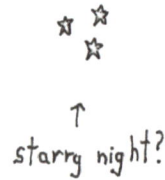

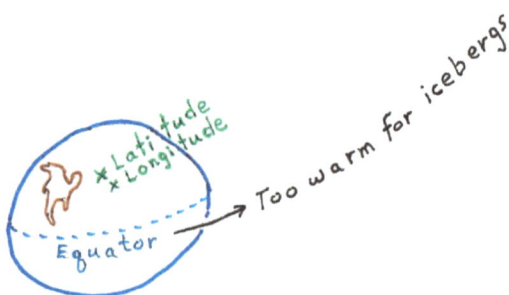

← iceberg

calm seas?   or   rough seas?

How does steel float on water?

full moon?   or   starry night?   or   fog?

x Latitude
x Longitude

Equator

→ Too warm for icebergs

omg

This wasn't mentioned in the brochure

← Kraken

dash dot

Morse code →

C
Come

Q
Quickly

D
Danger

"This is Titanic. CQD. Engine room flooded."

S
Save

O
Our

S
Souls

←(Only became popular after Titanic sank)

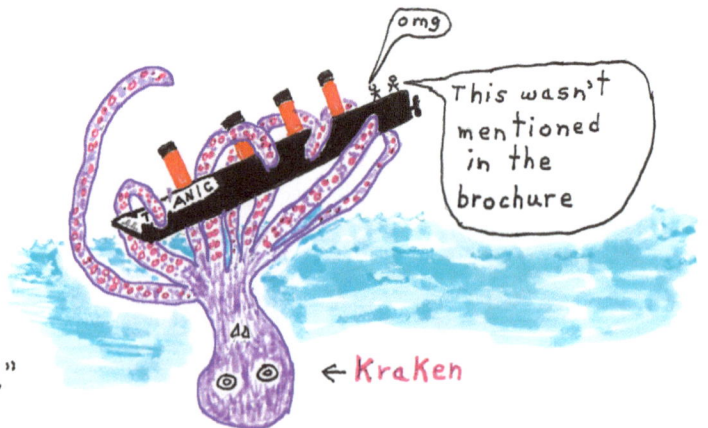

- A good investigator considers all possibilities

The Hidden Zoo Inside You is Allen Jones's fascinating, funny illustrated guide to microscopic organisms and the problems they can create. … Stuffed with an incredible amount of information, every page is enlightening … Warmth, humor, and enthusiasm permeate the hand-drawn and lettered book. … the net result is an effective and entertaining means of education. … *The Hidden Zoo Inside You* is a thorough, understandable graphic history of microbes and disease, presenting facts with a unique and appealing visual style.

— *Foreword Reviews*

Jones' artwork features hand-drawn sketches, accompanied by an array of in-the-margins notes that recall Randall Munroe's popular webcomic *xkcd*. … occasionally comedic … Each page in this manual contains a plethora of information, … there is a definite sense of thoroughness to the work that makes it unnecessary to be an expert in the subject matter to follow its many explanations. …. Like any good work of comic art, the subject dictates the reader's pace, and this is certainly a resource that one should take time to pore over and not rush through. Accompanying all of this historical information is the author's playful sense of humor. An expansive and informative epidemiological look at viruses.

— *Kirkus Reviews*

This is a monumental project admirably accomplished by a family physician … Medical and scientific jargon is either avoided or skillfully explained. … The content is surprisingly broad and detailed … The historical facts and scientific background have been well researched, and complex issues are clearly explained in layperson's terms for the non-medical reader. This book is primarily targeting teens and lay adults but is also a welcome review for healthcare professionals dealing with infectious diseases. The enlightening illustrations accompanied by ample humor make this volume much more interesting reading than cut and dried medical or scientific papers.

— Dr. Anthony W. Chow MD, FRCPC, FACP
Professor Emeritus
The University of British Columbia

A delightful approach to introducing complex scientific and technical subjects through sketches, diagrams, charts, even doodles! There's something in these pages for everyone, young and old, and you don't need to start at the beginning! Just open the book at any page; plunge in; and enjoy the drawings, the humour, and especially the puns while absorbing fascinating descriptions of the processes and criteria that contribute to epidemic illnesses, infections, diseases, remedies, parasites, and preventions. It's all here, and a lot more besides; don't be surprised if the route takes you through entomology, engineering, and meteorology! Enjoy the ride!

— Tim Sly, DPHI(UK), MSc, PhD(UK), CPHI(C)
Professor Emeritus (Epidemiology)
Toronto Metropolitan University

(Suggested) Options for reading this guide

Cut to the chase and head straight to the Coronavirus

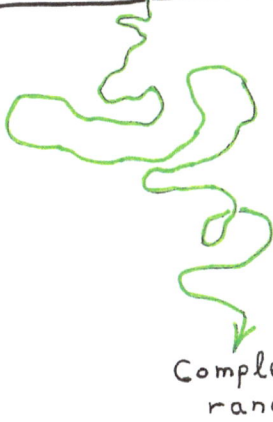

page 111

Completely random

Sort of random

Old School

Page 1 → Page 189
START   END

Just Keep on turning the pages

Dracula p.109

Cat-lover's page 72

Volcanoes
page 165-167

Lots o' bats
page 114-128

Check out my cool skeleton

Bronx Zoo lions p.133

Megalodon p. 16

p. 93
Virus ATTACK!

pangolin p.126

Bat skeleton p.114

Is a virus considered Life?
page 57

SMALLPOX page 21

BUBONIC PLAGUE + BLACK DEATH
page 9-14

Wuhan + Wuhan Institute of Virology
page 3-6

page, um, let me think ...I furget

Zombies

Anthrax p.58

R.I.P. - What Kills humans? p.38

N95 mask → page 155

Ebola. Eeek!
p. 18-20

TORCH infections during Pregnancy
page 84

1918 (Spanish) Influenza and the Amazing Alaska Roadtrip
pages 22-29

GANGRENE
p. 61

Typhoid Mary p.59

I have 1 hump
Camels p.125, p.138

FLESH-EATING DISEASE p.66

Old Yeller p.100

River Blindness 77 78 79

raindrops (p.165)

slurp, slurp
Tapeworms page 80

METRIC SYSTEM FOR NEWBIES p. 53

♀ - Are viruses real? Can they really spread to the whole world?

♂ - A question to your question. What is this?

♀ - A can of soup.

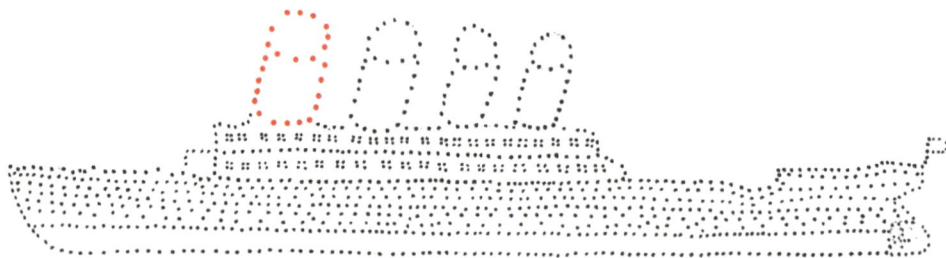

♂ - That was the correct <u>conclusion</u> based on 25 dots. But you need 975 more dots to get the right <u>answer</u>. It's the funnel of a ship.

` The answer to your virus questions requires more dots than you currently possess.

CONTENTS

♀ - Wait a second, you want
    me to melt Greenland?

♀ - Imagine the things
    we could learn.

☻ - There is way more
    detail on each chapter
    on the next pages

CHAPTER 1
THE COLD, HARD FACTS OF DEATH AND DISEASE

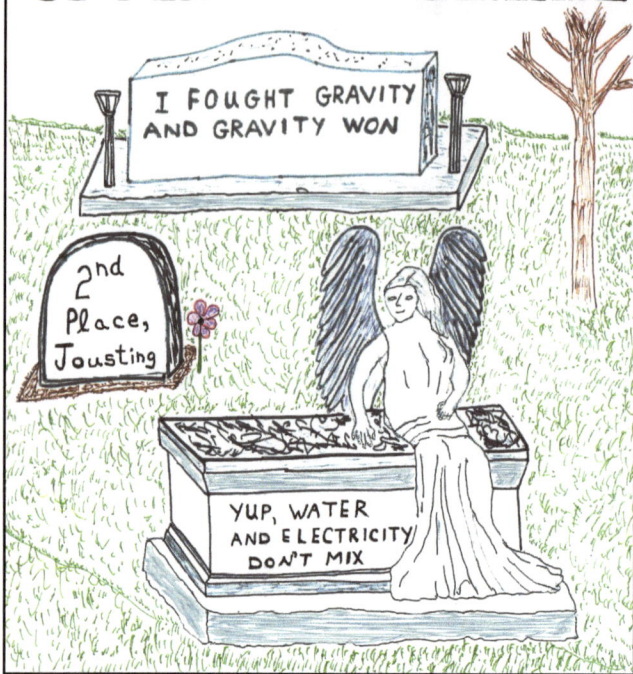

I FOUGHT GRAVITY AND GRAVITY WON

2nd Place, Jousting

YUP, WATER AND ELECTRICITY DON'T MIX

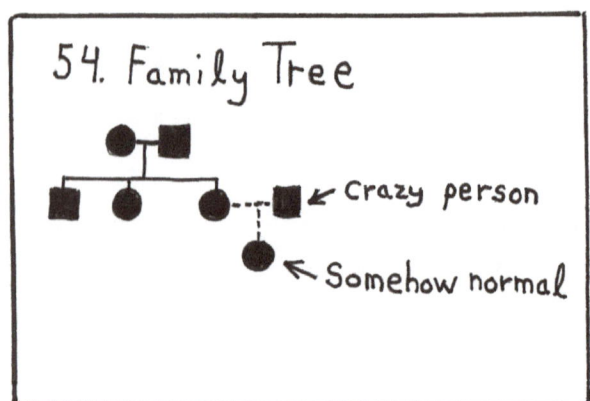

← Crazy person

← Somehow normal

Chapter 3
Meet the Viruses

Across

1   2   3   **Down**

1   2

```
¹C O R O N A V I R U ²S
   A                  M
 ²E B O L A           A
   I                  L
   E                  L
   S         ³P H A G E
             O
             X
```

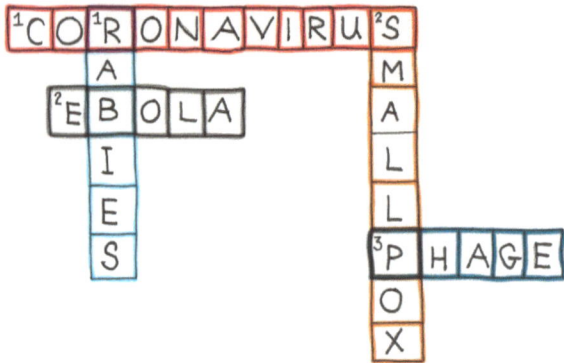

90. Pause for Station Identification

91. Virus versus Cell
92. Viral Geometry
93. Bacteriophages infect bacteria
    I ♡ this word
94. Matryoshka virus: From Russia with Love
95. Rembrandt Tulip-Breaking Virus.
    Say again?
96. Orsay virus: From France with Love

97.   Special Guest Appearance

98. 20 (twenty) viruses of humans.
  ☿ - Um, since there are 219 viruses
      that infect humans, isn't that
      a Short List?
          `Hello, viruses`
  ☿ - Affirmative

99. Polio virus
100. Rabies virus

101-110   `BATS ON TRIAL`
        ↳Rabies Inquest
101. State Your Full Name
102. JAWS
103. Vampire bat
104. What are fangs?
105. Bram Stoker's *Dracula*
106. ⎫ 99 dogs : 1 bat
107. ⎭
108. The Most Important Book
109. HOLLYWOOD
110. Reduction to absurdity

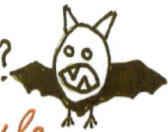

Chapter 4

Coronavirus –
it has more personality
than you thought

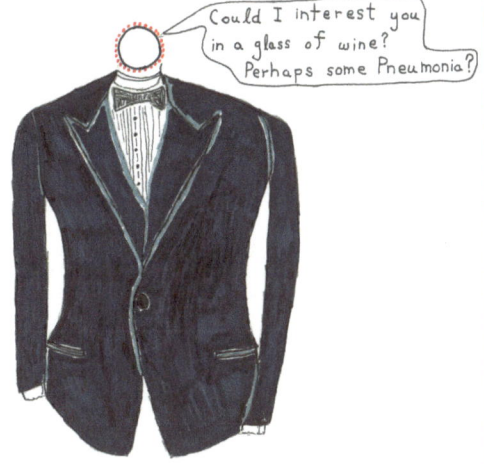

Could I interest you in a glass of wine? Perhaps some Pneumonia?

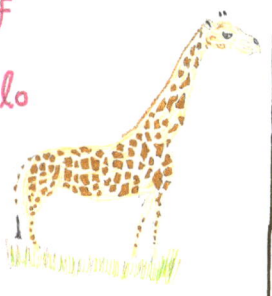

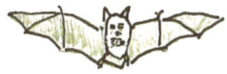

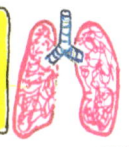

CHAPTER 5

THE **HORRENDOUSLY** CONFUSING 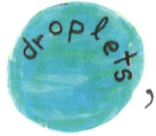 WORLD OF droplets, aerosols,

P.A.R.T.I.C.L.E.S, 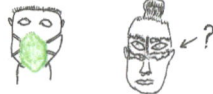 MASKS, ←?

AND SOCIAL DISTANCING.

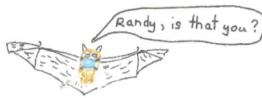 Randy, is that you?

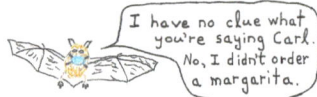 I have no clue what you're saying Carl. No, I didn't order a margarita.

CHAPTER 6
OMG WHAT A DISASTER

WHAT CAN THE TITANIC,

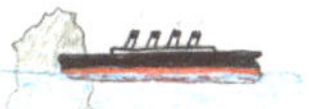

A NUCLEAR ACCIDENT,

A PLANE CRASH,

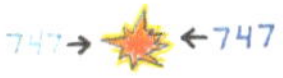

AND COW INTESTINES

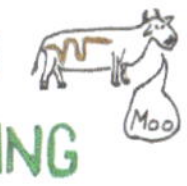

TEACH US ABOUT MANAGING

A PANDEMIC?

How huge?

Seriously huge

HUGE

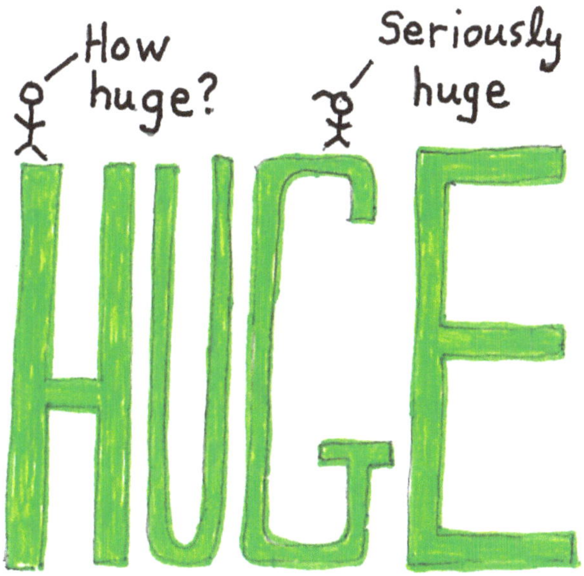

Want more information? There is a huge bibliography on allenjonesmd.com where the key points of every source used in this guide are summarized in bulleted points.

You may not know this, but you can memorize vast amounts of information using the simple tools described on page 189.

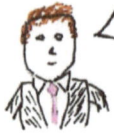

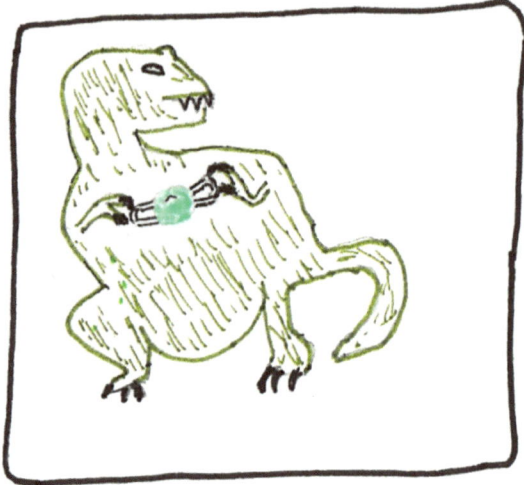

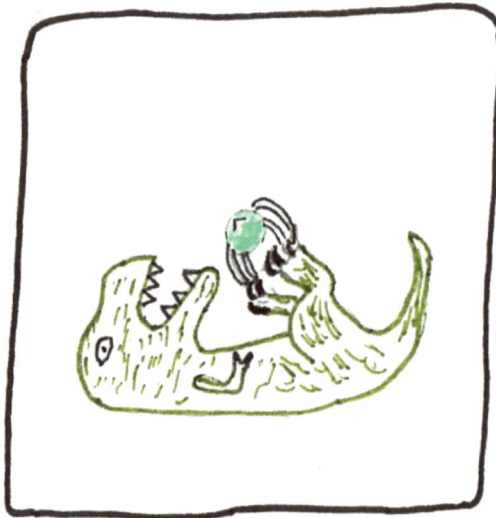

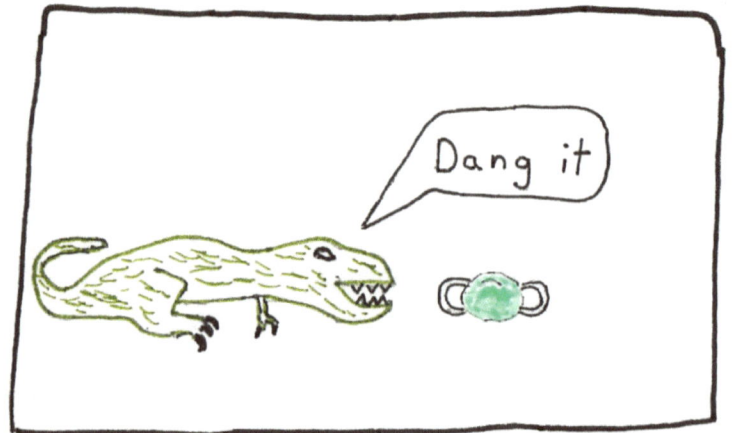

T. rex was killed by Coronavirus because its itty-bitty arms were too short to put a mask on its face.

CHAPTER 1
THE COLD, HARD FACTS
OF DEATH AND DISEASE

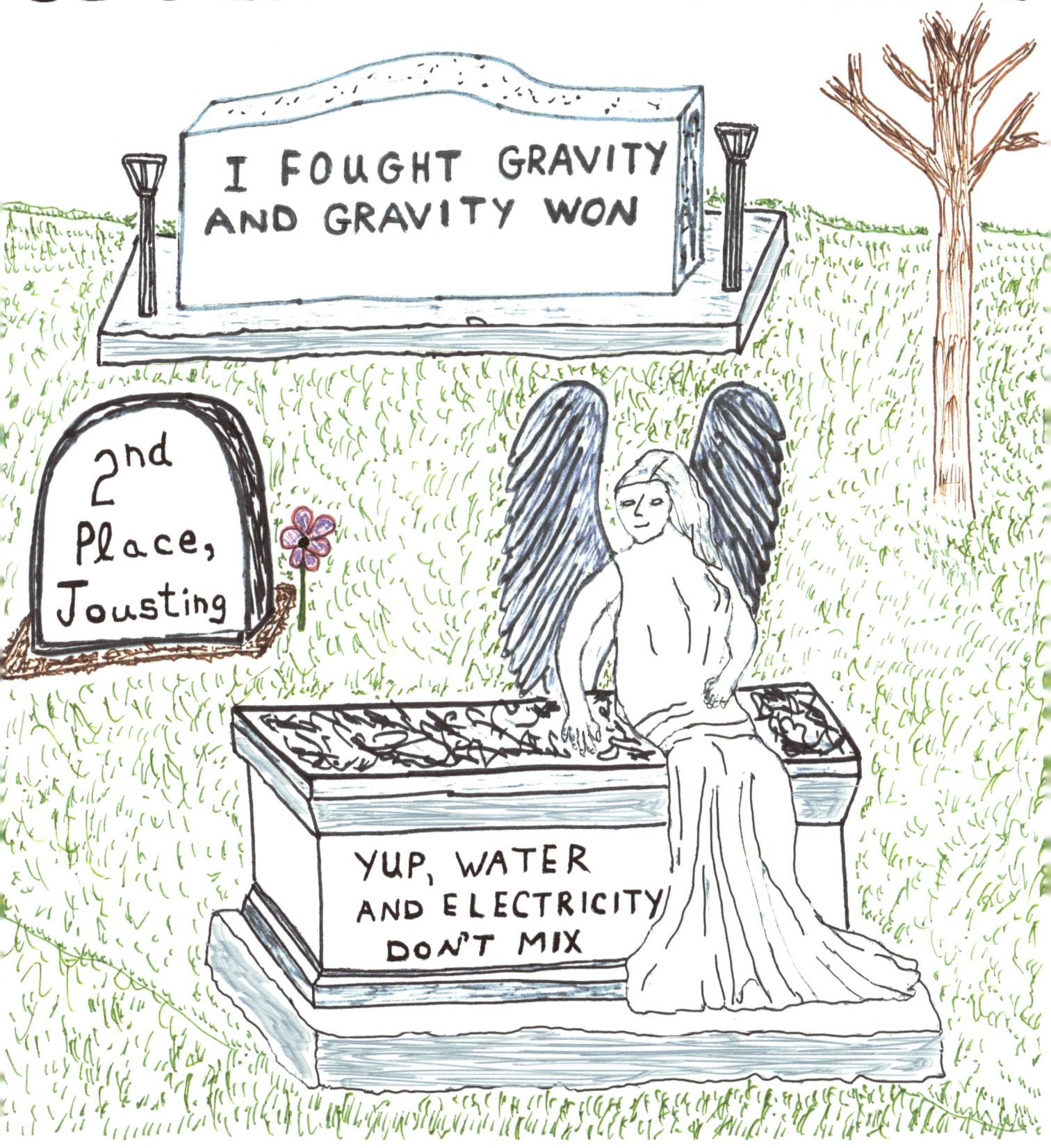

I FOUGHT GRAVITY
AND GRAVITY WON

2nd
Place,
Jousting

YUP, WATER
AND ELECTRICITY
DON'T MIX

- If we agree on definitions, life is a bit easier

Endemic
= Constant presence of disease (for example, Malaria) in this community or region.

Epidemic
= Sudden increase in disease above what is expected.

Pardon me, would you have any Gray Poupon?

← Billionaire on superyacht

← Emperor penguin 4 feet tall

- Is that a flat Earth?
- Yes. The other side has no coronavirus.

Pandemic
= the epidemic spreads to other countries or continents.

- Epidemiology is the study of patterns of disease.

  - This is what the folks at the CDC (Centers for Disease Control and Prevention) do all day, every day.

    This is good   This is better

"Epid ee me all aw jee"

SOMPOO SAYS

Hollywood Outbreak

OUTBREAK (2005, Warner Brothers)

"We got 19 dead, 100 more infected. It's spreading like a bush fire."

Dustin Hoffman (trying to prevent outbreak from turning into a pandemic)

Outbreak: Motaba River village

- An 'outbreak' is an Epidemic in a limited geographic area.

Real Outbreak : ☼ Coronavirus

Origin : Seafood market, Wuhan, Hubei, China
          city   province country

"A novel coronavirus from patients with pneumonia in China"
New England Journal of Medicine
24 January 2020
Authors: Zhu et al
                    'and others' (Latin)

Patient #1: 49 year-old ♀ (Female)
⊙ Retailer in seafood market
⊙ 23 December 2019: cough, chest pain
⊙ 4 days later: worse
⊙ CT chest: Pneumonia
⊙ Discharged (sent home)

Patient #2: 61 year-old ♂ (male)
⊙ Frequent visitor to seafood market
⊙ 20 December 2019: cough, fever
⊙ Respiratory Distress
⊙ Ventilator
⊙ 9 January 2020: Died

- Let's pay a visit to Wuhan

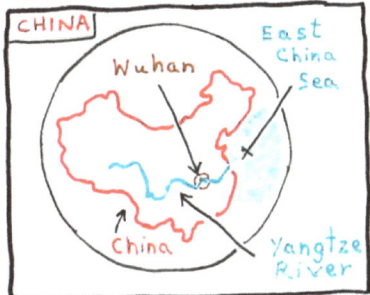

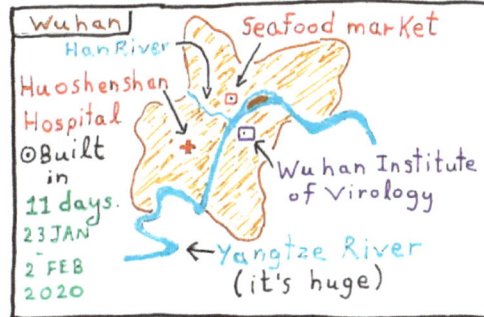

CHINA

Wuhan
East China Sea
Yangtze River
China

Wuhan
Han River
Seafood market
Huoshenshan Hospital
◎ Built in 11 days.
23 JAN - 2 FEB 2020
Wuhan Institute of Virology
← Yangtze River (it's huge)

○ Wuhan has 11 million people.
○ The (mighty) Yangtze River flows through Wuhan, en route to the East China Sea.

○ NYC — 7 a.m.   London — 12 noon   China (all of it) — 8 p.m.

- Wuhan has 13 districts, and a metro with 9 lines, and 4 ring roads, and interesting bridges.
- 3 towns merged to become Wuhan:

1. Hankou
   ◎ North of the Yangtze River
   ◎ Now made of 3 districts

   QIAOKOU DISTRICT
   JIANGHAN DISTRICT ◎ Seafood market is here
   JIANG'AN DISTRICT

2. Hanyang
   ◎ West of the Han River

3. Wuchang
   ◎ South of the Yangtze River
   ◎ Wuhan Institute of Virology is here

- Coronavirus does not infect lobsters
← shellfish
← hedgehogs
← badgers   Live in the market at time of Samples
← snakes
← turtle doves

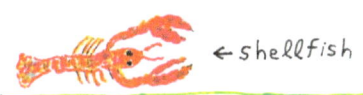

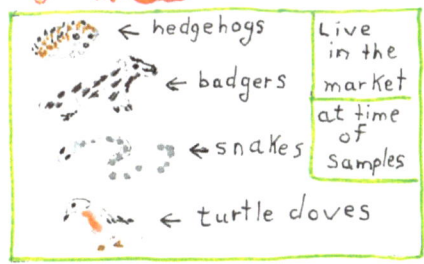

The Seafood market is the size of 3 Walmarts.
It is closed down on 1 JANUARY 2020.

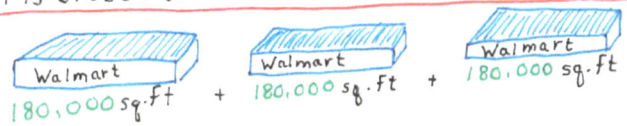

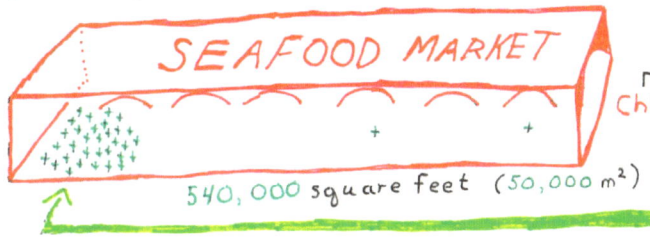

Walmart 180,000 sq. ft + Walmart 180,000 sq. ft + Walmart 180,000 sq. ft

SEAFOOD MARKET
540,000 square feet (50,000 m²)

→ (Different from USA CDC)
China CDC takes 585 samples from January 1-12
◎ 33 are ☣ Coronavirus positive
└→ 31 of these are from the west end where there is wildlife

- The Seafood Market is at the intersection of 2nd Ring Road @ Xinghua Road

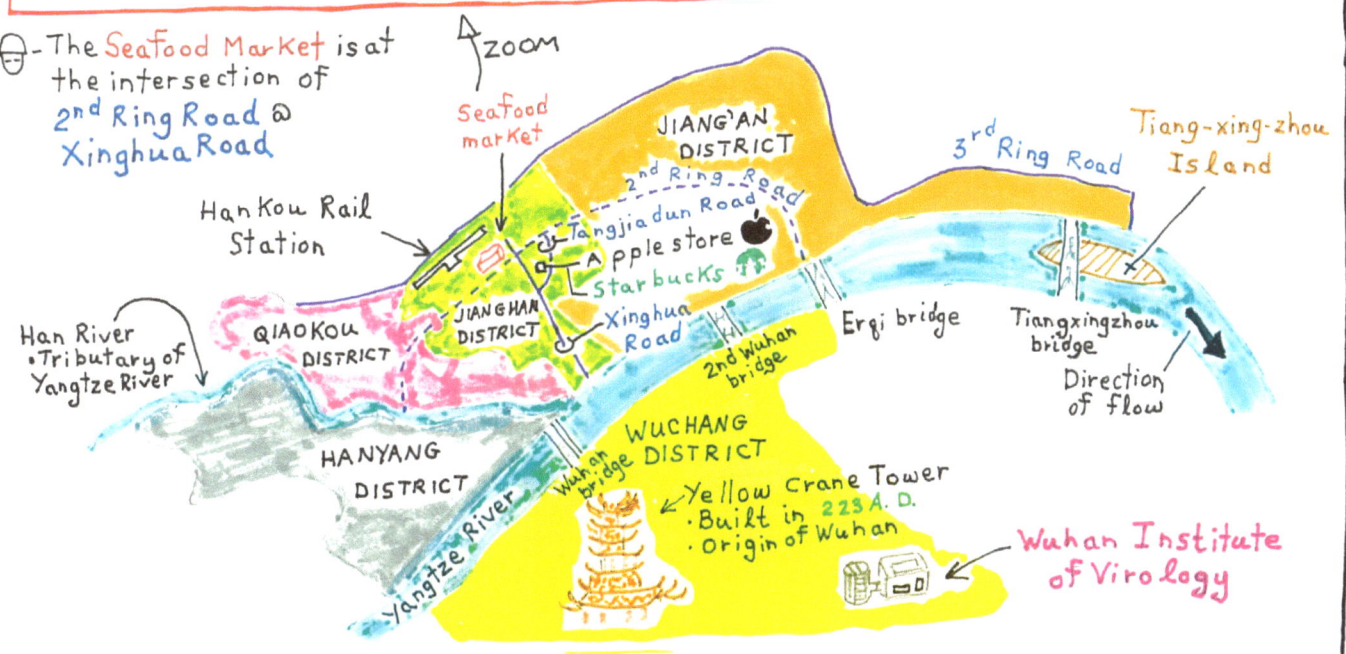

↑ ZOOM

Seafood market
JIANG'AN DISTRICT
2nd Ring Road
3rd Ring Road
Tiang-xing-zhou Island

Hankou Rail Station
Tangjiadun Road
Apple store
Starbucks
Xinghua Road
JIANGHAN DISTRICT

Han River
• Tributary of Yangtze River
QIAOKOU DISTRICT

Ergi bridge

2nd Wuhan bridge
Tiangxingzhou bridge
Direction of flow

HANYANG DISTRICT
Yangtze River
Wuhan bridge
WUCHANG DISTRICT

Yellow Crane Tower
• Built in 223 A.D.
• Origin of Wuhan

Wuhan Institute of Virology

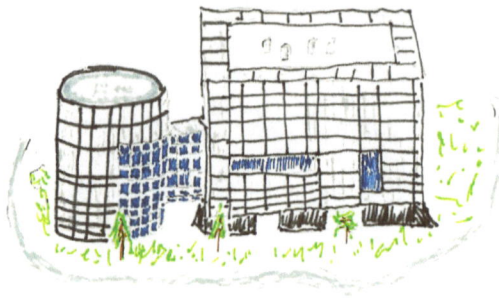

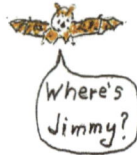

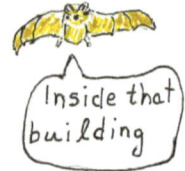

"Where's Jimmy?"

"Inside that building"

Wuhan **Virus** **Institute**

武汉　病毒　研究所

wǔhàn　bìngdú　yánjiū suǒ

"woo han"　"bing doo"　"yenchoo sue ah"

♀ - Isn't it called the Wuhan Institute of Virology?

♂ - Yes, but the Chinese symbols are arranged as Wuhan Virus Institute.

☼ **Corona** **virus**

新　病毒

xīnguān　bìngdú

"sing gwon"　"bing doo"

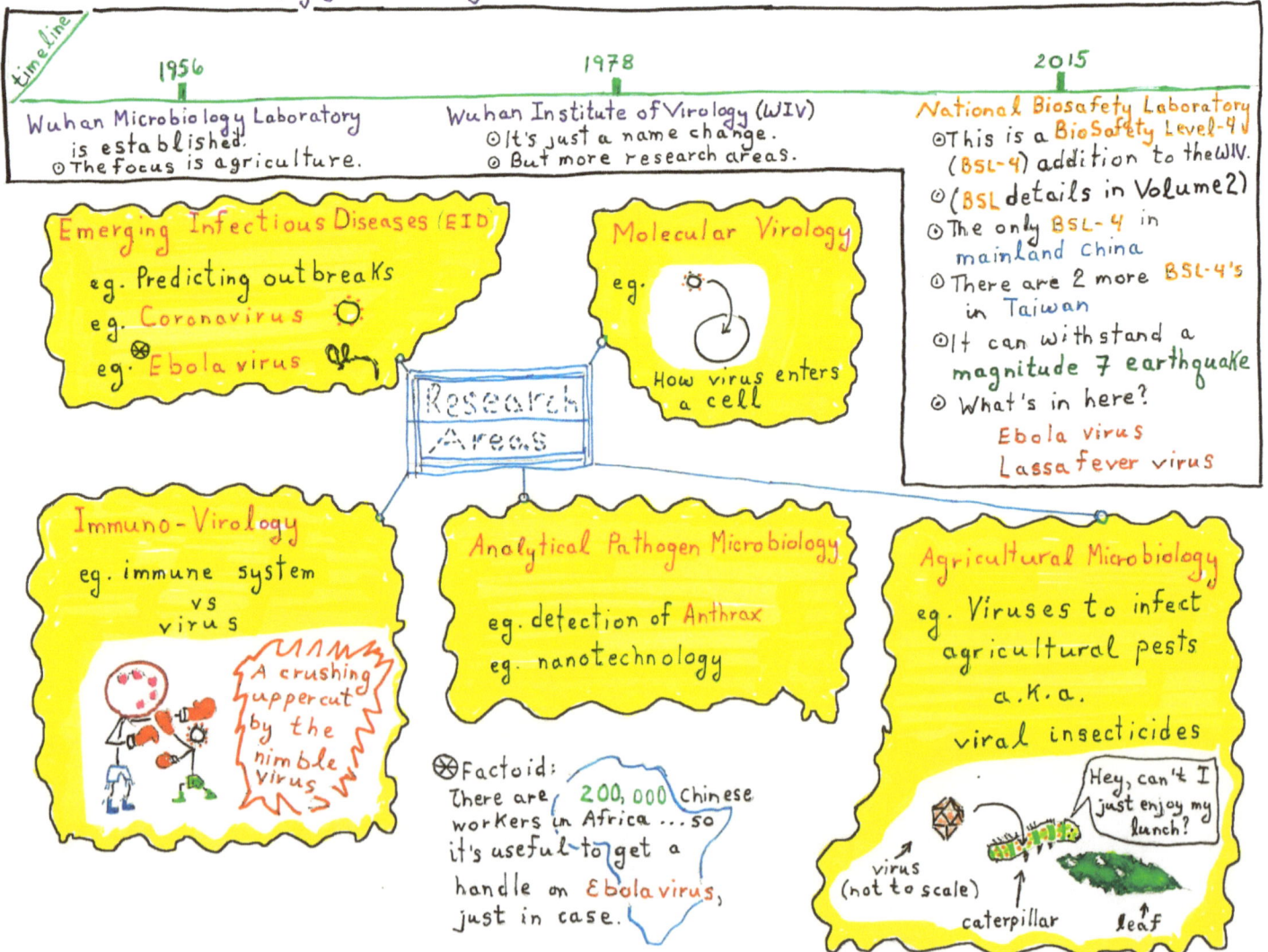

- "bing doo" sounds like a harmless children's game ... until your eyeballs start dissolving

timeline

1956
Wuhan Microbiology Laboratory is established.
⊙ The focus is agriculture.

1978
Wuhan Institute of Virology (WIV)
⊙ It's just a name change.
⊙ But more research areas.

2015
National Biosafety Laboratory
⊙ This is a BioSafety Level-4 (BSL-4) addition to the WIV.
⊙ (BSL details in Volume 2)
⊙ The only BSL-4 in mainland China
⊙ There are 2 more BSL-4's in Taiwan
⊙ It can withstand a magnitude 7 earthquake
⊙ What's in here?
Ebola virus
Lassa fever virus

Emerging Infectious Diseases (EID)
eg. Predicting outbreaks
eg. Coronavirus ☼
eg. Ebola virus

Molecular Virology
eg.
How virus enters a cell

Research Areas

Immuno-Virology
eg. immune system vs virus

A crushing uppercut by the nimble virus

Analytical Pathogen Microbiology
eg. detection of Anthrax
eg. nanotechnology

� Factoid:
There are 200,000 Chinese workers in Africa ... so it's useful to get a handle on Ebola virus, just in case.

Agricultural Microbiology
eg. Viruses to infect agricultural pests a.k.a. viral insecticides

"Hey, can't I just enjoy my lunch?"

virus (not to scale)

caterpillar

leaf

- Since we're visiting, let's check out those bridges...

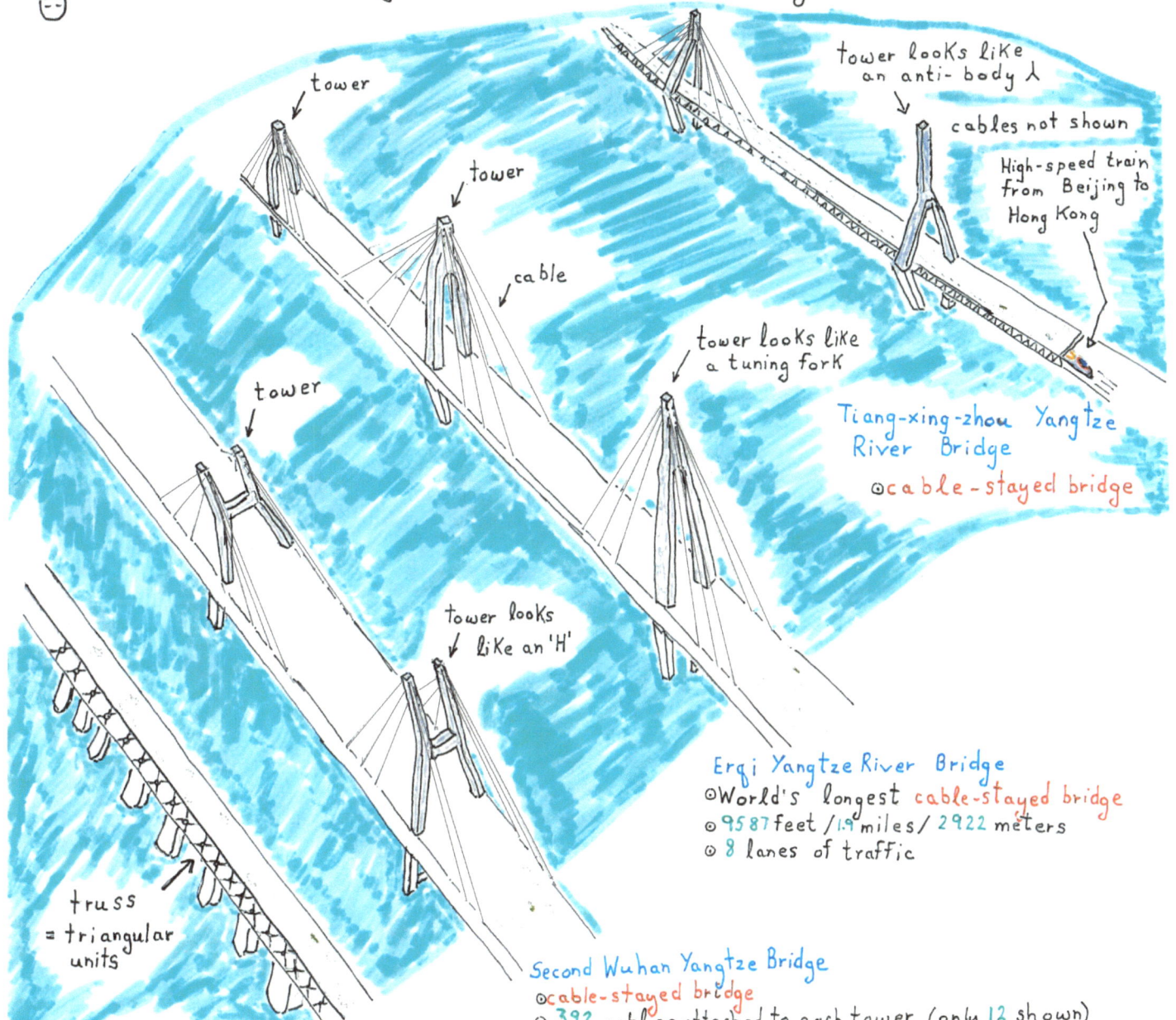

tower

tower

cable

tower

tower looks like
an anti-body λ

cables not shown

High-speed train
from Beijing to
Hong Kong

tower looks like
a tuning fork

Tiang-xing-zhou Yangtze
River Bridge
◎ cable-stayed bridge

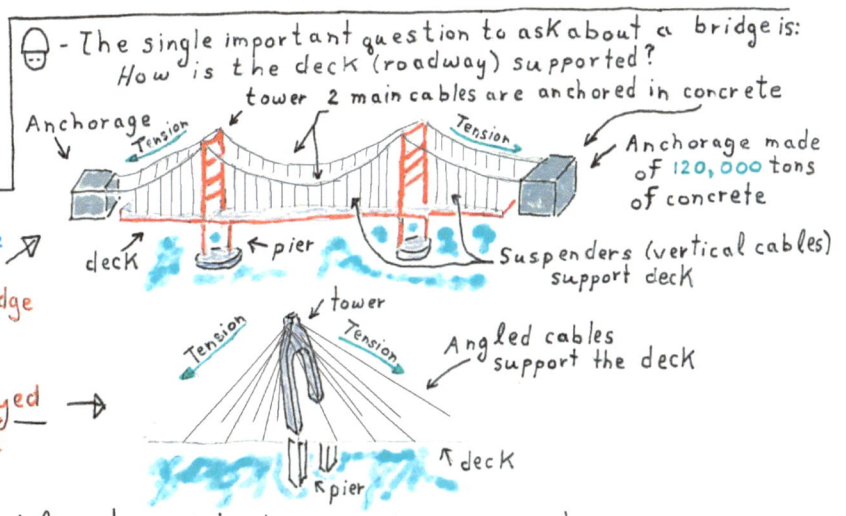

tower looks
like an 'H'

Erqi Yangtze River Bridge
◎ World's longest cable-stayed bridge
◎ 9587 feet / 1.9 miles / 2922 meters
◎ 8 lanes of traffic

truss
= triangular
units

Second Wuhan Yangtze Bridge
◎ cable-stayed bridge
◎ 392 cables attached to each tower (only 12 shown)

Wuhan Yangtze Bridge
◎ Truss bridge is old school.
◎ 1st bridge in China to span
   the Yangtze River
◎ Built in 1957

- The single important question to ask about a bridge is:
  How is the deck (roadway) supported?
  tower 2 main cables are anchored in concrete

Anchorage   Tension   Tension   Anchorage made
                                           of 120,000 tons
                                           of concrete
deck   pier   Suspenders (vertical cables)
                          support deck

- And the relevance
  to coronavirus
  is ... ?

- Be patient

Golden Gate
Bridge is
a suspension bridge

cable-stayed →
bridge

tower
Tension   Tension   Angled cables
                          support the deck
                    deck
         pier

- Get it? A cable-stayed bridge requires no anchorages.

- How do you lockdown a city of 11 million people?

Conversely, what are all the ways an infected person can leave, and where to?

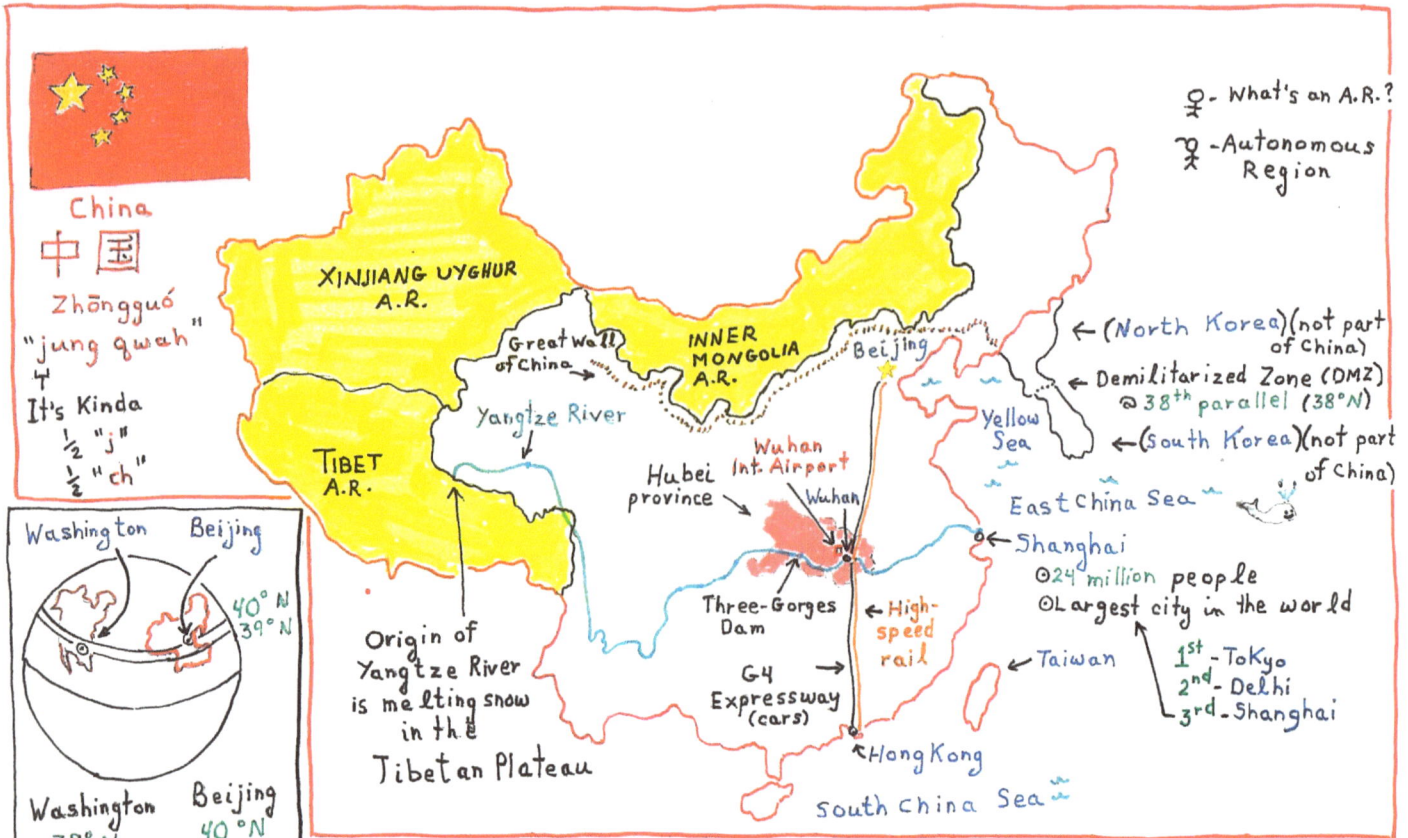

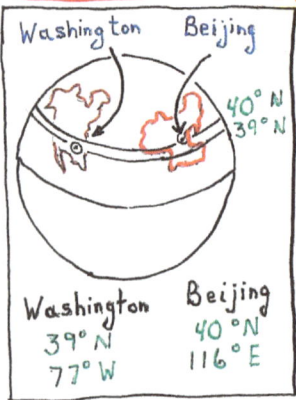

♀ - What's an A.R.?

☿ - Autonomous Region

China

中国

Zhōngguó

"jung qwah"

4

It's Kinda ½ "j" ½ "ch"

XINJIANG UYGHUR A.R.

INNER MONGOLIA A.R.

TIBET A.R.

Great Wall of China →

Beijing ★

Yangtze River

Hubei province →

Wuhan Int. Airport

Wuhan

← (North Korea) (not part of China)

← Demilitarized Zone (DMZ) @ 38th parallel (38°N)

← (South Korea) (not part of China)

Yellow Sea

East China Sea

○ Shanghai
○ 24 million people
○ Largest city in the world

1st - Tokyo
2nd - Delhi
3rd - Shanghai

Three-Gorges Dam

← High-speed rail

G4 Expressway (cars)

Origin of Yangtze River is melting snow in the Tibetan Plateau

← Taiwan

Hong Kong

South China Sea

Washington   Beijing

40° N
39° N

Washington
39° N
77° W

Beijing
40° N
116° E

Attention!
Go home
No cars
No trains
No planes
No skinny dipping in the Yangtze

Wuhan ✈

International flights

Moscow
London
Rome   Istanbul   Dubai

Osaka
Seoul
Singapore
Bali

San Francisco (SFO)

NYC

G4 Beijing - Hong Kong Expressway
- Goes through Wuhan
- 2272 Km

High Speed rail

Aluminum body to ↓ weight

electric motor

"Harmony" train

300 Km/hour
186 miles/hour

M Wuhan Metro

track gauge 4 FT 8½" same as:

228 stations

UNDERGROUND
London

NYC Subway

M Paris Metro

M Moscow Metro
4 FT 11 27/32"

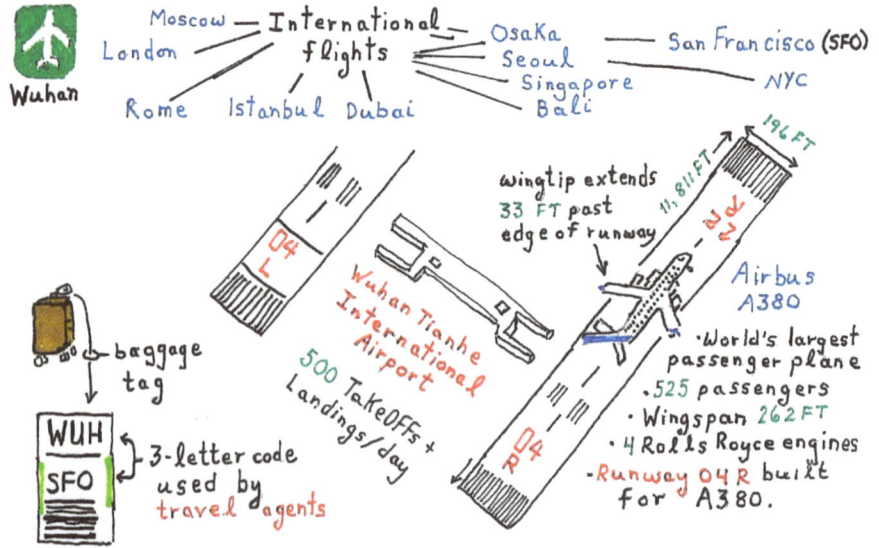

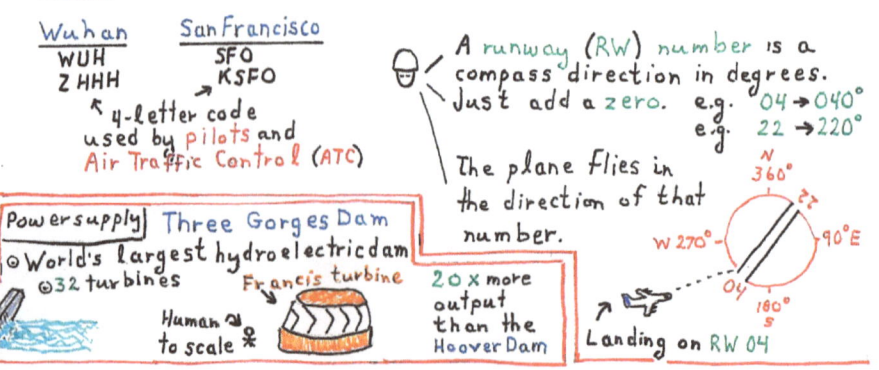

baggage tag

WUH
SFO

3-letter code used by travel agents

Wuhan
WUH
Z HHH

San Francisco
SFO
KSFO

4-letter code used by pilots and Air Traffic Control (ATC)

Wuhan Tianhe International Airport

500 TakeOffs + Landings/day

wingtip extends 33 FT past edge of runway

196 FT

Airbus A380

· World's largest passenger plane
· 525 passengers
· Wingspan 262 FT
· 4 Rolls Royce engines
- Runway 04R built for A380.

A runway (RW) number is a compass direction in degrees. Just add a zero. e.g. 04 → 040° e.g. 22 → 220°

The plane Flies in the direction of that number.

N 360°
W 270°
90° E
180° S

Landing on RW 04

Power supply Three Gorges Dam
○ World's largest hydroelectric dam
○ 32 turbines

Francis turbine

Human to scale

20 x more output than the Hoover Dam

YANGTZE RIVER →

- Plagues and pandemics are the constant companion of humankind.

PLAGUE YEARBOOK

Typhus
Class of 430 B.C.
Enjoys terrifying strangers

Bubonic Plague
Voted most likely to kill multiple times

Smallpox
Voted most likely to wipe out civilizations

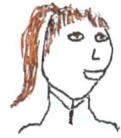

Influenza
Has always wanted to visit Spain

Cholera
Voted most likely to kill by diarrhea

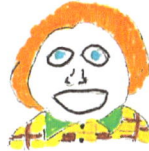

Yellow Fever
Crazy about mosquitoes

Ebola
A self-admitted loner who scares even the principal

27

28

Everyone on the Left page is a bacteria.
- Everyone on the Right page is a virus.

Let's explore them to create some context for what coronavirus is up to.

Plague of Athens

430 B.C.

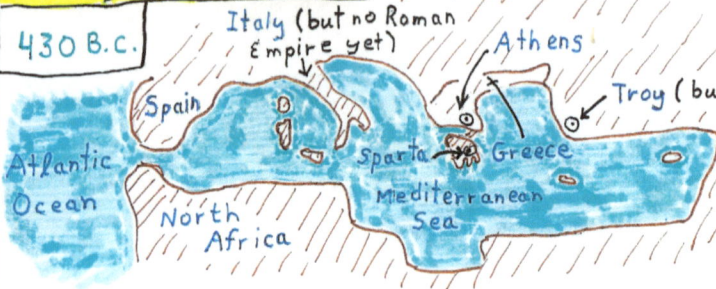

Italy (but no Roman Empire yet)
Athens
Troy (but the Trojan War, starring Brad Pitt and Eric Bana, was way earlier, ~ 1200 B.C.)
Spain
Atlantic Ocean
Sparta
Greece
Mediterranean Sea
North Africa

- Okay, so it's 430 B.C.
- Athens is at war with Sparta (and FYI that famous battle of the 300 Spartans against the Persians was 50 years earlier in 480 B.C.)

- And nasty Typhus comes along.
  ○ Here is the account by Thucydides, an Athenian general + historian:

"It struck the healthy without warning, starting with high fever in the head. ... Sneezing and sore throats followed, and soon the trouble descended to the chest, causing a severe cough. ... Pain was acute, for most were affected by a hollow retching accompanied by violent spasms which lasted for different times in different cases. ... Most, then, died from the internal fever on the seventh or ninth day with their bodily strength unimpaired. ... The disease never attacked the same man twice, at least not fatally. ... In addition to it's other effects, the plague caused a great increase in lawlessness."

Thucydides
born 460 B.C., so age 30 during the plague

SOMPOO SAYS
"Thoo Koo thee thees"
└ th like the

R.I.P. 75,000 - 100,000 deaths.

- Was that a pandemic or an epidemic?
- It seemed to stay in Athens, so it was an epidemic. If it spread, say to Italy and Spain, then it would be a pandemic.

Life cycle	Louse - borne Typhus

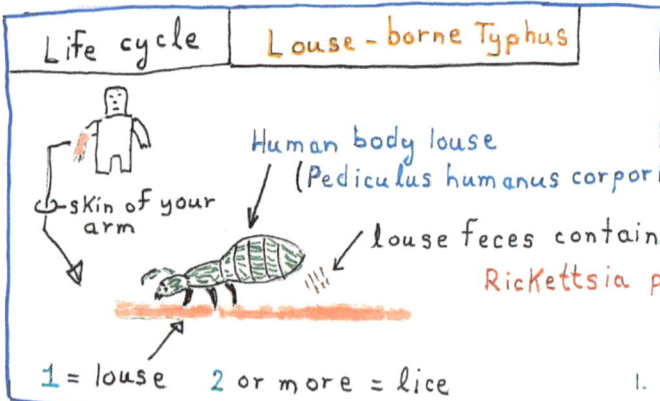

skin of your arm

Human body louse
(Pediculus humanus corporis)

louse feces contain bacteria with a crazy name:
Rickettsia prowazekii

1 = louse   2 or more = lice

Steps to Kill human:
1. Louse bites your skin
2. Louse craps on you
3. Bacteria is in the crap (feces)
4. You scratch the bite
5. The bacteria gets into the wound
6. The bacteria enters the blood
7. You die

- The illness is also called Epidemic Typhus
- It's rare today but overcrowding spreads it.
- The treatment is the antibiotic called doxycycline.
- Okay, the Plague of Athens in 430 B.C. is thought to be caused by Typhus. That's a best guess.
- Typhus is not Typhoid Fever (it's later on).

Anne Frank died of Typhus. I read her book, The Diary of Anne Frank, at the Bergen-Belsen concentration camp where she died. It was a powerful, solemn experience.

PRECISION OF SPEECH

IS THE

LUBRICATION

OF SCIENCE

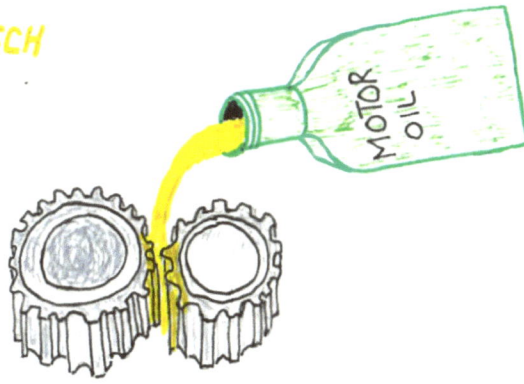

☺ - Before proceeding, let's get some terms straight.

'Plague' in its broadest sense means torment.

Cheryl, you are a plague upon this team

Cheryl Right Fielder

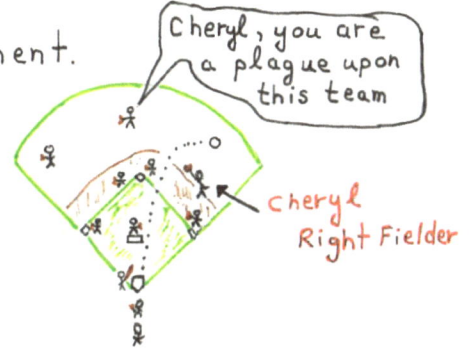

'Plague' in a biblical sense means punishment.

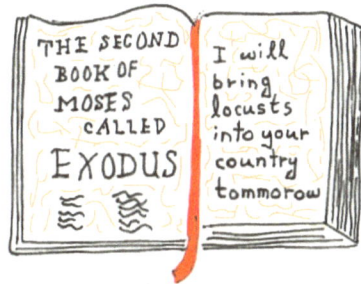

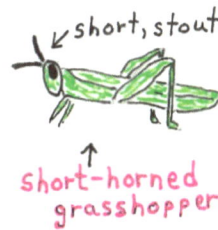

THE SECOND BOOK OF MOSES CALLED EXODUS

I will bring locusts into your country tommorow

↙ short, stout antenna

When grasshoppers swarm they are called locusts

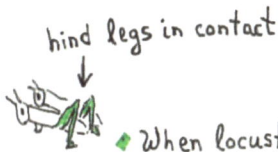

Short-horned grasshopper

hind legs in contact

◆ When locusts crowd together there is tactile stimulation of their hind legs ... ... which causes serotonin release in their nervous system ... which causes them to change color, eat more, and breed more ... plague of locusts

◆ The largest swarm was 12 trillion locusts ... say goodbye to your crops (famine)

'Plague' in a loose medical sense means any nasty infection on a mass scale. e.g. Plague of Athens

'Plague' in a strict medical sense means Bubonic-Plague (next page).
Pneumonic   Septicemic

'Pestilence' is a loosey-goosey synonym for Plague.

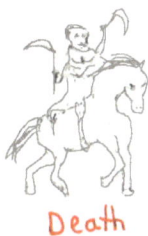

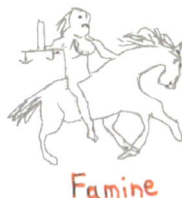

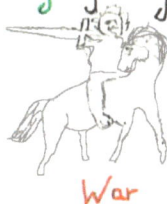

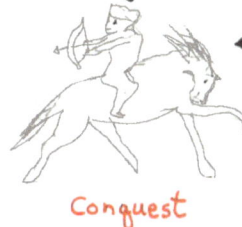

← The Four Horsemen of the Apocalypse

⊙ Pestilence is somehow tossed in there.

Death   Famine   War   Conquest

- The Bubonic Plague is, well, plain ol' horrible.

Horrible Menu

Bubonic Plague $9

⊙ Comes with your choice of:

Pustule = pus-filled blister (where flea bit you)

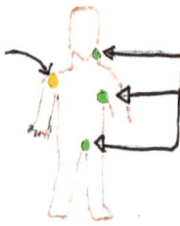

Swollen, painful *lymph nodes* in neck, armpit, groin ↖ #1 site

50-90% fatal

⊙ May burst (rupture) → release of foul-smelling pus

- 'Boubon' is the Greek word for groin. 'Bubo' for short. Because lymph nodes in the groin swell, it's called 'bubonic'.

Pneumonic Plague $15
100% fatal

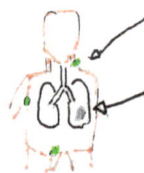

Swollen *lymph nodes* (optional)

Pneumonia
⊙ That means <u>bacteria</u> are growing in the lungs.

- The year is 1348 A.D.
- Has the microscope been invented yet?
No.
No one has a hot clue what bacteria are or why people are dropping dead.

Septicemic Plague $12
25% Fatal

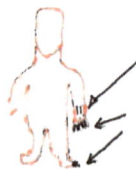

Blackened skin (bleeding in skin)

Gangrene (dead flesh) of fingers and toes

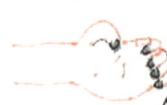

Hence, "Black Death"

- Notice the similarity to 'septic'?
- Septicemia means bacteria multiplying in your blood

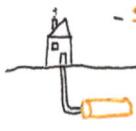

↖ septic tank

↑ Black, dying fingertips

Gluten-free Plague upon request

SOMPOO SAYS
- "bew bon ick" ⌐ rhymes with you
- "new mon ick"
- "sep tah seem ick"
- "sep tah seem ee ah"

Plot Spoiler: Plague is caused by a bacteria. The location determines the menu choice.
Bacteria in Lymph nodes → Bubonic Plague
Bacteria in Lungs → Pneumonic Plague
Bacteria in Blood → Septicemic Plague

Collectively, this is called 'Plague'.

- Here's a description of Plague:
"For it began in England in Dorsetshire in the year of our Lord 1348, and immediately advancing from place to place it attacked men without warning and for the most part those who were healthy. Very many of those who were attacked in the morning it carried out of human affairs before noon. And no one whom it willed to die did it permit to live longer than three or four days."

- So 1348 would be a year to avoid in a time machine
- I concur

Plague Recipe

Ingredients:

↑ bacteria

↙ flea

↙ rat (black rat preferred but brown acceptable)

↗ human

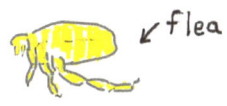

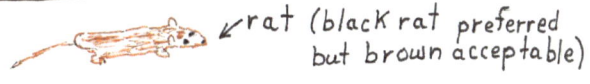

Plague Instructions
(think, sequence of events)

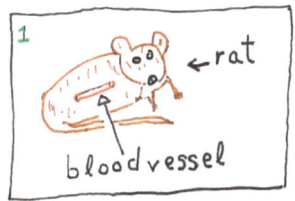

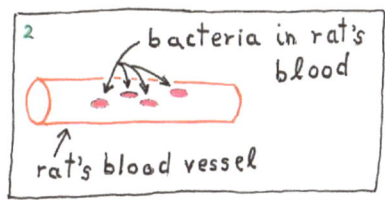

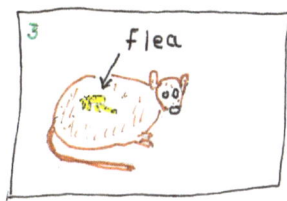

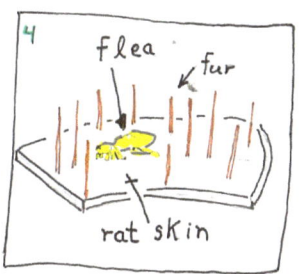

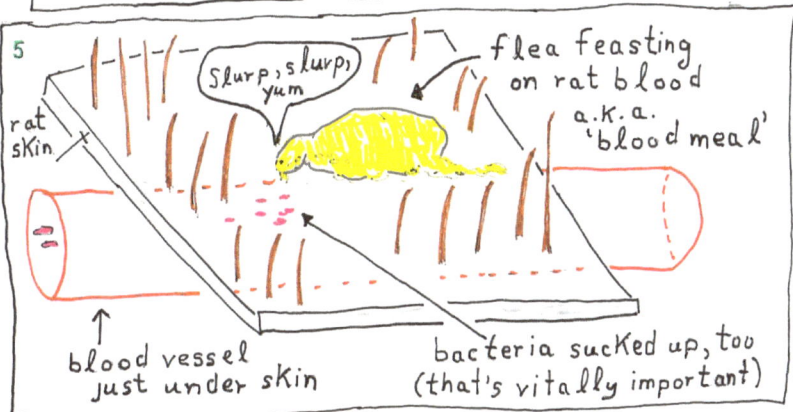

1 ←rat
blood vessel

2 bacteria in rat's blood
rat's blood vessel

3 flea

4 flea ↓ fur
rat skin

5
Slurp, slurp, yum
flea feasting on rat blood a.k.a. 'blood meal'
rat skin
blood vessel just under skin
bacteria sucked up, too (that's vitally important)

- Now things take an unexpected turn, which requires an understanding of flea digestive anatomy (which you probably had no idea you were going to learn today).

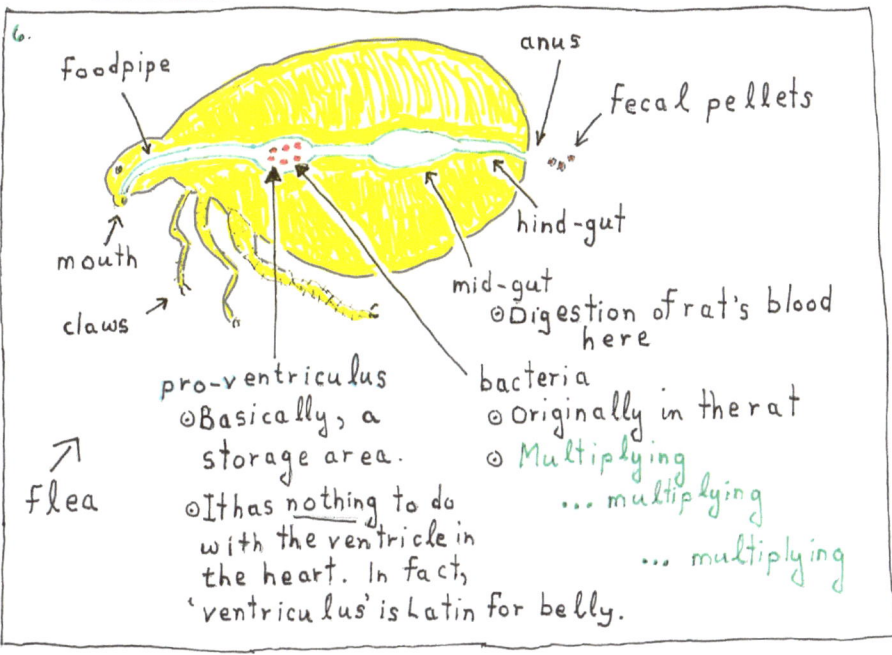

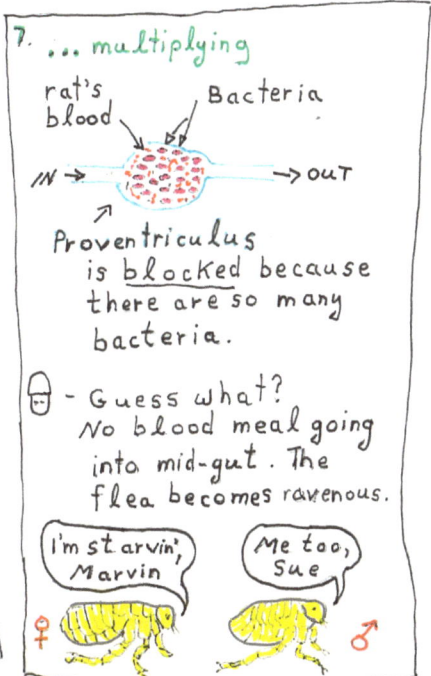

6.
foodpipe
anus
Fecal pellets
mouth
claws
hind-gut
mid-gut
⊙ Digestion of rat's blood here
pro-ventriculus
⊙ Basically, a storage area.
⊙ It has nothing to do with the ventricle in the heart. In fact, 'ventriculus' is Latin for belly.
flea
bacteria
⊙ Originally in the rat
⊙ Multiplying
... multiplying
... multiplying

7. ... multiplying
rat's blood   Bacteria
IN →   → OUT
Proventriculus is blocked because there are so many bacteria.

- Guess what? No blood meal going into mid-gut. The flea becomes ravenous.

I'm starvin', Marvin
Me too, Sue

8

starving flea

rat

human

Humans and rats are always in close proximity

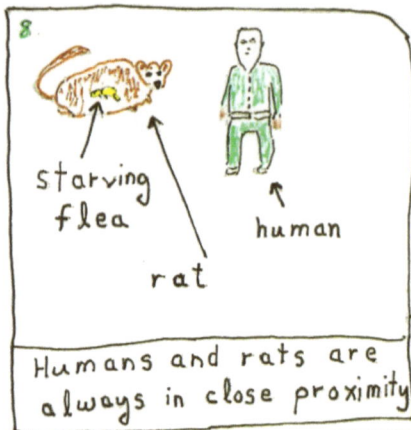

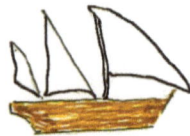

Maybe a sailboat

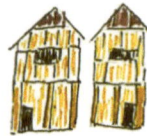

Maybe a crowded medieval city

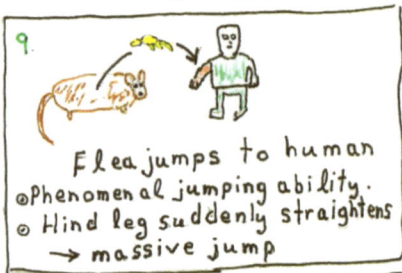

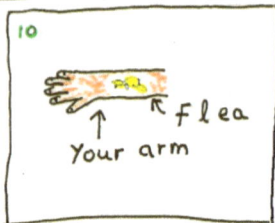

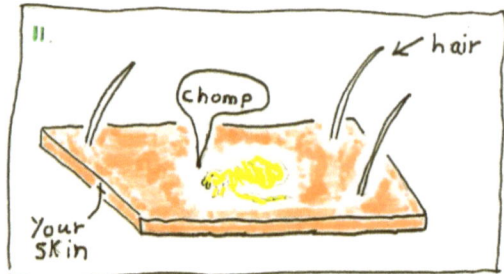

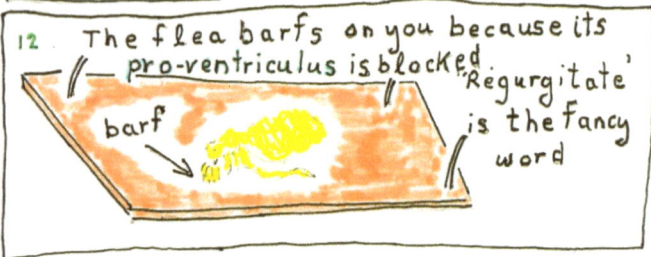

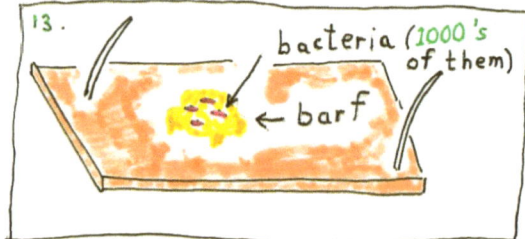

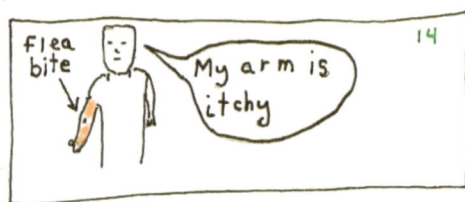

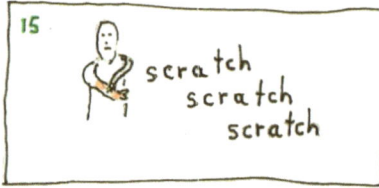

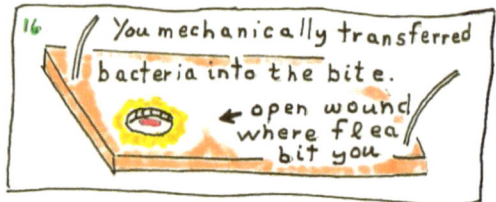

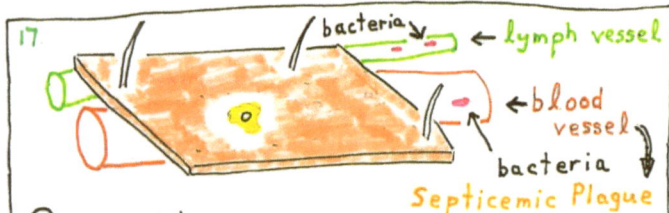

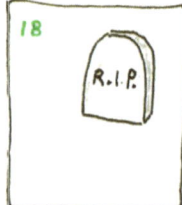

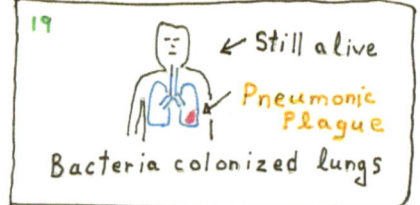

9

Flea jumps to human
◉Phenomenal jumping ability.
◉ Hind leg suddenly straightens → massive jump

10

Your arm

← flea

11

← hair

chomp

Your skin

12 The flea barfs on you because its pro-ventriculus is blocked. 'Regurgitate' is the fancy word

barf

13.

bacteria (1000's of them)

← barf

14

flea bite

My arm is itchy

15

scratch
scratch
scratch

16 You mechanically transferred bacteria into the bite.

← open wound where flea bit you

17

bacteria ↘

← lymph vessel

← blood vessel

bacteria
Septicemic Plague

18

R.I.P.

or

19

← Still alive

Pneumonic Plague

Bacteria colonized lungs

☺ - Key points:

1. Lymph vessels flow nearby blood vessels.
2. Lymph vessels are filled with lymphatic fluid, which is kinda like blood minus all the contents.
3. Lymph vessels empty into lymph nodes.
4. Bacteria end up in lymph nodes ... which swell ... Bubonic Plague.
5. In a completely different scenario, cancer cells can spread via the lymph vessels. This is called 'lymphatic spread.' This is precisely why a surgeon dissects the lymph nodes in a woman's armpit - to see if Breast Cancer cells spread there.

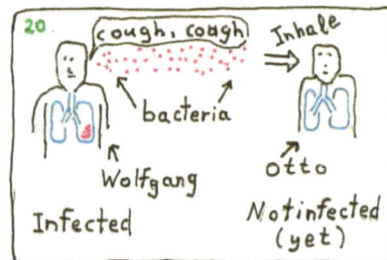

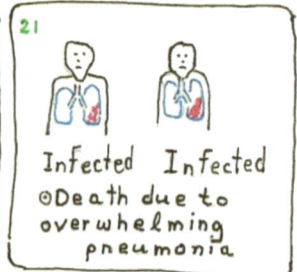

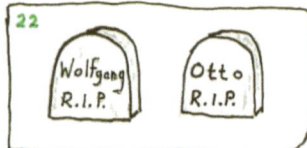

20 cough, cough

Inhale

bacteria

Wolfgang

otto

Infected

Not infected (yet)

21

Infected Infected
◉Death due to overwhelming pneumonia

22

Wolfgang R.I.P.

Otto R.I.P.

☺ - How many other people did Wolfgang and Otto infect before they died? That's the R_0 ("R not") (R naught) number. Details later.

(as in, Bubonic / Pneumonic / Septicemic Plague)

- Plague ✓ has caused epidemics at least 50 times.
And colossal ⟨pandemics⟩ at least 3 times.

- The point of the 3 maps below is that Plague has been plaguing humans since 541 A.D. (in fact, since 1850 B.C.)

- ☀ How many coronavirus pandemics have we had? 3

2003
2012
2019-2020-2021

Will there be another in the year 2028?
2280?
2820?

Who Knows?
800 years is about 32 generations of humans from now.

Plague epidemics from 541 A.D. to 2018 A.D.

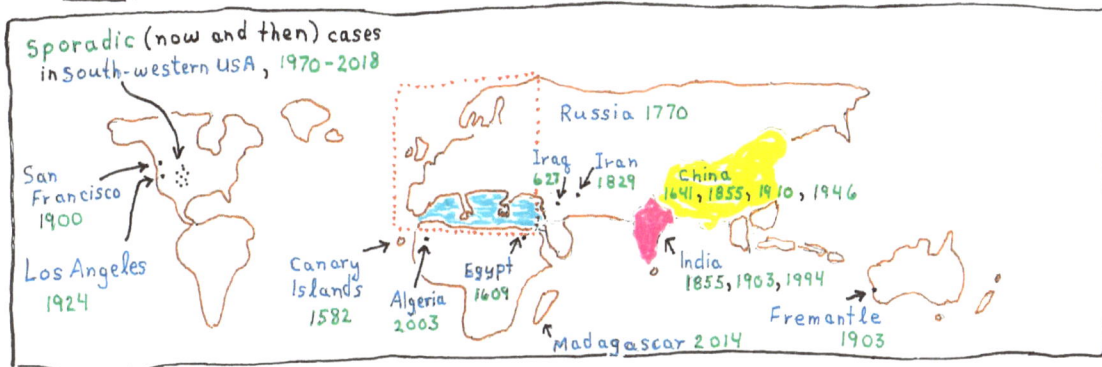

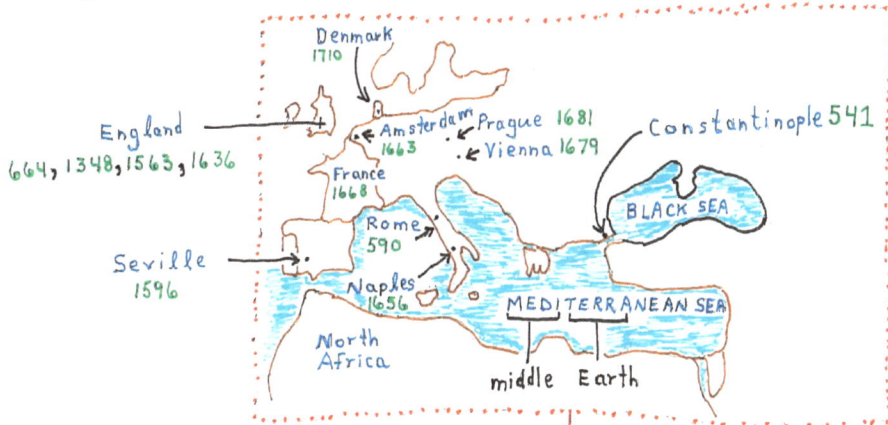

Sporadic (now and then) cases in South-western USA, 1970-2018

San Francisco 1900

Los Angeles 1924

Canary Islands 1582

Algeria 2003

Egypt 1609

Russia 1770

Iraq 627   Iran 1829

China 1641, 1855, 1910, 1946

India 1855, 1903, 1994

Madagascar 2014

Fremantle 1903

Denmark 1710

England 664, 1348, 1563, 1636

Amsterdam 1663   Prague 1681
Vienna 1679

France 1668

Constantinople 541

Rome 590

BLACK SEA

Seville 1596

Naples 1656

MEDITERRANEAN SEA

North Africa

middle Earth

Plague of Justinian 1st
◉ 541 A.D.
◉ Basically, all this region.
◉ Justinian I is the Roman Emperor
◉ 25 million deaths
◉ 5000 deaths per day in Constantinople (modern-day Istanbul, amazing city! Go visit!)
◉ This was a pandemic.

Black Death 2nd
◉ 1348 A.D. (officially 1346-1353)
◉ Basically, all this region.
◉ 75 million deaths (the numbers vary from 50-200m)
◉ All 3 forms of Plague.
◉ This was a pandemic = spreads to other countries or continents

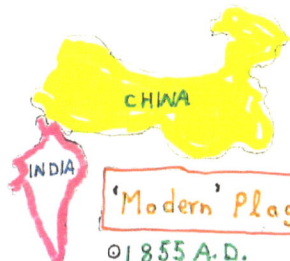

CHINA

INDIA

'Modern' Plague 3rd
◉ 1855 A.D.
◉ 12 million deaths
◉ This was a pandemic.

- Let's recap.
  We started with rat-to-human transmission of the bacteria.
  Well, more like rat-to-flea-to-human

  ` Then we progressed to human-to-human transmission

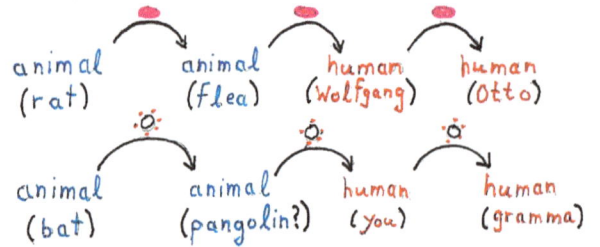

animal (rat) → animal (flea) → human (Wolfgang) → human (Otto)

animal (bat) → animal (pangolin?) → human (you) → human (gramma)

  ` See a similarity to ☼ coronavirus?

- Some official names

← Yersinia pestis
  ⊙ Cause of Plague.
  ⊙ Rod shape.
  ⊙ Survives with or without oxygen. Thrives in blood.
  ⊙ Is it a pest? Yes, that's an understatement.
  ⊙ Is it a pestilence? Yes.
  ⊙ So its species name is 'pestis.'

← Alexandre Yersin
  ⊙ What year was he born? 1863 (in Switzerland)
  ⊙ Did he have a microscope? Yes.
  ⊙ He discovers the Plague bacteria, which is named after him.

  old-school microscope →

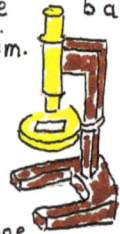

  ⊙ Very first, ghetto microscope was in 1608.

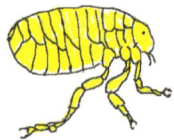

← Oriental rat flea
  ⊙ It likes rats.
  ⊙ Humans, if necessary
  ⊙ 'Resilin' is the elastic protein responsible for the huge jumps.
  ⊙ If a human was a flea, the world record for long jump would be 300FT.

2.5 mm
1/10th inch

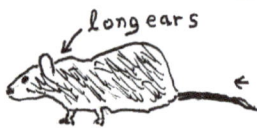

long ears

← Black rat (Rattus rattus)
  ⊙ Probably brought Plague from Asia to Europe
  ⊙ Seems to transmit Plague better than brown rat.

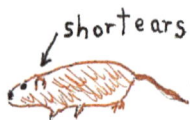

short ears

← Brown rat (Rattus norvegicus)
  a.k.a. Norway rat
  a.k.a. wharf rat
  a.k.a. laboratory rat
  a.k.a. fancy rat (pet rat)

  ⊙ It replaced the black rat in Europe.

Homo sapiens
  ⊙ Dies, in this story.

- Relevant Trivia:
  Yersinia pestis is stored/studied today in BioSafety Level 4 (BSL-4) labs.
  ⊙ If you get Septicemic Plague, you can develop (and die of) Adult Respiratory Distress Syndrome (ARDS). Same problem with ☼ coronavirus.

  ⊙ Today, we treat plague with streptomycin.

  Fascinatingly, streptomycin is made by a soil bacteria called Streptomyces.

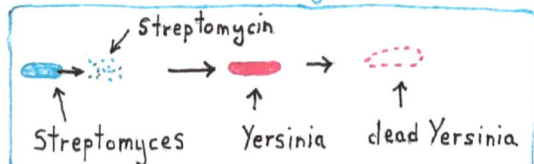

  Streptomycin

  Streptomyces   Yersinia   dead Yersinia

  In other words, bacteria kill other bacteria. It's a cruel world, at all levels.

SOMPOO SAYS "Strep toe my sin" "Strep toe my sees"

- Yellow Fever ... let's keep it to 1 page, shall we?

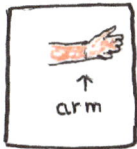

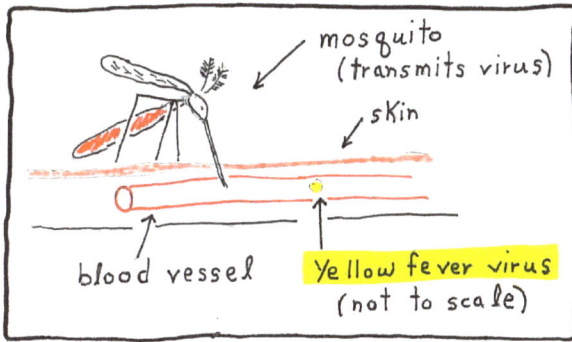

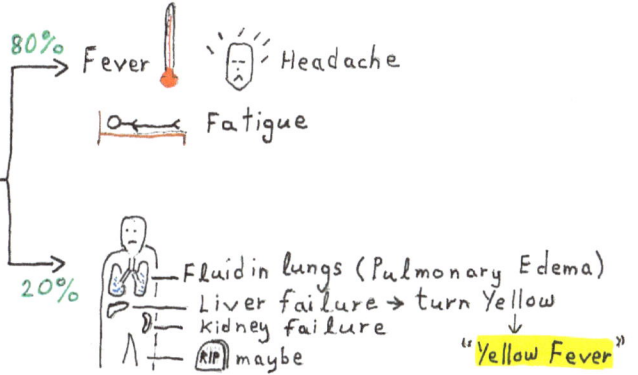

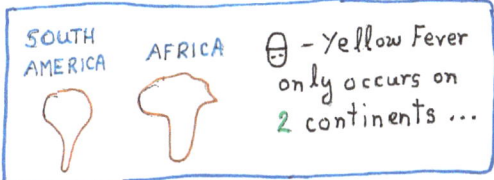

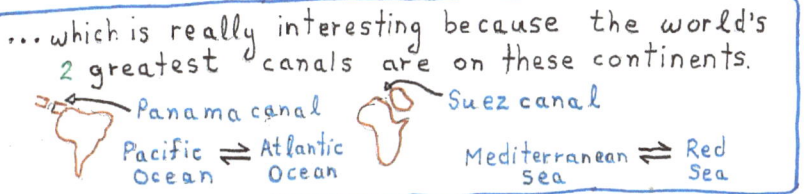

↑ arm

mosquito (transmits virus)
skin

blood vessel

Yellow fever virus (not to scale)

80% → Fever | Headache
Fatigue

20% → Fluid in lungs (Pulmonary Edema)
Liver failure → turn Yellow
kidney failure   ↓
RIP maybe   "Yellow Fever"

SOUTH AMERICA   AFRICA   - Yellow Fever only occurs on 2 continents ...

... which is really interesting because the world's 2 greatest canals are on these continents.

Panama canal   Suez canal
Pacific ⇌ Atlantic   Mediterranean ⇌ Red
Ocean   Ocean   Sea   Sea

- I know, Panama is in Central America. Let's pretend it's part of South America. Don't ruin my story.

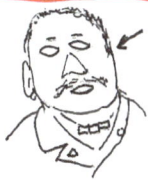

Ferdinand de Lesseps
⊙ World's greatest engineer
⊙ 1869 - Builds Suez canal.
⊙ 1874 - Asked to build Panama canal.

⊙ 1881 - Construction begins.
EPIC FAIL   Yellow Fever kills RIP 22,000 French workers
⊙ 1889 - Construction abandoned.
- de Lesseps returns to France in ignominy

♀ - ignominy?
♀ - uber-shame

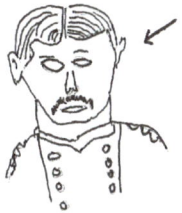

Major Walter Reed, M.D.
⊙ US Army Medical Corps
⊙ 1900 - Identifies the Aedes aegypti mosquito as the cause of yellow fever.
⊙ The famous Walter Reed Medical Center a.k.a. Bethesda Naval Hospital is named after him. And JFK's autopsy was done there in 1963.

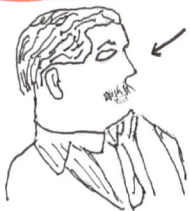

Dr. William Crawford Gorgas
⊙ US Chief Sanitary Officer
⊙ 1904 - He is tasked with clearing the mosquito from 500 square miles of ∨ jungle in the (as yet unbuilt) Panama canal zone.
swampy!

The Plan

shovel dirt   or   spray insecticide
· 120 tons used (108 metric tonnes)

or   spray oil to mess up mosquito larva in water
600,000 gallons

4000 men in 'mosquito brigades'

'standing' water where mosquitoes breed

← workers live here

← mesh on doors and windows to stop mosquitoes

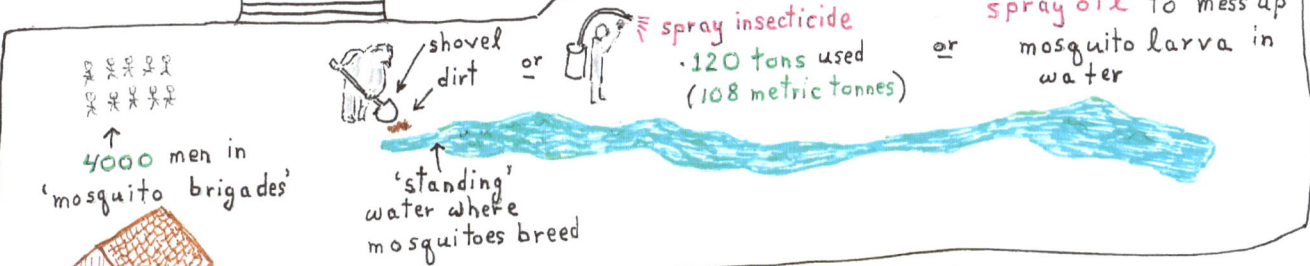

1906 November - No Yellow Fever in canal zone.
Construction begins.
Success

1914 - Panama canal opens.
⊙ It's a classic American 'Anything Is Possible' project.

"A man. A plan. A canal. Panama."
↖ Famous palindrome (reads same ⇌)

- I lied. 2 pages.

Central American Seaway

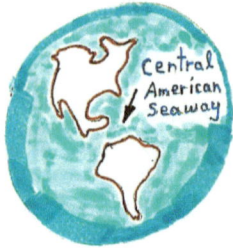

10 million years ago there was no Panama. Water flowed freely between the Pacific Ocean and Atlantic Ocean via the Central American Seaway.

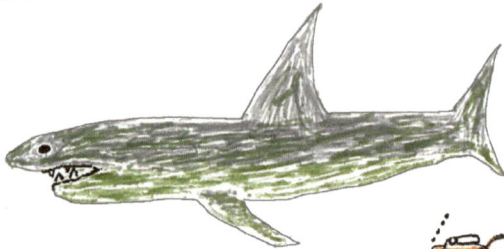

← Megalodon
o It would have swum through the Central American Seaway

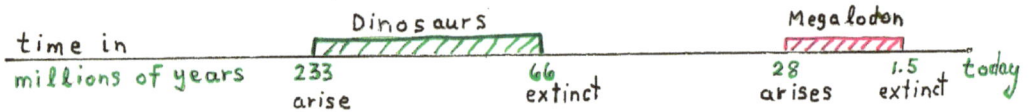

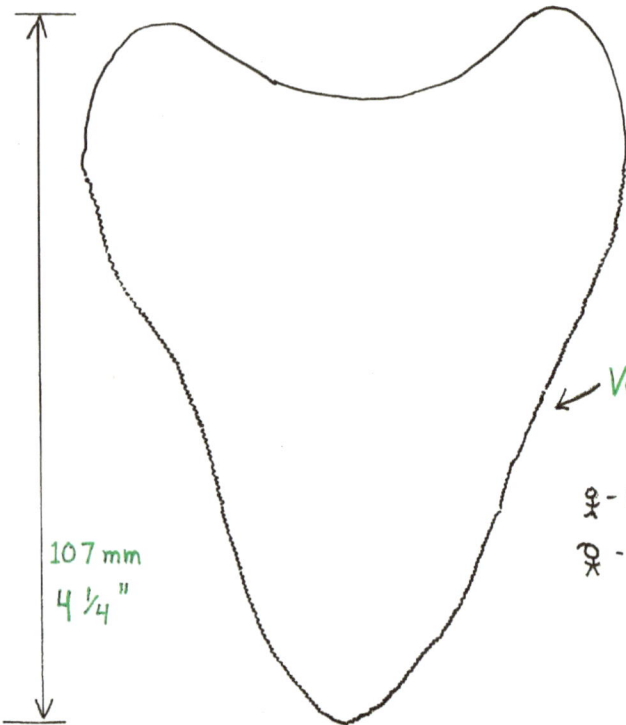

time in millions of years

Dinosaurs
233 arise   66 extinct

Megalodon
28 arises   1.5 extinct   today

← Outline of Megalodon tooth (that I bought at Mr. Wood's Fossils in Edinburgh, Scotland)

← Very fine serrations (whereas a Great White Shark tooth has coarse serrations)

♀ - How did this Apex predator go extinct?

♂ - When the Central American Seaway closed 3 million years ago, the end result was cooler water. It is thought that Megalodon preferred (or evolved in) warmer waters.

107 mm
4 ¼"

- Guess what?
Sharks contain a substance called squalamine that may interfere with the ability of the Yellow Fever virus to enter a host cell.

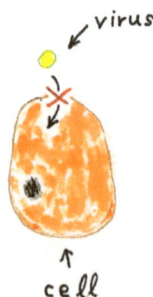

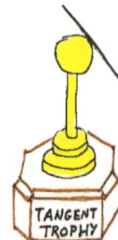

← virus

↑ cell

TANGENT TROPHY

"And the Tangent Trophy goes to Al Jones for putting Megalodon in a graphic novel about Coronavirus."

- Let's pause our tour of the **PLAGUE YEARBOOK** and identify some patterns and principles.

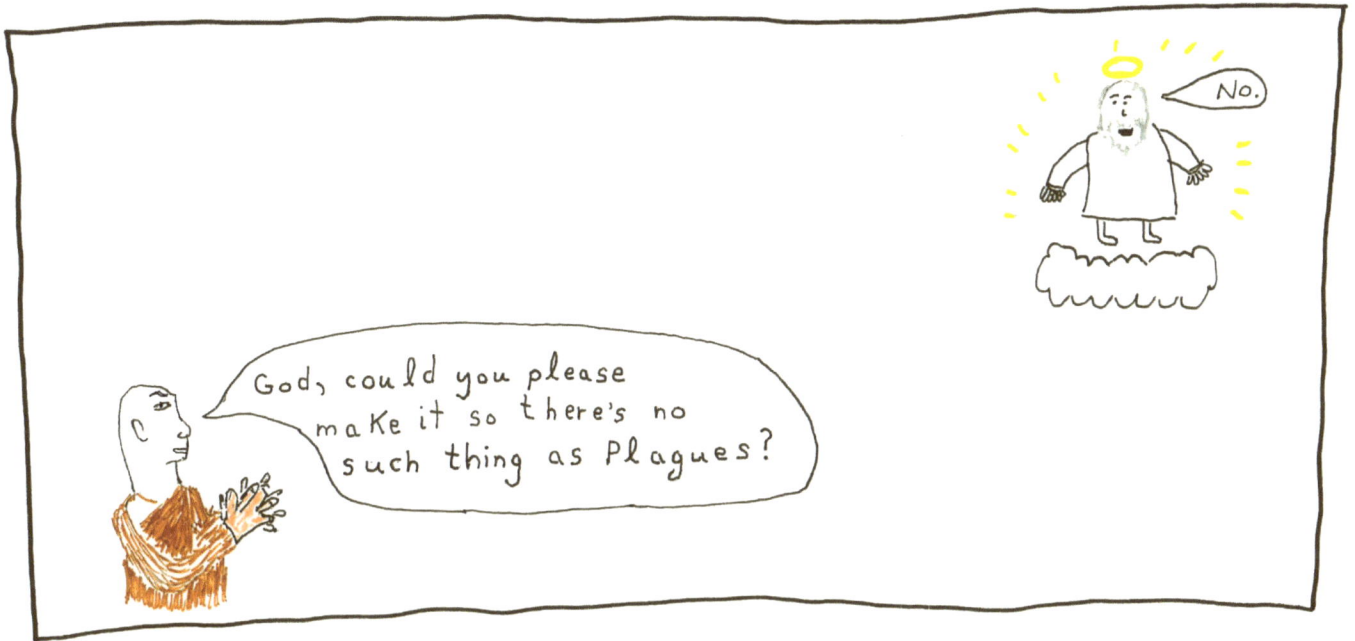

No.

God, could you please make it so there's no such thing as Plagues?

- OK, so much for that idea.
  - Let's look for our first pattern:

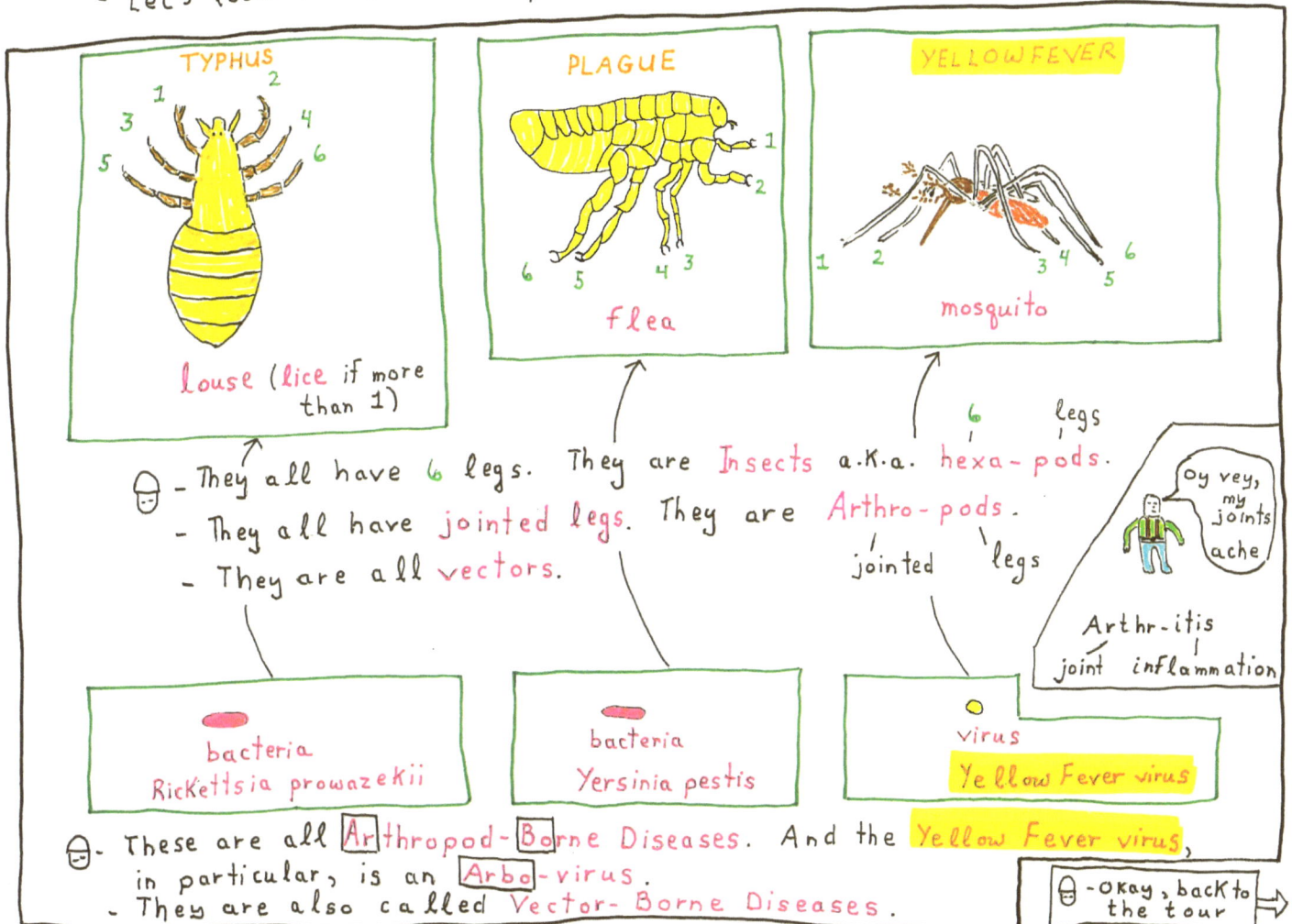

TYPHUS

1 2 3 4 5 6

louse (lice if more than 1)

PLAGUE

1 2 6 5 4 3

flea

YELLOW FEVER

6 legs

1 2 3 4 5 6

mosquito

- They all have 6 legs. They are Insects a.k.a. hexa-pods.
- They all have jointed legs. They are Arthro-pods.
- They are all vectors.

jointed legs

Oy vey, my joints ache

Arthr-itis
joint inflammation

bacteria
Rickettsia prowazekii

bacteria
Yersinia pestis

virus
Yellow Fever virus

- These are all Arthropod-Borne Diseases. And the Yellow Fever virus, in particular, is an Arbo-virus.
  - They are also called Vector-Borne Diseases.

- Okay, back to the tour →

Ebola

← Ebola virus
⊙ Looks like a piece of string
⊙ It's magnified 160,000 times

♀ - What's that font?

♂ - Braggadocio. Created in 1930 for Monotype Corporation.

☻ - There are 4 big rivers in Africa.

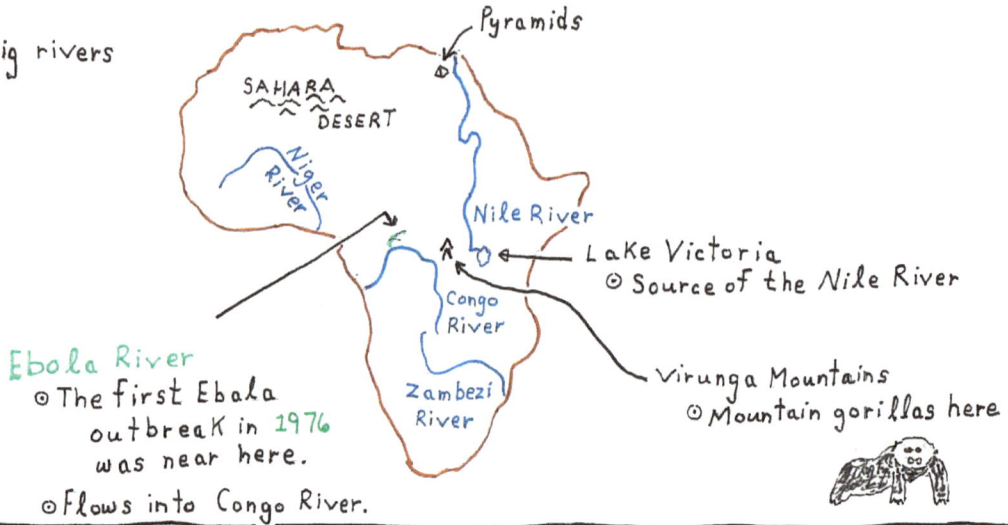

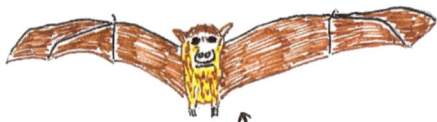

Pyramids

SAHARA DESERT

Niger River

Nile River

Lake Victoria
⊙ Source of the Nile River

Congo River

Zambezi River

Ebola River
⊙ The first Ebala outbreak in 1976 was near here.
⊙ Flows into Congo River.

Virunga Mountains
⊙ Mountain gorillas here

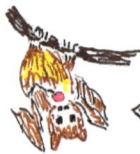

← eating fruit upside down

fruit bat
⊙ It carries the Ebola virus but is not harmed.
⊙ This is a best guess. The exact bat is not known.

☻ - Who is harmed?

humans

monkeys

chimpanzee

gorilla

human primate

non-human primates

Primates

☻ - How does Ebola kill primates?

In doctorspeak ⟨ Septic Shock

Disseminated Intra-vascular Coagulation (DIC)
+
Consumptive Coagulopathy

Translation
Death by low blood pressure

Blood clots all over the place.

Clotting factors run out ... now internal bleeding

(☻ - There are 13 clotting factors in the blood, numbered I to XIII.)

☺ - How does Ebola spread? It's complicated.

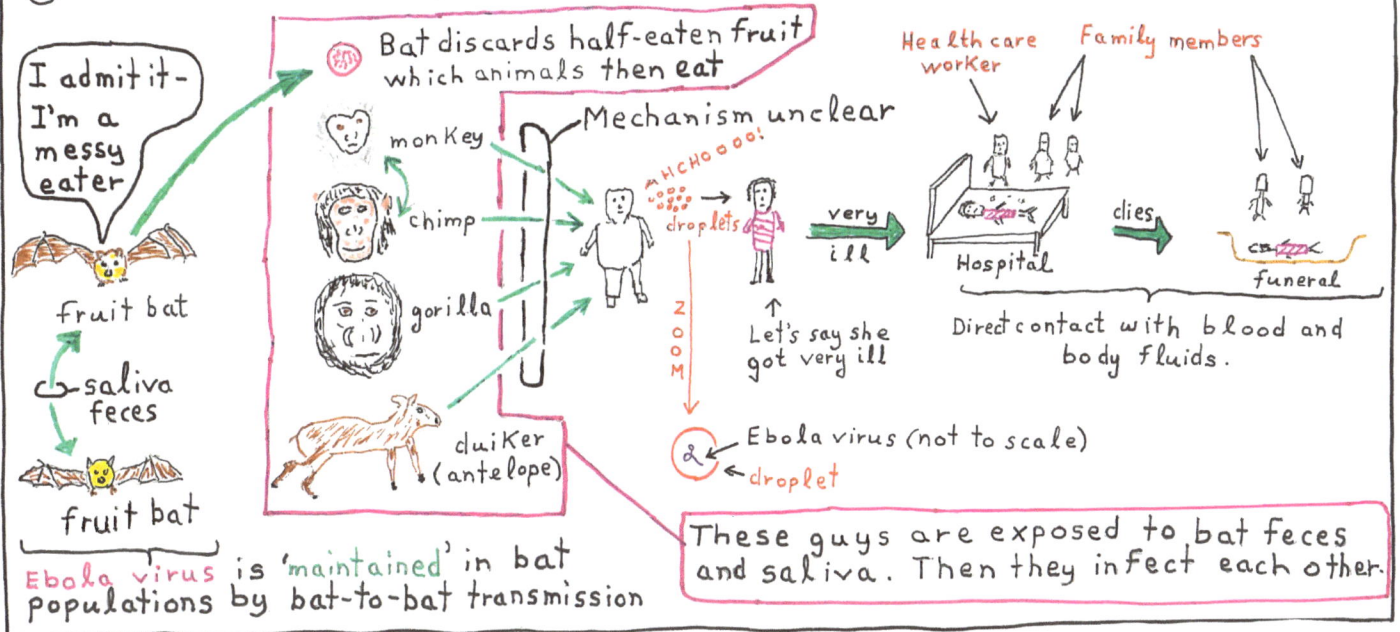

"I admit it - I'm a messy eater"

fruit bat

saliva feces

fruit bat

Ebola virus is 'maintained' in bat populations by bat-to-bat transmission

Bat discards half-eaten fruit which animals then eat

monkey
chimp
gorilla
duiker (antelope)

Mechanism unclear

AHCHOOOO! droplets

ZOOM

Let's say she got very ill

Ebola virus (not to scale)
droplet

very ill

Hospital

Health care worker   Family members

dies

funeral

Direct contact with blood and body fluids.

These guys are exposed to bat feces and saliva. Then they infect each other.

☺ - Ebola outbreaks have occurred every few years from 1976 to 2018, usually with 50-250 deaths. And the outbreak lasts 3-4 months.
- The worst outbreak, by far, was in 2014, with ~11,000 deaths.

1976 - Original outbreak
⊙Patient #1 - Headmaster at a school.
⊙Also, a Belgian nun whose blood is sent to the CDC in Atlanta.

♀ - Why is Ebola so scary?
♂ - Because every time there's an outbreak, about 50% of those infected will die

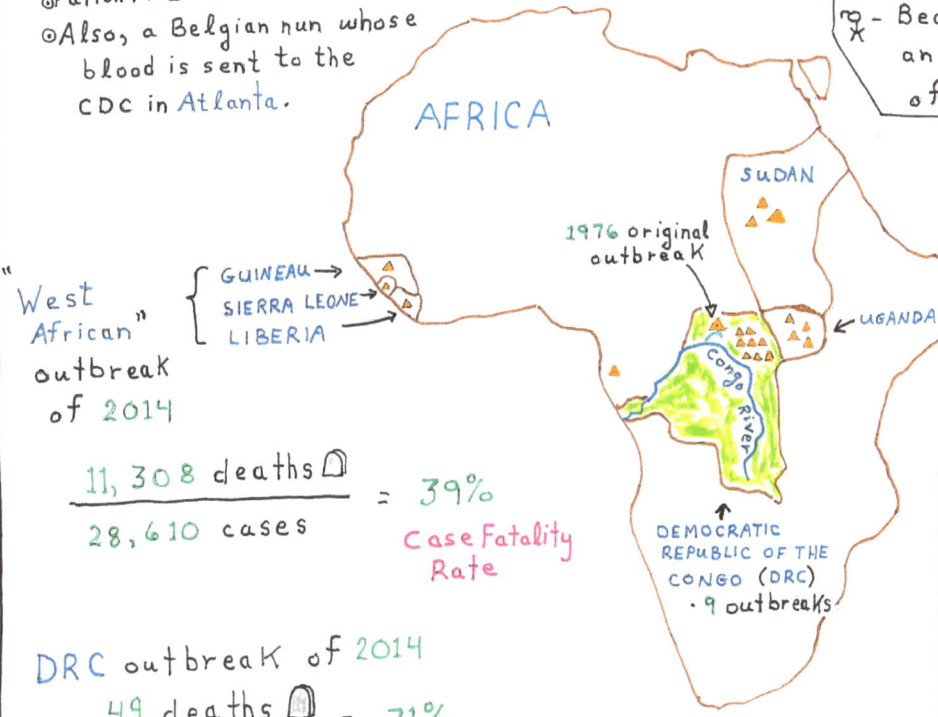

AFRICA

SUDAN

1976 original outbreak

GUINEAU
SIERRA LEONE
LIBERIA

UGANDA

Congo River

"West African" outbreak of 2014

$\frac{11,308 \text{ deaths}}{28,610 \text{ cases}}$ = 39% Case Fatality Rate

DEMOCRATIC REPUBLIC OF THE CONGO (DRC)
· 9 outbreaks

DRC outbreak of 2014
$\frac{49 \text{ deaths}}{69 \text{ cases}}$ = 71% Case Fatality Rate

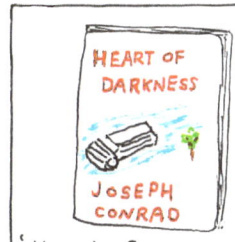

Interesting name changes
⊙ Congo Free State 1885-1908
⊙ Belgian Congo 1908-1960
⊙ Zaire 1971-1997
⊙ Democratic Republic of the Congo (DRC) 1997 to present

HEART OF DARKNESS
JOSEPH CONRAD

'Heart of Darkness', written in 1889, is about a perilous journey up the Congo River. It was the inspiration for Francis Ford Coppola's film, 'Apocalypse Now.'

Q - How did the 2014 Ebola outbreak get out of control? Specifically, why were there 28,000 cases in West Africa, versus the usual 200-300 cases?

① 'Porous' borders between countries.

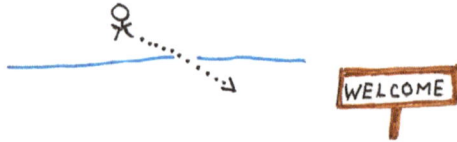

WELCOME

② Internal Expertise lacking

n = 17

- There were, at the time, only 17 medical doctors graduating per year in Liberia.

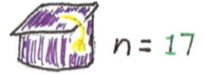

HCW

- 20% of Health Care Workers (HCW) died.

- Health systems collapsed.

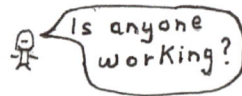

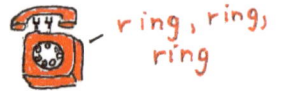

Is anyone working?

ring, ring, ring

③ External Expertise lacking

- Getting international experts to outbreak zone is difficult.

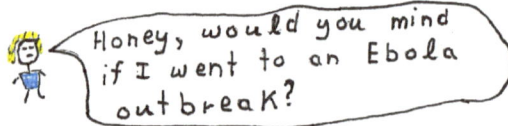

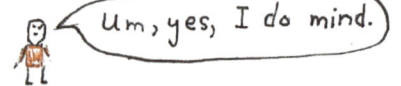

Honey, would you mind if I went to an Ebola outbreak?

Um, yes, I do mind.

- Majority don't go.
- Spouse says, No.
- Department Chair at University says, No.
- Discouraged by 3 week quarantine when return home.
- Who ends up going? Really brave, selfless people.

④ Personal Protective Equipment (PPE) unKnowns

- It was unclear how people were dying so it was unclear what PPE to use.

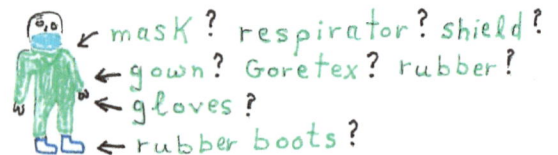

mask? respirator? shield?
gown? Goretex? rubber?
gloves?
rubber boots?

⑤ Transparency to share knowledge was subpar.

⑥ Poor political response ... Africa is neglected.

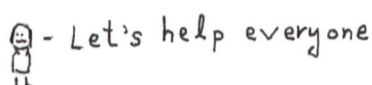

- Let's help everyone   - Let's not

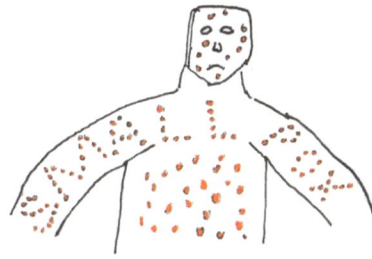

smallpox virus
Ironically, it kind of resembles the skin of an infected person.

- Smallpox is horrible. It definitely qualifies as a plague.
- Smallpox is a virus.

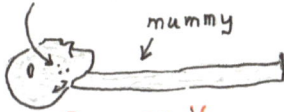

A pox on you

Old English 'poc' means skin lesion. And 'pox' means the same.

Smallpox scars
mummy
Ramses V
• Pharoah of Egypt in 1157 B.C. (the pyramids were built earlier, in 2575 B.c.)
• He died, it is thought, of Smallpox.

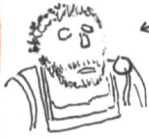

Marcus Aurelius Antoninus
• Emperor of Rome 161-180 A.D.
• He's the aging emperor in 'Gladiator.'
• Smallpox epidemic from 165-180 A.D. is the 'Antonine Plague.'
   • 2000 deaths per day in Rome.

← Emperor Sompoo
I just wanted to try that name on for size.
Okay, all told, Smallpox has killed about 500 million people.

◇ The Crusades ✚ brought more Smallpox to Europe.
◇ The Spaniards brought Smallpox to South America and Central America, wiping out the non-immune Aztecs and Incas in a single generation.

- Smallpox ravages the skin.

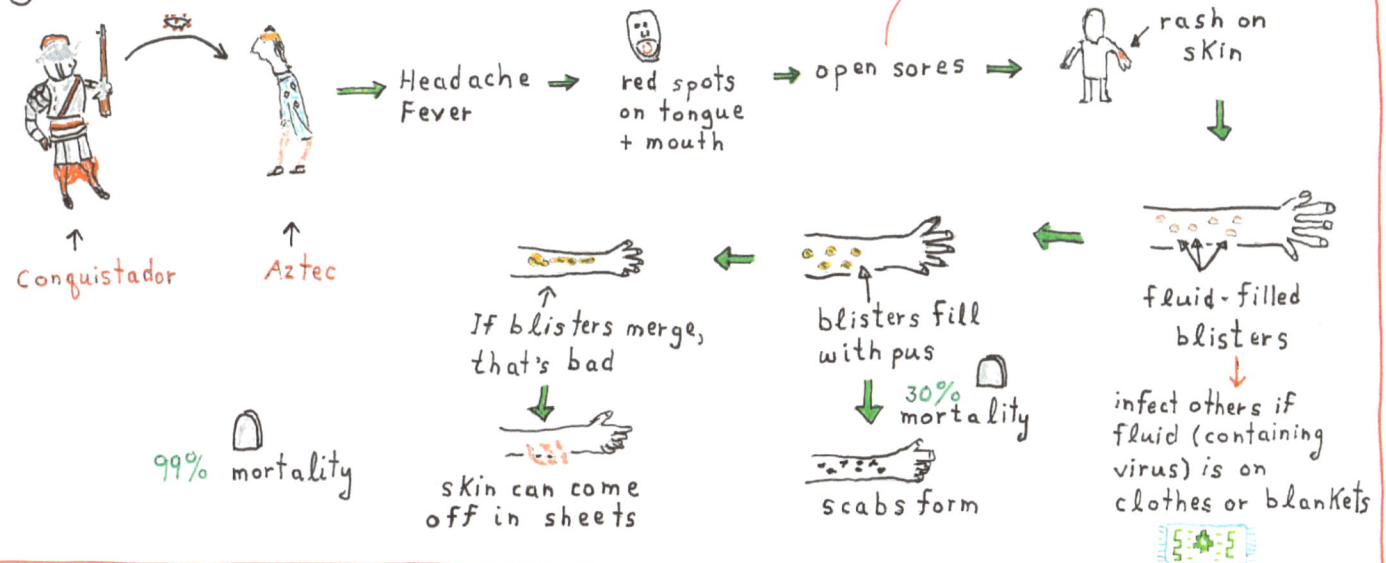

Conquistador   Aztec

Headache Fever → red spots on tongue + mouth → open sores → rash on skin

infect others

fluid-filled blisters
infect others if fluid (containing virus) is on clothes or blankets

blisters fill with pus
30% mortality
scabs form

If blisters merge, that's bad
skin can come off in sheets

99% mortality

Spanish Influenza

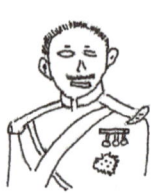

Queen Eugenie
- Better Known as 'Ena'
- Granddaughter of Queen Victoria of England
- Hangs around Buckingham Palace as a child.
- Born in Scotland, 1897.

King Alfonso XIII
- King of Spain
- Born at Royal Palace of Madrid, 1896.

- But first, the backstory ... In 1905, 19-year old Alfonso meets 18-year old Ena in London at a ball ... but Alfonso has poor English, Ena speaks no Spanish, so they converse in French ... they are smitten ♡♡ ... They are married in 1906 in Madrid with much pomp and circumstance (minus the bomb thrown at the wedding procession 💥) ... Ena has a son in 1907 who is, by nationality, ½ Spanish and ½ British.

- Geo-politics → Spain somehow ends up being neutral in World War I (1914-1918) Jul 28 Nov.11
  ↳ No censorship of the press in Spain during WWI.

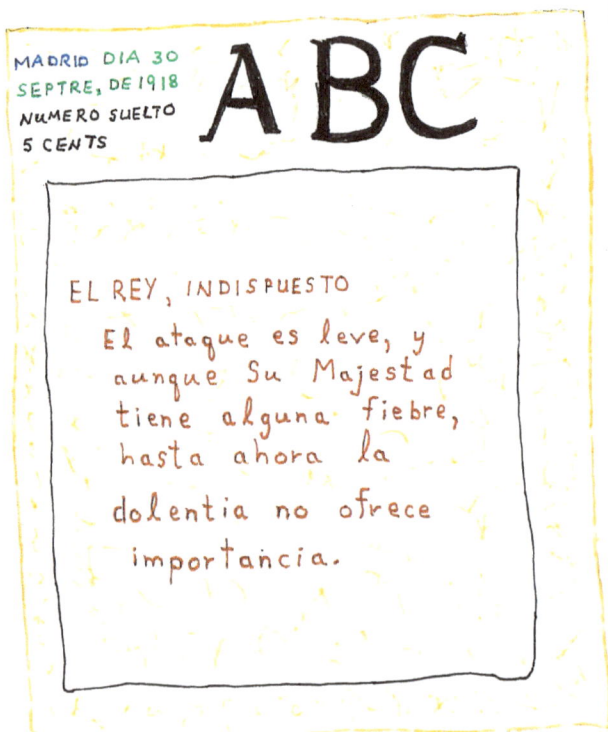

ABC is Spain's oldest daily newspaper, and continues to this day.

On 30 September 1918, it reports:

THE KING, INDISPOSED
The attack is slight, and although His Majesty has some fever, so far the pain is not important.

MADRID DIA 30 SEPTRE, DE 1918
NUMERO SUELTO 5 CENTS

ABC

EL REY, INDISPUESTO
El ataque es leve, y aunque Su Majestad tiene alguna fiebre, hasta ahora la dolentia no ofrece importancia.

(Muchas gracias to ABC)

- That's how it became Known as the 'Spanish Influenza.'

In fact, it was a global pandemic.

Population: 1.5 billion (1918)
Infected: 500 million
Deaths: 50 million

- The word 'flu' first appeared in 1839.
- And 'influenza' may be derived from the Latin, 'influentia'. That's a guess.

- The official name today is:
  1918 Influenza Pandemic

O ← Influenza virus
 ⊙ That's the view from an electron microscope →

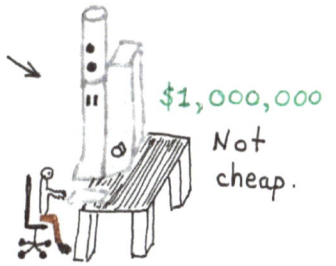

$1,000,000
Not cheap.

O - There are 4 types of Influenza virus (a.k.a. flu virus):
[Type A]
 ⊙ This guy infects ⎯ - humans
 ⎯ - birds
 ⎯ - pigs

⊙ Influenza Type A has a high rate of mutation. Every year it's a different virus. 1918 was a bad year.

⊙ And it has sub-types with weird names like H1N1 or H3N2 that sound like the license plates of a tiny country.

⊙ 'Influenza Type A: subtype H1N1' caused the Spanish Influenza a.k.a. 1918 Influenza Pandemic. It probably jumped from bird to human.

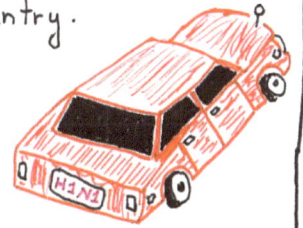

You can ignore B, C and D
[Type B]
 ⊙ Milder illness
 ⊙ Only humans
[Type C]
 ⊙ Rarely occurs

[Type D]
Moo
 ⊙ Affects cattle, not humans

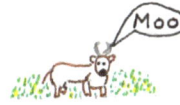

Influenza Type A is the one that concerns us. And the flu vaccine protects against it.

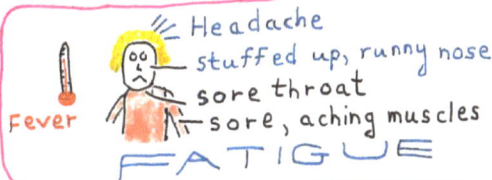

Headache
stuffed up, runny nose
sore throat
sore, aching muscles
Fever
FATIGUE

← This is what the flu (Influenza) feels like.
So do a ton of other illnesses, so they are called 'flu-like symptoms'

↳ Of the 450 million survivors of the 500 million infected in 1918, most felt like this. In a word, crappy.

♀ - So why did 50 million people die?
♀ - The virus beat up the lungs which were then susceptible to an infection by bacteria.

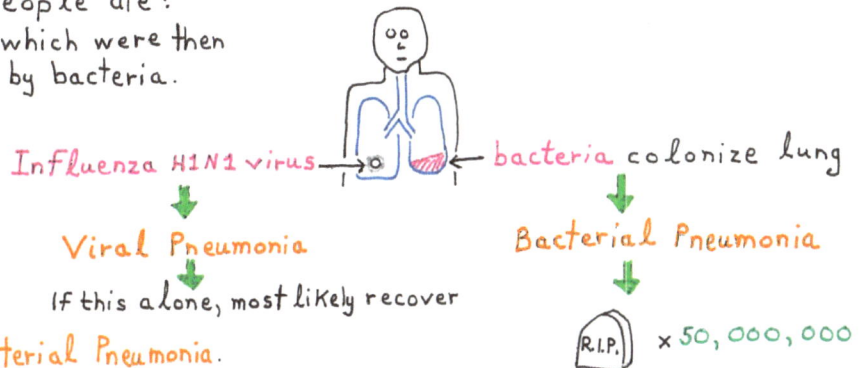

Influenza H1N1 virus → ← bacteria colonize lung

Viral Pneumonia
If this alone, most likely recover

Bacterial Pneumonia

R.I.P. × 50,000,000

- Get it? They died of Bacterial Pneumonia. They did not die of Viral Pneumonia.

- This is called a 'super-infection.'
 ! This use of 'super' does not mean super-strong, like Superman.

 ! It means something (bacteria) on top of something else (virus).

- You're already familiar with 'super' meaning on top.

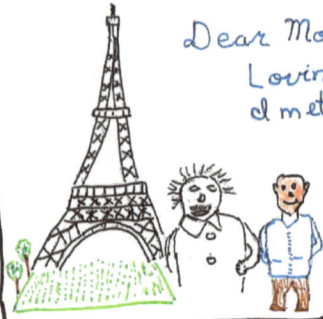

Dear Mom and Dad,
Loving Paris.
I met Albert Einstein.
your loving son,
Carl
p.s. Send $ for relativity experiments

Images can be super-imposed.

- The Bacterial 'super'-infection of the was figured out 90 years later.

ARMED FORCES INSTITUTE OF PATHOLOGY

- What's pathology?
- The study of diseased tissues under a microscope

1918 Influenza Pandemic

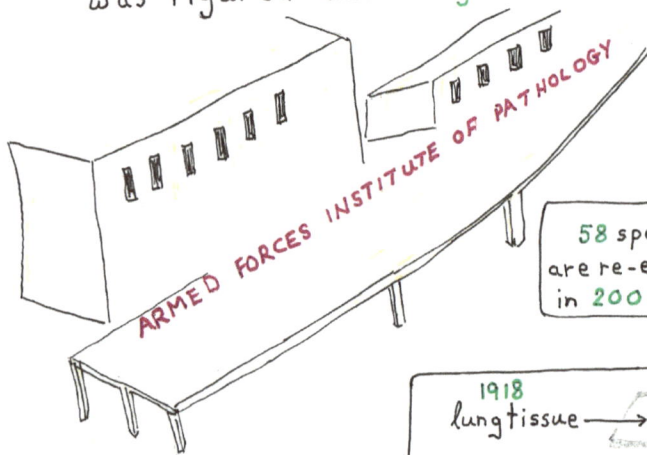

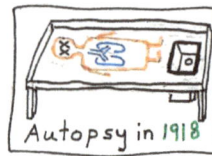

Autopsy in 1918

chop, chop → Sample of lung tissue is cut out

Stored in preservative (that kills virus) at the National Tissue Repository of the Armed Forces Institute of Pathology (AFIP)

58 specimens are re-examined in 2008

1918 lung tissue → ← glass slide

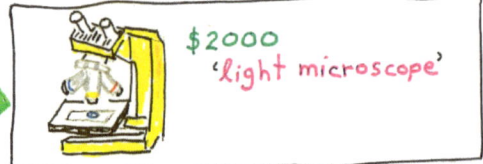

$2000 'light microscope'

massive numbers of bacteria
Lung tissue
← view in microscope
Large numbers of white blood cells (they fight bacteria)

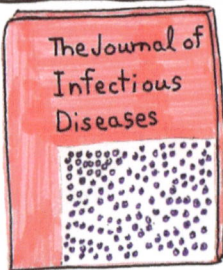

The Journal of Infectious Diseases

Volume 198
Issue 7
Pages 962-970
1 October 2008

- The findings are reported in a paper titled:

Predominant Role of Bacterial Pneumonia as a Cause of Death in Pandemic Influenza: Implications for Pandemic Influenza Preparedness

Authors: David Morens, Jeffrey Taubenberger, Anthony Fauci
↑ Recognize that name?

Conclusions
1. If this virus returns, it's bad news.
2. Pandemic Planning must go beyond preventing the virus alone.

Virus
Anti-viral drugs   Vaccine

Bacteria
Stockpiles of anti-biotics   Vaccine

A for Effort
A for Alaska

The remarkable story of how the deadly 1918 Influenza virus was buried, dug up, and resurrected.

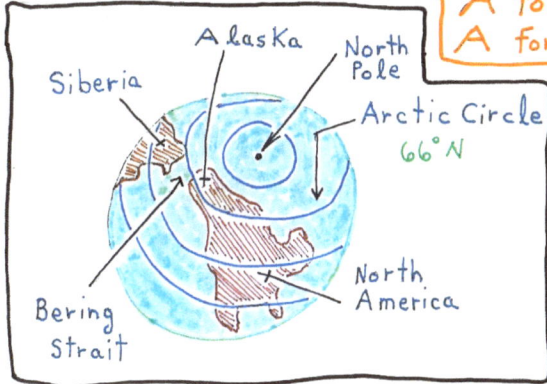

Globe illustration:
Siberia • Alaska • North Pole • Arctic Circle 66°N • North America • Bering Strait

Alaska map:
Arctic Circle 66°N
ALASKA
Brevig Mission
⊙ Coastal village in Alaska
⊙ 65°N, 166°W
Anchorage
⊙ 72 of 80 villagers die of the 1918 Influenza virus in 5 days, from November 15-20, 1918.
⊖ - Why such high mortality? They are native Inuit and have no immunity, reminiscent of the Aztecs having no immunity to the Smallpox virus.

gold miner   pick axe
⊙ Gold miners dug a mass grave for the 72 bodies

perma-frost
⊙ Permafrost is completely frozen ground made of ice, rocks, soil and dead plants.

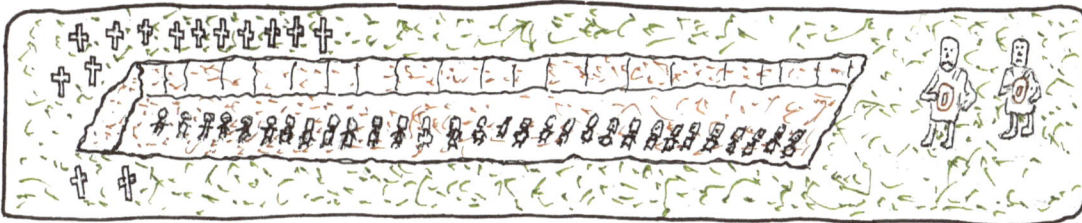

33 years later, in 1951

Scientists go to Brevig Mission with the goal of recovering and studying the virus.

Brevig Mission → ⊙ ALASKA

I will recover the virus
Johan Hultin, PhD
⊙ micro-biologist
↳ studies micro-scopic organisms with a micro-scope

I will open the chest cavity to expose the lungs
Jack Layton, MD
⊙ pathologist
↳ Doctor who examines dead people

I have experience digging up mammoth bones in permafrost
Otto Geist
⊙ paleontologist
↳ studies fossils. Lots of digging.

Camp fire
7 Feet of perma-frost
frozen bodies
A fire is lit for 2 days to thaw the perma-frost

The first body is a little girl in a blue dress and with red ribbons in her hair. That's sad.

Exhumed bodies are side by side

SNIP   scissors
snippets of lung tissue are placed inside a thermal jar
frozen lungs

Dr. Layton exposes the lungs

Johan Hultin
CO_2 fire extinguisher
Thermal jar is kept frozen with CO_2.

The lung specimens must remain frozen for the journey to the science lab

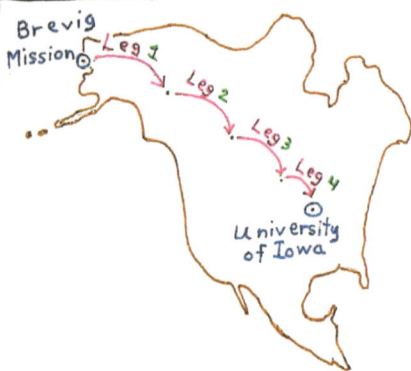

Brevig Mission
Leg 1
Leg 2
Leg 3
Leg 4
University of Iowa

Douglas Commercial
DC-3 →
- Twin-propeller plane
- 30 passengers
- 207 miles per hour cruise speed
- 1500 mile range
- 23,000 foot ceiling
- Made by Douglas Aircraft which later becomes McDonnell Douglas which later merges with Boeing.

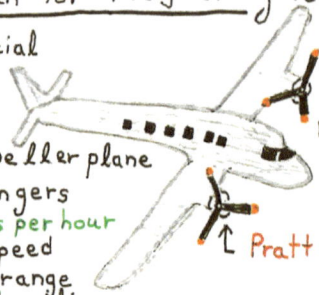

Propeller is 11 feet in diameter

Pratt & Whitney 14-cylinder engine

The journey is 3232 miles. The aircraft range is 1500 miles so 1000 mile "Legs" are safe so there's always leftover fuel. [I'm guesstimating 1000 miles. Maybe more. Maybe less.] Point is, at each refueling stop, Johan Hultin sprays the thermal jar with his CO_2 fire extinguisher to keep the lung tissue frozen. And all the other passengers are like, "Who the hell is that guy?!"

Science Lab University of Iowa

chicken egg →
chicken embryo →
Johan Hultin →

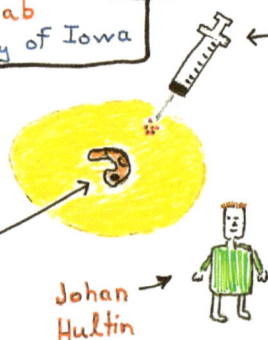

← Syringe injects thawed lung tissue into a chicken egg.
- The hypothesis (proposed explanation) is that the 1918 Influenza virus in the lung tissue can be brought back to life (bearing in mind it's debatable whether viruses are 'Life') ... and will kill the chicken inside the egg. I know, sounds kind of grim - resurrect the virus to kill an unborn chicken.

- Waaaaal, the experiment didn't really work. Too bad, so sad. A lot of grave digging for nothing. And the chicken probably ended up in an omelette.

Bear in mind, the year is 1951.
It isn't until 1953 that the DNA double helix is discovered by Francis Crick, James Watson, and Rosalind Franklin, heralding a revolution in the understanding of genetics (essentially, the code that creates all living things, including viruses - so maybe they are 'Life'. We'll get into that later).

Wouldn't you know it? Johan Hultin is a persistent scientist. He goes back to Alaska 45 years later, in 1995, because of huge advances in genetics.

Johan exhumes an obese woman at Brevig Mission
† †
of note, all the crosses are gone, so Johan erects 2 new ones, which is respectful

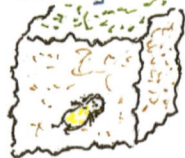

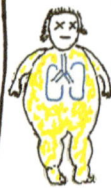

The good news is that the woman's fat insulated her lungs during warm periods when the perma-frost thawed (in the upper layer). This probably prevented her lungs from decomposing.

The next steps in the quest are coordinated by **Dr. Jeffrey Taubenberger, M.D., PhD** who is the **Chief of Viral Pathogenesis and Evolution** at the **National Institute of Allergy and Infectious Disease** (the same place where **Dr. Fauci** works)

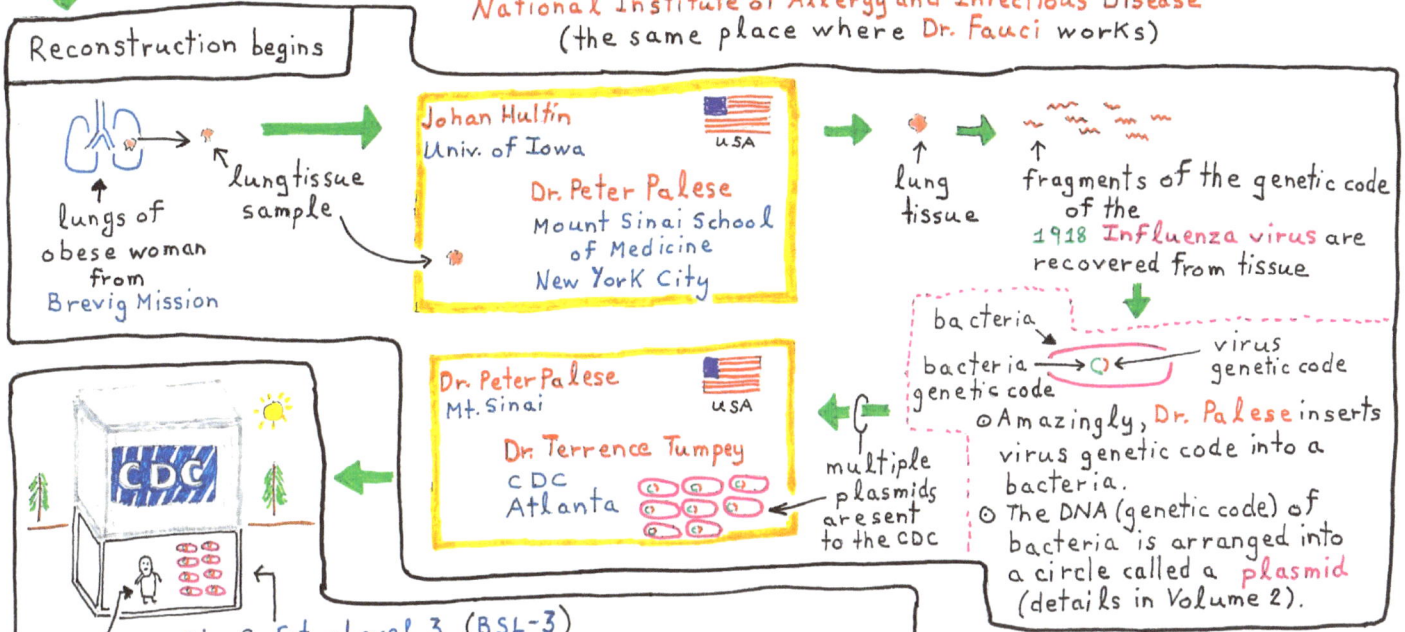

Reconstruction begins

lungs of obese woman from **Brevig Mission**

lung tissue sample

Johan Hulfin
Univ. of Iowa   USA

Dr. Peter Palese
Mount Sinai School of Medicine
New York City

lung tissue

fragments of the genetic code of the **1918 Influenza virus** are recovered from tissue

bacteria
bacteria genetic code → virus genetic code

○ Amazingly, **Dr. Palese** inserts virus genetic code into a bacteria.
○ The DNA (genetic code) of bacteria is arranged into a circle called a **plasmid** (details in Volume 2).

Dr. Peter Palese
Mt. Sinai   USA

Dr. Terrence Tumpey
CDC
Atlanta

multiple plasmids are sent to the CDC

CDC

CDC Bio-Safety-Level 3 (BSL-3)

Dr. Terrence Tumpey
○ PhD in micro-biology

Here is his **CONTRACT** →

"check the boxes if you agree to the terms"

☑ You are going to reconstruct the virus that killed 50 million people.

☑ Only 1 person will do the experiments: **Terrence Tumpey**

☑ You only work after hours, when all other **CDC** employees have left the facility and gone home.

☑ Fingerprint scan to enter BSL-3

☑ Iris scan to remove virus genetic material from freezer

☑ If you become infected, you will be permanently quarantined, cut off from the outside world.

The 8 genes of the virus are reunited

Experiment #1

Experiment #2

Reconstructed 1918 Influenza virus
↳ ○

Mouse infected with virus

↓

Very dead mouse

(details on next page)

The Return of the Chicken

Step 1. **Obtain** egg
← 10-day old chicken egg
Live embryo (developing organism)

Step 2. **Disinfect** egg surface (shell)
iodine

Step 3. **Drill** hole in shell

Step 4. **Inject** **Reconstructed** 1918 virus into hole a.k.a. inoculation

Step 5. **Seal** hole with paraffin wax

Step 6. **Incubate** at 36°C (97°F) for 3 days

Step 7. **Crack** egg open

Step 8. **Inspect**

Virus is lethal to chicken embryo

Membranes surrounding chicken have **pocks (lesions)** where virus grew

Why do all of this?
To prepare for another ○ **1918 Influenza Virus** ... that will make ○ **Coronavirus** look like a walk in the park.

θ – Let's recap

○ ←Genetically-engineered 1918 Influenza Pandemic virus.

⊙ The CDC recreated the virus to learn more about it.

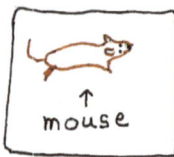

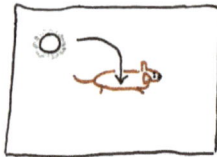

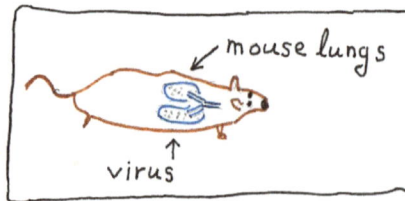

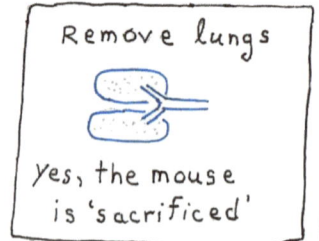

↑ mouse

mouse lungs

virus

Remove lungs

Yes, the mouse is 'sacrificed'

Findings

1. The virus beat the crap out of the mouse lungs.

2. 39,000 times more virus in mouse lungs than with 'ordinary' influenza viruses.

3. The protective mucous layer inside the airways (details later) breaks down
... bacteria have easier colonization of lungs, leading to lethal super-infection.

θ – So in conclusion, the 1918 Influenza Pandemic virus seemed to kill because of bacterial super-infections made easier by lung damage due to the virus.

– And by the way, sometimes we say this:

Primary (1°) infection = the virus

Secondary (2°) infection = the bacterial super-infection

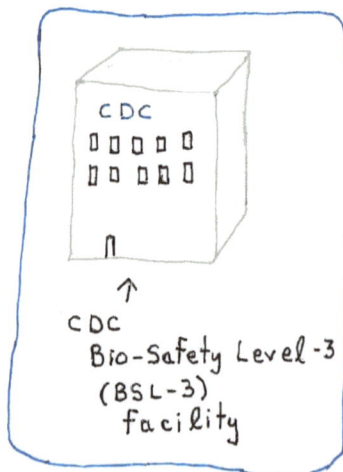

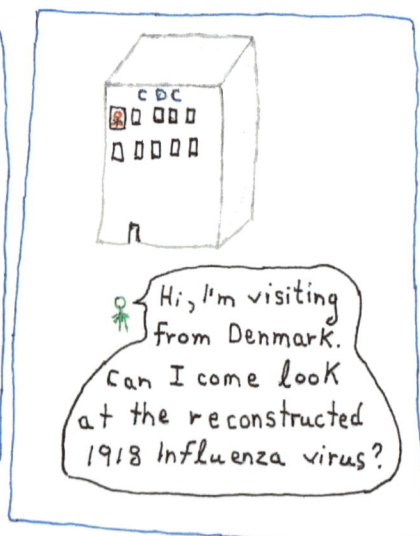

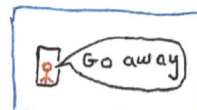

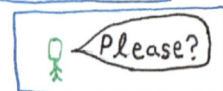

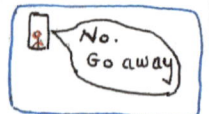

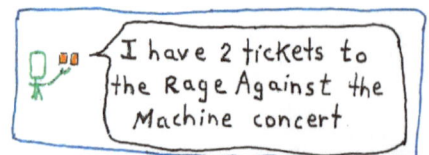

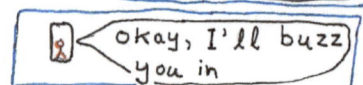

CDC
↑
CDC
Bio-Safety Level-3
(BSL-3)
facility

CDC

Hi, I'm visiting from Denmark. Can I come look at the reconstructed 1918 Influenza virus?

Go away

Please?

No. Go away

I have 2 tickets to the Rage Against the Machine concert.

okay, I'll buzz you in

⊖ - Points of clarity for people obsessed with details

Remember, Influenza virus comes in 4 Types

A ← This concerns us
B
C
D

Type A

Human Influenza A virus ○
↑ human
→ 1918 Spanish Influenza (Spanish Flu)
  └ sub-type H1N1
→ 1957 Asian Flu
→ 1968 Hong Kong Flu
⊙ It can also infect pigs. *oink oink*

⊖ - There is a 'seasonal flu' every year.

3 pandemics — It's just that 1918, 1957 and 1968 were bad years.

Avian Influenza A virus ○
↑ bird
⊙ It infects: chicken *cluck cluck* turkey *gobble gobble* duck *quack quack* goose *honk honk* + 100 other birds

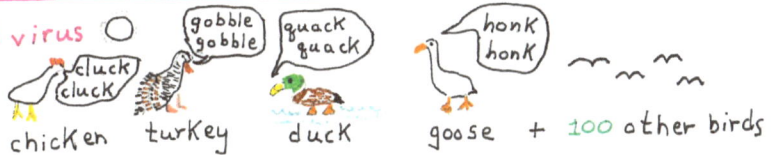

Sick bird ↘ nasal secretions ⊙ contains virus
↑ Feces ⊙ contains virus

→ ⊙ Infect more birds. They can die.

→ ⊙ This is rare
⊙ Can be severely ill
⊙ The naming is very confusing
  ⌐If the bird is sick, it's called: Avian Influenza
  ⌐If the human is sick, it's called: Avian Flu Bird Flu

⊙ Yes, the bird virus can also infect a pig.

Swine Influenza A virus ○
↑ Pig
cough, cough I can't breathe
⊙ Infected pigs have respiratory issues.
⊙ Rarely infects humans.
⊙ Again, confusing terminology:
  Sick pig = Swine Flu, Swine Influenza
  Sick human = Swine Flu, Swine Influenza

- Can I just say, 'I have the flu'?
- Sure

⊖ - Get it? These Influenza Type A viruses jump all over the place like it's Cirque de Soleil.

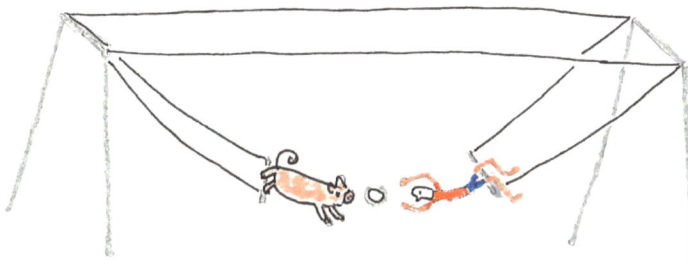

- So the Influenza virus jumps from animals to humans just like coronavirus?
- Probably even more

CHOLERA

cholera bacteria

- **Cholera** causes death by Diarrhea.

Thinking simply, food goes in, poop (stool) comes out.

Thinking mechanically, stool has to be <u>soft</u> in order to be pushed out.

And how is softness achieved? By <u>water</u>.

- Are we really going to talk about diarrhea and feces?
- Yup

My digestive tract is basically a tube from start to finish

← foodpipe
← stomach

→ water
→ Cholera-infected water

Small Intestine (S.I.) (small bowel)
- ☐ Food digested here.
- ☐ Cholera attacks here.

☐ It is 'small' because it is narrow.

= 10 FEET long

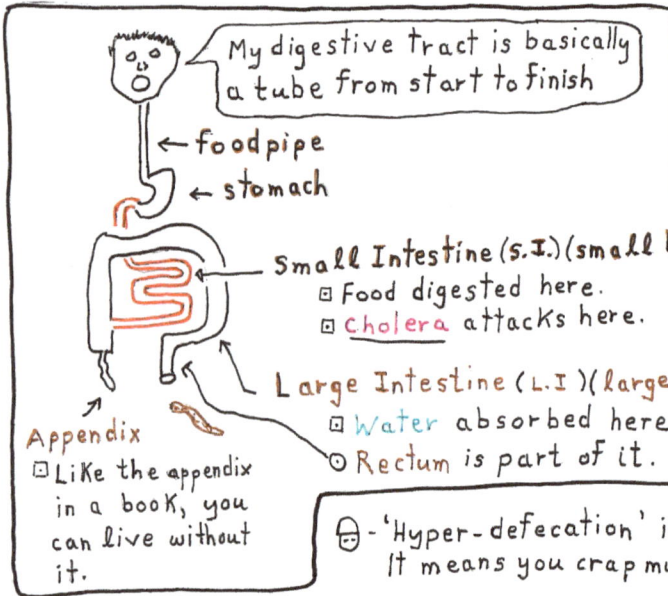

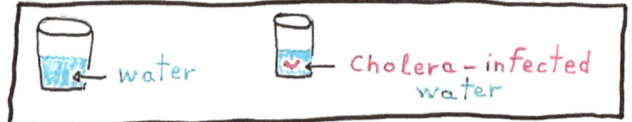

15 FEET of intestines packed into you way better than any suitcase

Large Intestine (L.I) (large bowel) (colon) = 5 FEET long
- ☐ Water absorbed here.
- ○ Rectum is part of it.

↑ Appendix
☐ Like the appendix in a book, you can live without it.

- 'Hyper-defecation' is not diarrhea. It means you crap multiple times per day.

Cholera bacteria → produces → Cholera Toxin (CTX)

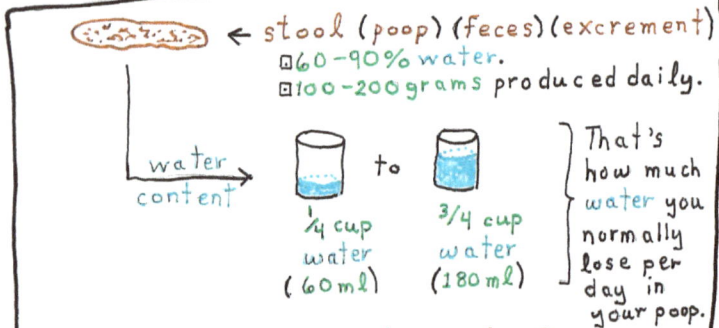

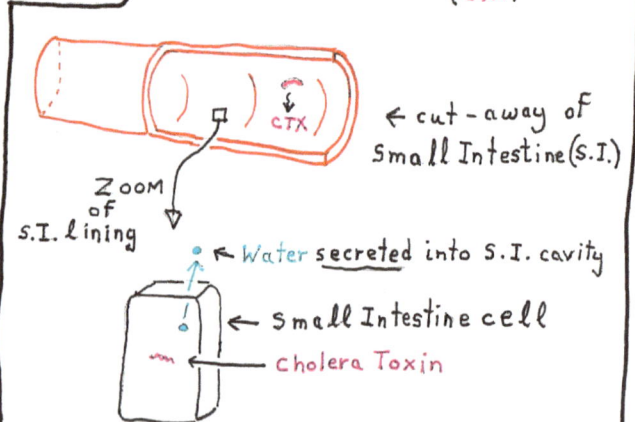

← stool (poop) (feces) (excrement)
- ☐ 60-90% water.
- ☐ 100-200 grams produced daily.

water content

¼ cup water (60ml) to ¾ cup water (180ml)

That's how much water you normally lose per day in your poop.

CTX

← cut-away of Small Intestine (S.I.)

Zoom of S.I. lining

← Water secreted into S.I. cavity
← Small Intestine cell
← Cholera Toxin

- Diarrhea is watery stool.
- Basically, ↑ water content so it changes from the familiar soft into a liquid splatter.

- The Cholera Toxin causes small intestine cells to secrete water.

- The diarrhea of Cholera is extreme.

4 cups per hour (1000 ml/h) (1 liter/h)
⇩
Massive fluid loss + dehydration
⇩
R.I.P. Can die in a matter of hours from Shock.

98 cups per day (24,000 ml/day) (24 liters/day) =

☺ - Cholera killed 1,000,000 Russians from 1846 to 1860.
- But the most famous Cholera outbreak only killed 616 people.
 Let's visit London ...

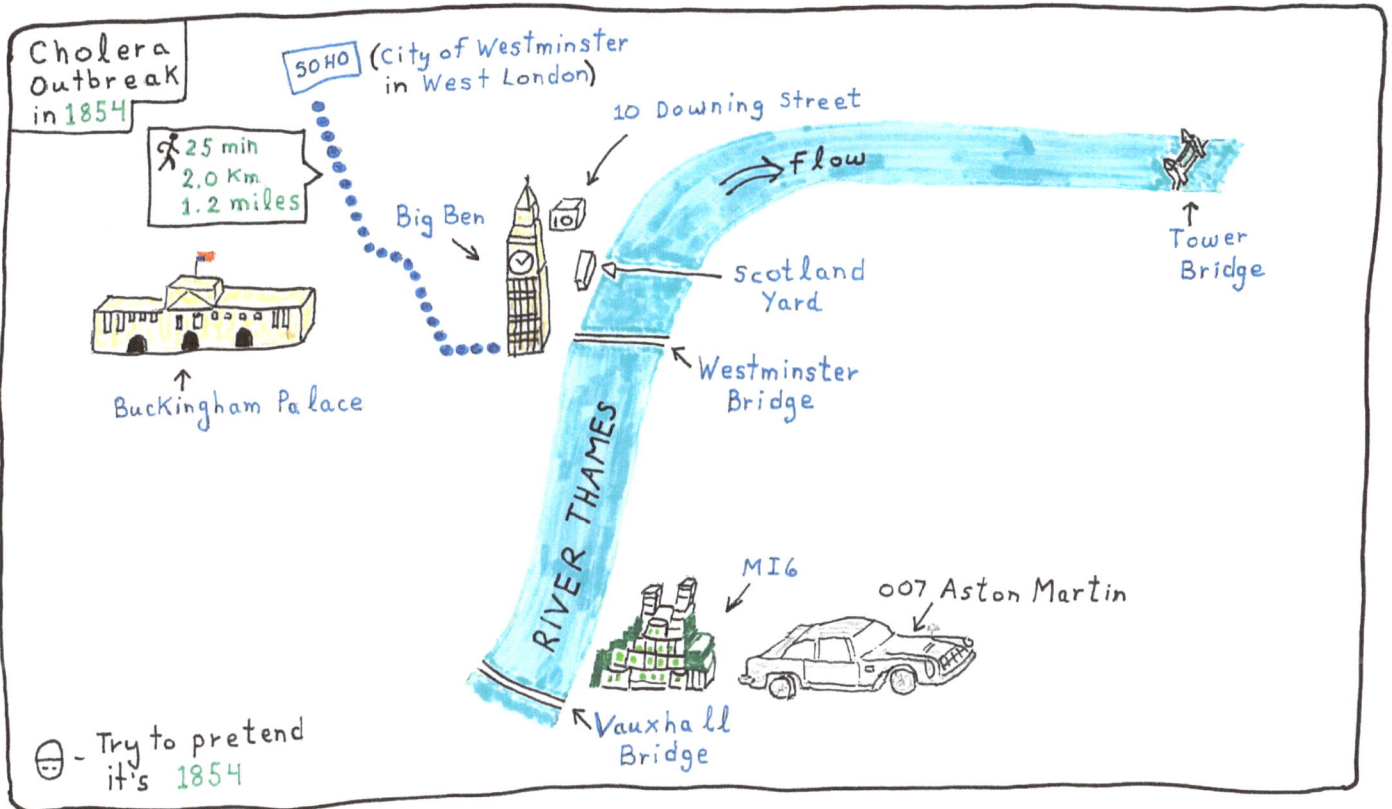

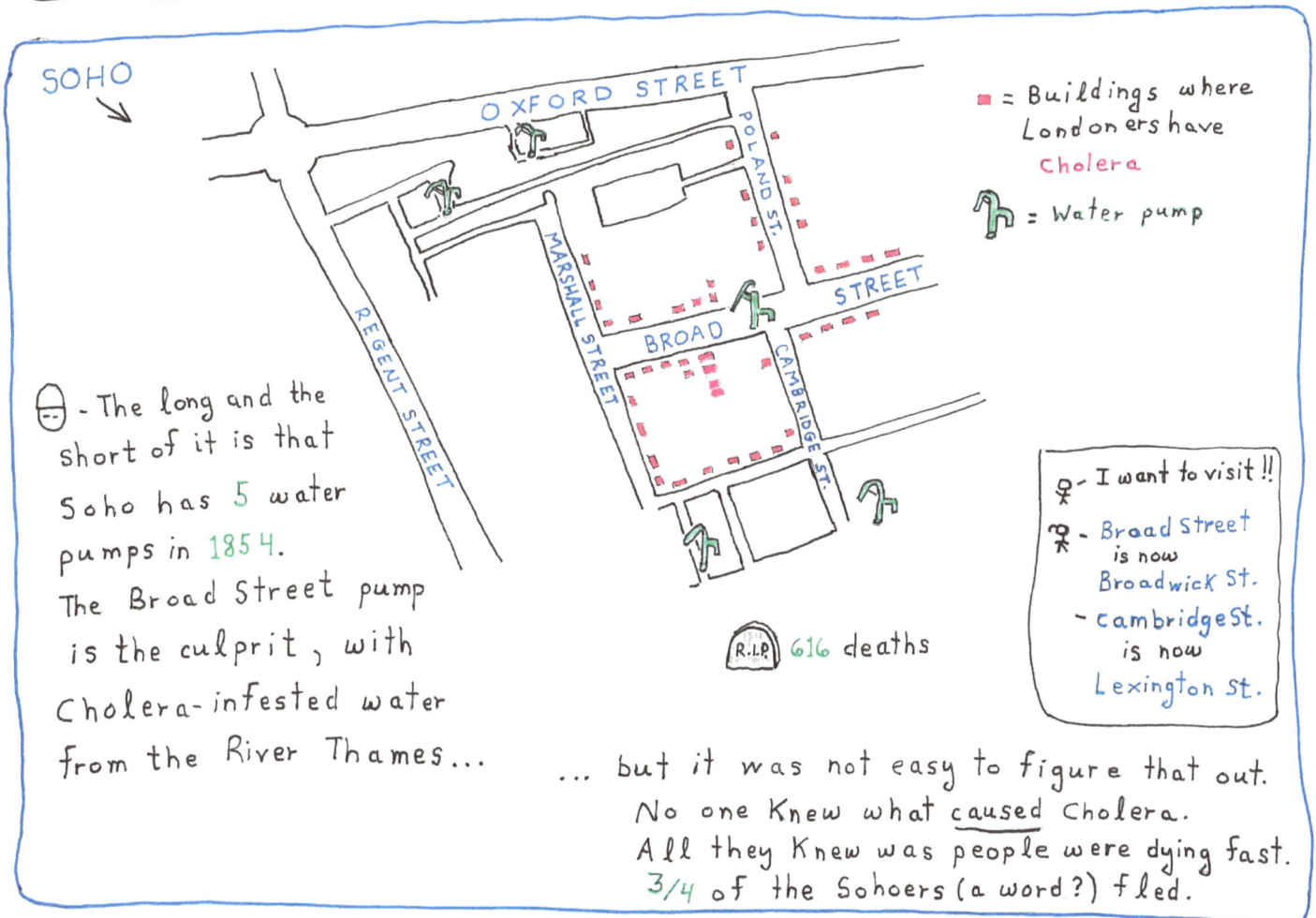

Cholera Outbreak in 1854

SOHO (City of Westminster in West London)

🚶 25 min
2.0 Km
1.2 miles

Big Ben

10 Downing Street

→ Flow

Tower Bridge

Buckingham Palace

Scotland Yard

Westminster Bridge

RIVER THAMES

MI6

007 Aston Martin

Vauxhall Bridge

☺ - Try to pretend it's 1854

SOHO →

OXFORD STREET

POLAND ST.

MARSHALL STREET

REGENT STREET

BROAD STREET

CAMBRIDGE ST.

■ = Buildings where Londoners have Cholera

🚰 = Water pump

☺ - The long and the short of it is that Soho has 5 water pumps in 1854.
The Broad Street pump is the culprit, with Cholera-infested water from the River Thames...

R.I.P. 616 deaths

- I want to visit !!
- Broad Street is now Broadwick St.
- Cambridge St. is now Lexington St.

... but it was not easy to figure that out.
No one knew what <u>caused</u> Cholera.
All they knew was people were dying fast.
3/4 of the Sohoers (a word?) fled.

"The most terrible outbreak of cholera which ever occurred in this Kingdom."

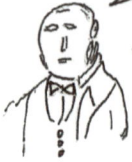

← Dr. John Snow

He goes seriously CSI on things.
- He doubts that air causes Cholera, as was supposed.
- He investigates the 4 water companies that pump water from the River Thames. SOHO RIVER THAMES
  - 2 of them are good. Ⓐ Ⓐ
  - 2 of them are sketchy. Ⓕ Ⓕ
    ↳ Their 'filtered' water contains animal hair. Nice. And all kinds of crap and corruption.

- He visits everyone who is sick → draws a map (previous page)
  → everyone is clustered around the Broad Street pump.

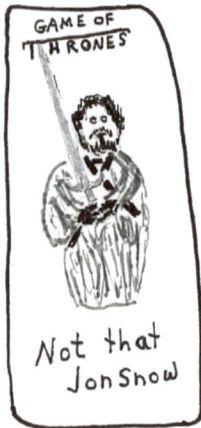

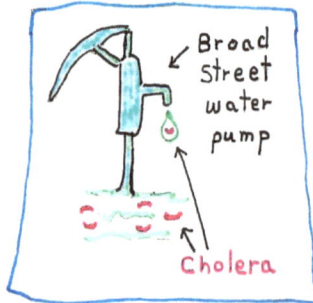

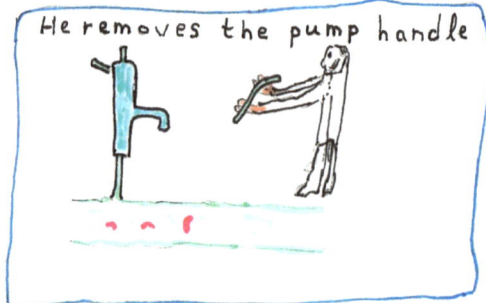

GAME OF THRONES

Not that Jon Snow

Broad Street water pump
Cholera

He removes the pump handle

No more Cholera. Hurrah.

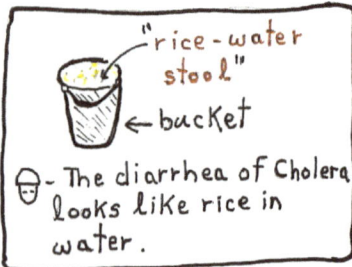

"rice-water stool"
← bucket
- The diarrhea of Cholera looks like rice in water.

- Of note, Dr. Snow, has only deduced scuzzy water is the cause.
  - He does not have wi-fi.
  - He does not know the bacteria has been identified in Florence.

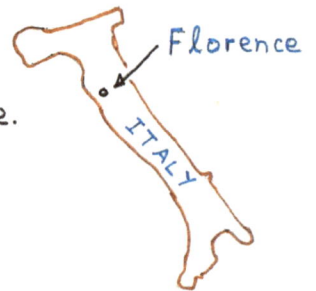

Florence
ITALY

Vibrio cholera
· Lives in water.

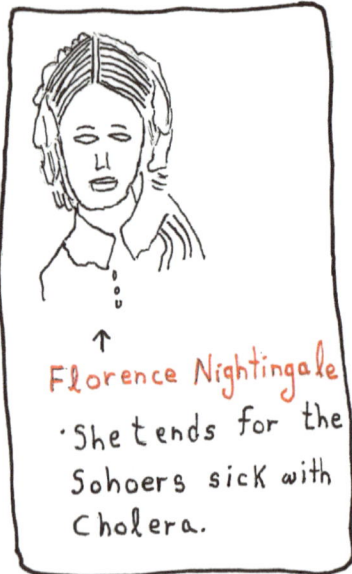

Florence Nightingale
· She tends for the Sohoers sick with Cholera.

- Dr Snow is a founder of Epidemiology. His 'dot map' is the forerunner of the very popular Johns Hopkins University ☼ Coronavirus dashboard created by the engineer Dr. Lauren Gardner.

SOMPOO SAYS · "Vib ree oh" "collar ah"

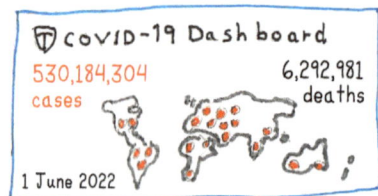

COVID-19 Dashboard
530,184,304 cases
6,292,981 deaths
1 June 2022

- If you enter 'John Snow' into Google Maps or Apple Maps you'll find the culprit pump but it's not there anymore, just a marker.

- With that brief tour of the **PLAGUE YEARBOOK** complete, let's identify more patterns and principles.

We humans have been under attack for thousands of years.

BACTERIA ← ⋮ → VIRUSES

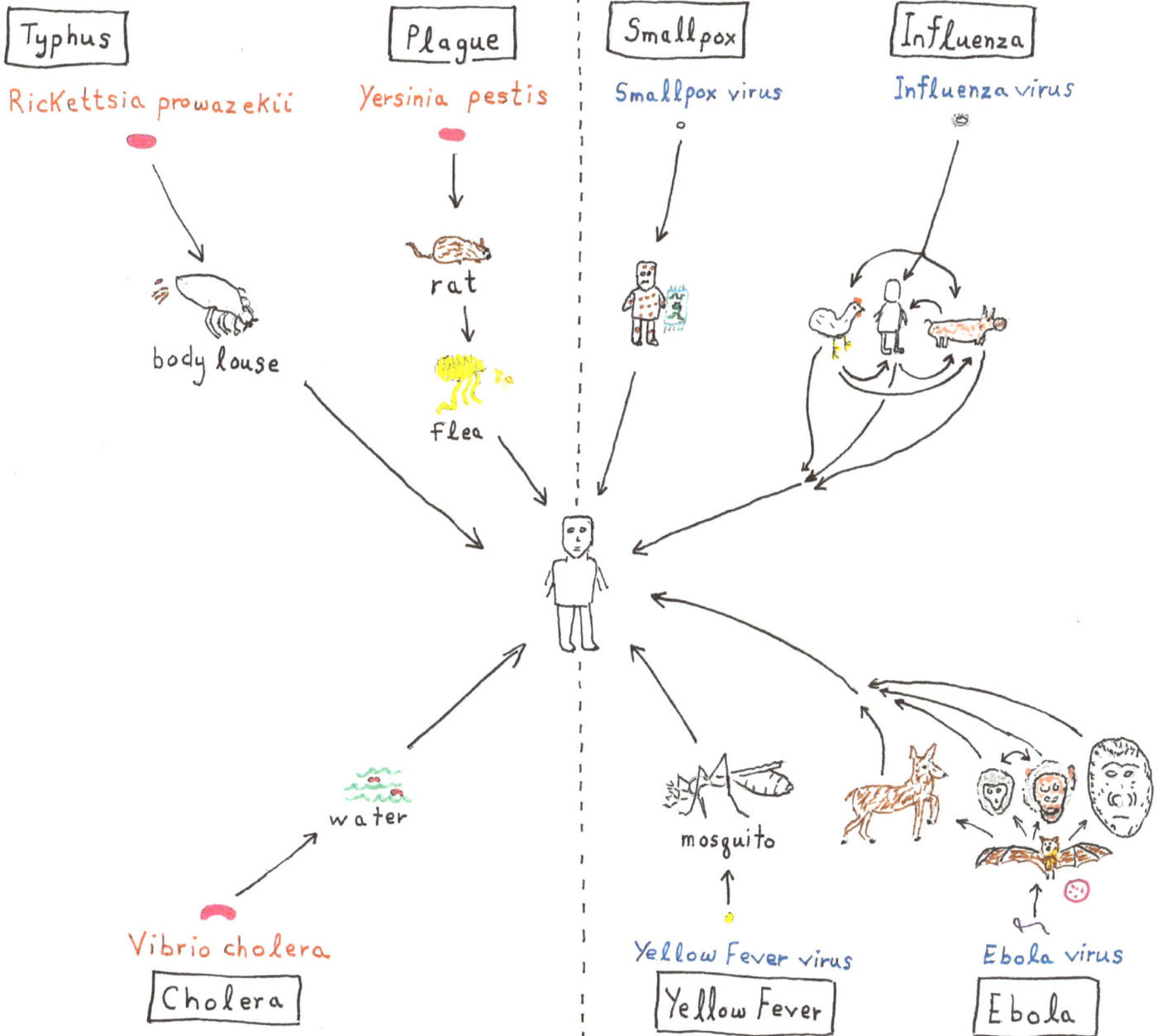

Typhus

Rickettsia prowazekii

body louse

Plague

Yersinia pestis

rat

flea

Smallpox

Smallpox virus

Influenza

Influenza virus

water

Vibrio cholera

Cholera

mosquito

Yellow Fever virus

Yellow Fever

Ebola virus

Ebola

- But this is hardly the *full* extent of things ...

☻ – Humans are attacked by 1424 species of pathogens.

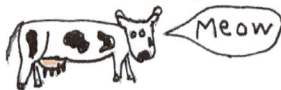
♀ – What's a pathogen?

☂ – An umbrella term for everything on this page.
↘ So are:
· germ
· microbe
· micro-organism
· agent
· infectious agent
· bug
  (Kinda informal)

BACTERIA
538

VIRUSES
219

AMOEBAS
57

FUNGI
317

WORMS
287

PRIONS   (for example,
            Mad Cow Disease)
6
                    Meow

☻ – Not all of these pathogens are scary.
↘ For example, the fungus that causes athlete's foot is not scary (well, maybe the smell is scary), whereas the fungus that causes a super-infection (on top of) ☀Coronavirus Viral Pneumonia is definitely a nasty Fungal Pneumonia. And of the 538 species of bacteria, there are about 60 species that do most of the damage.

☺ - Let's think abstractly.

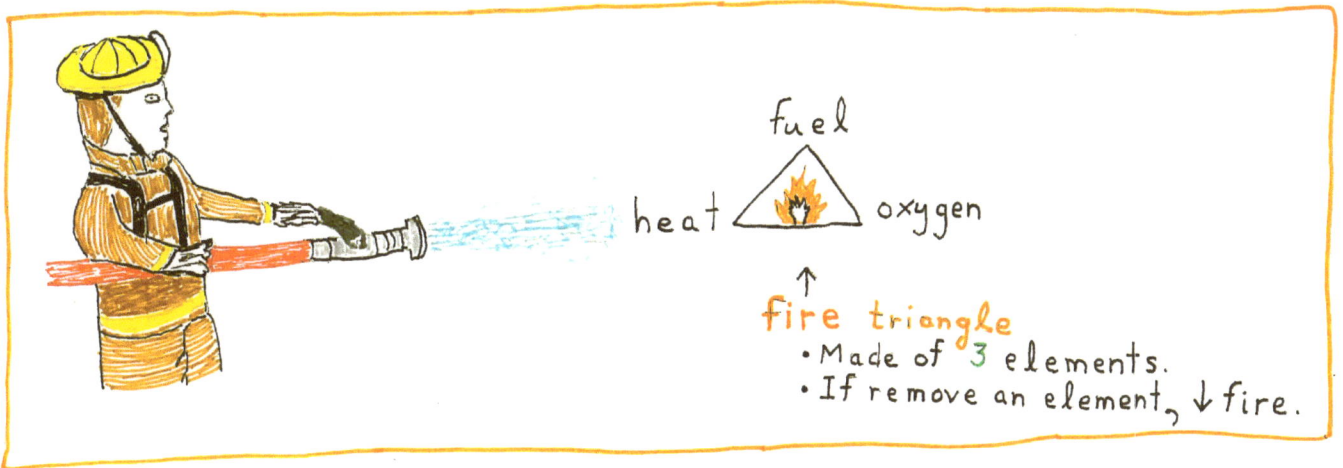

fuel

heat △ oxygen

↑
fire triangle
• Made of 3 elements.
• If remove an element, ↓ fire.

... likewise

Host 👤

Vector

Agent   Environment

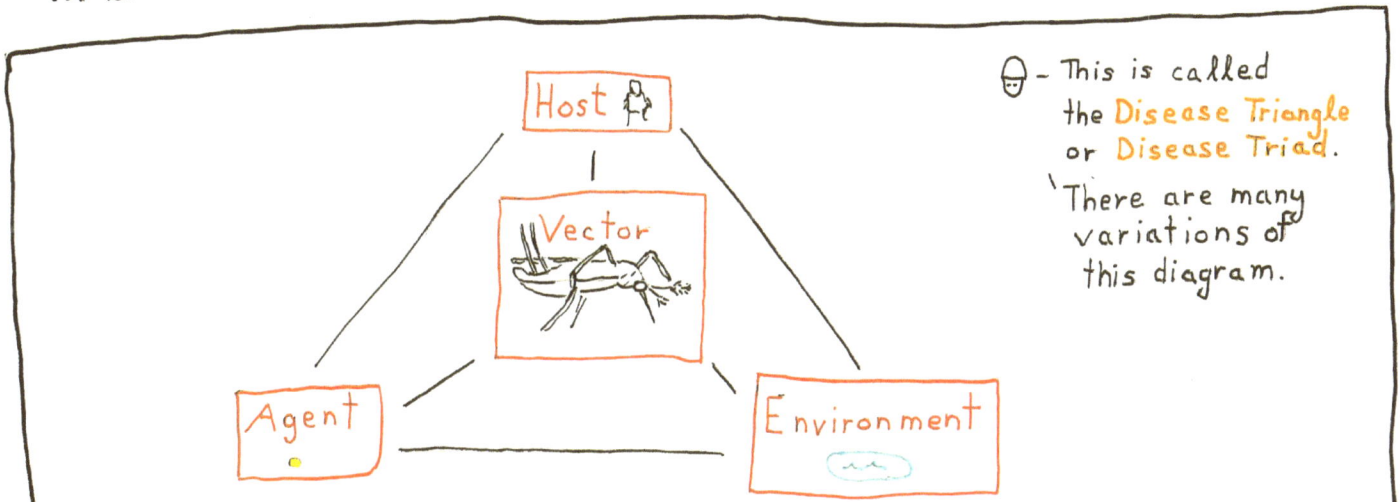

☺ - This is called
the Disease Triangle
or Disease Triad.
`There are many
variations of
this diagram.

☺ - We can remove an element here to ↓ 'infectious fire.'
` Let's think about removal of the elements of Yellow Fever.

Host
• Never apply for a job working on the Panama canal in 1881.
• Yellow Fever vaccine
• Intact immune system

Vector
• Wear mosquito repellant
• Insecticide to kill mosquitoes

Agent (infectious agent)
• Very hard to actually
remove the Yellow
Fever virus

Environment
• Drain swamps where
mosquitoes breed

(Thank you to Dr. Timothy Sly, Professor of Epidemiology and Public Health at Ryerson University, Toronto, for permission to use this diagram.)

- Time to get the view from 30,000 feet.

We started out like this

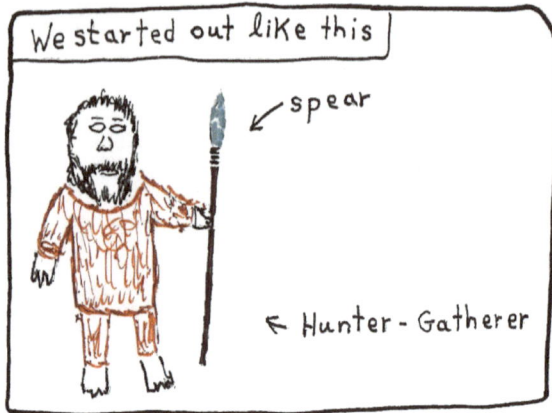

spear

← Hunter - Gatherer

... time passed

...

8000 B.C., give or take

farm

domesticated animals

farmer → pitchfork

hut

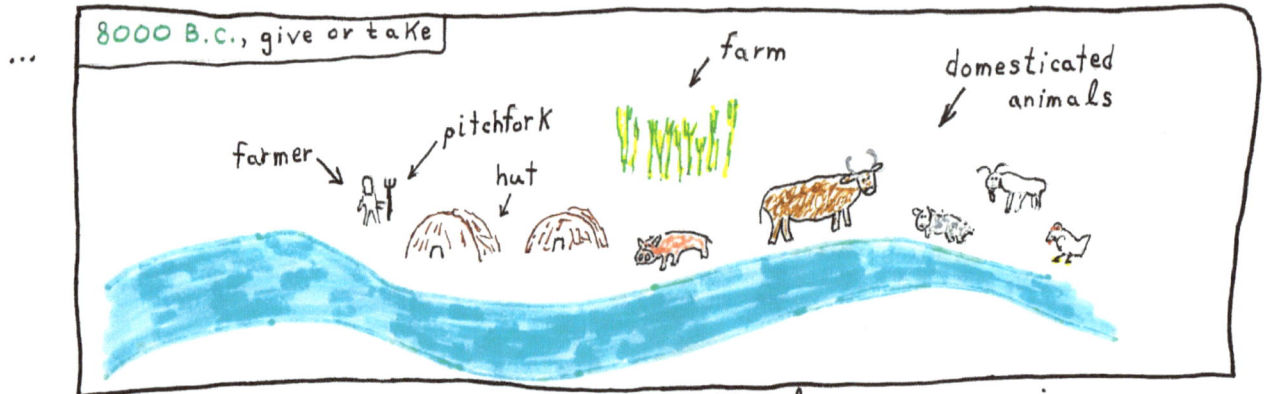

- Agriculture, which usually comes with living near a river, is a defining aspect of 'civilization'.

- Agriculture is also a great way for humans, animals, bacteria, viruses, and other germs to all be in the same place.

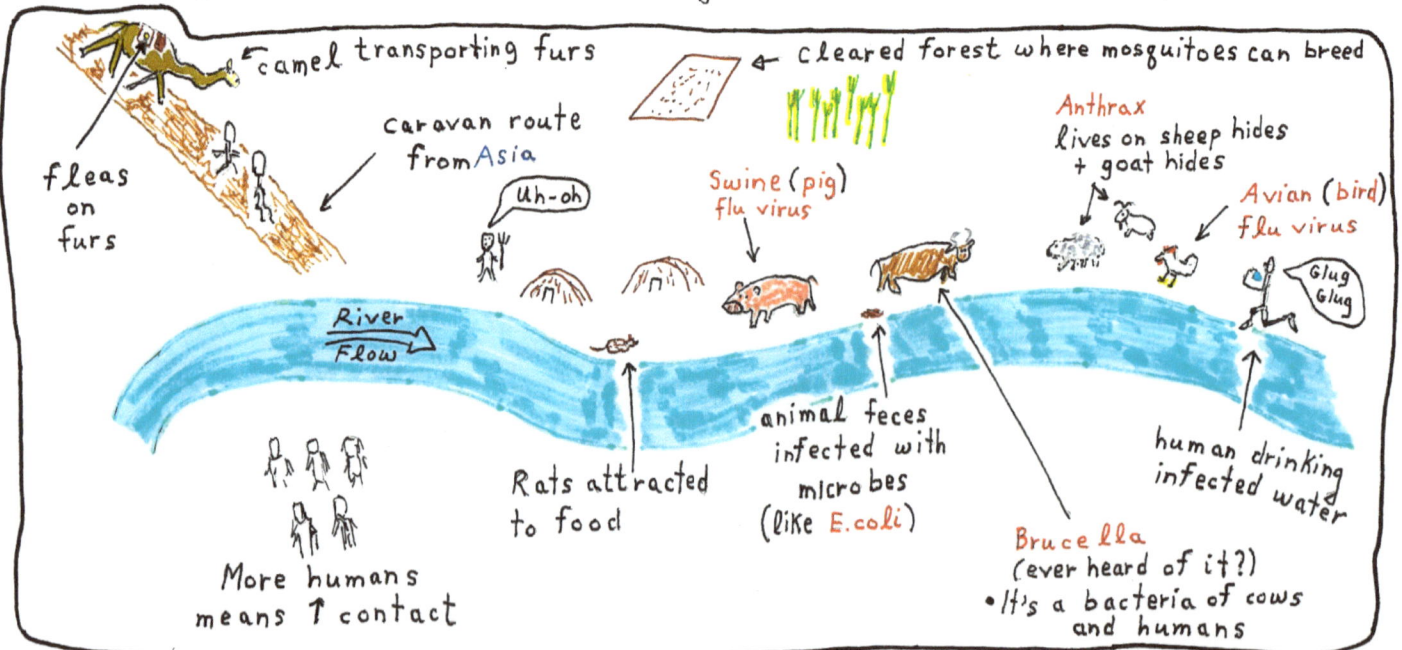

camel transporting furs

← cleared forest where mosquitoes can breed

caravan route from Asia

Anthrax lives on sheep hides + goat hides

fleas on furs

Uh-oh

Swine (pig) flu virus

Avian (bird) flu virus

Glug Glug

River Flow

Rats attracted to food

animal feces infected with microbes (like E.coli)

human drinking infected water

More humans means ↑ contact

Brucella (ever heard of it?) • It's a bacteria of cows and humans

- Agriculture, hence civilization itself, is a risk factor for epidemics of disease.

- How is it we are even alive, surrounded as we are by all these pathogens?

Let's consider a <u>hypothetical</u> worst virus ever...

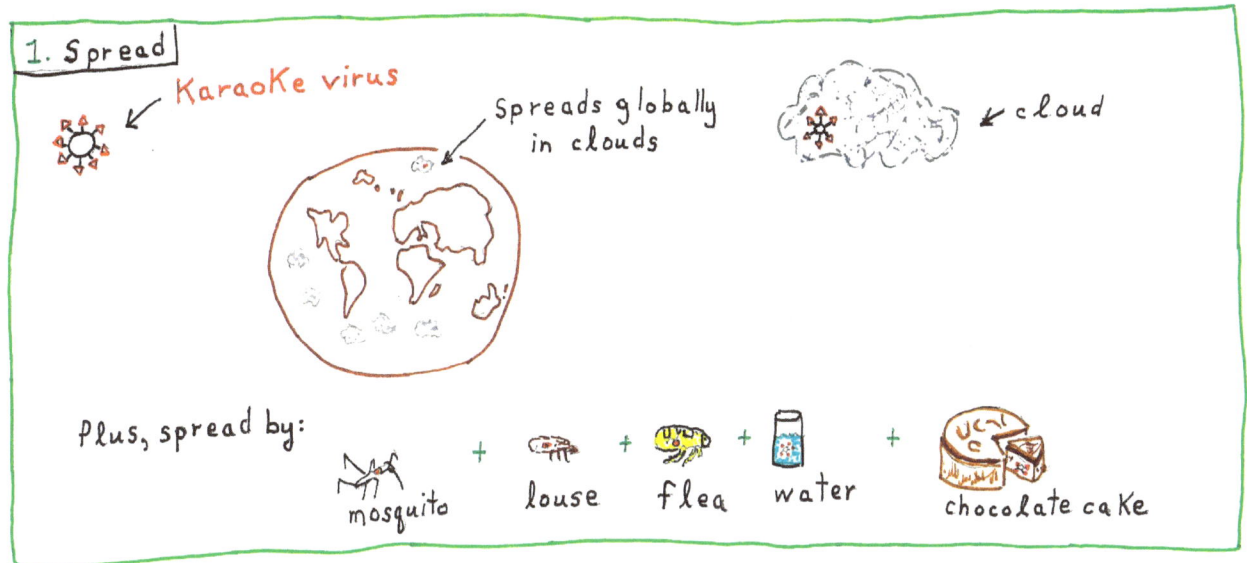

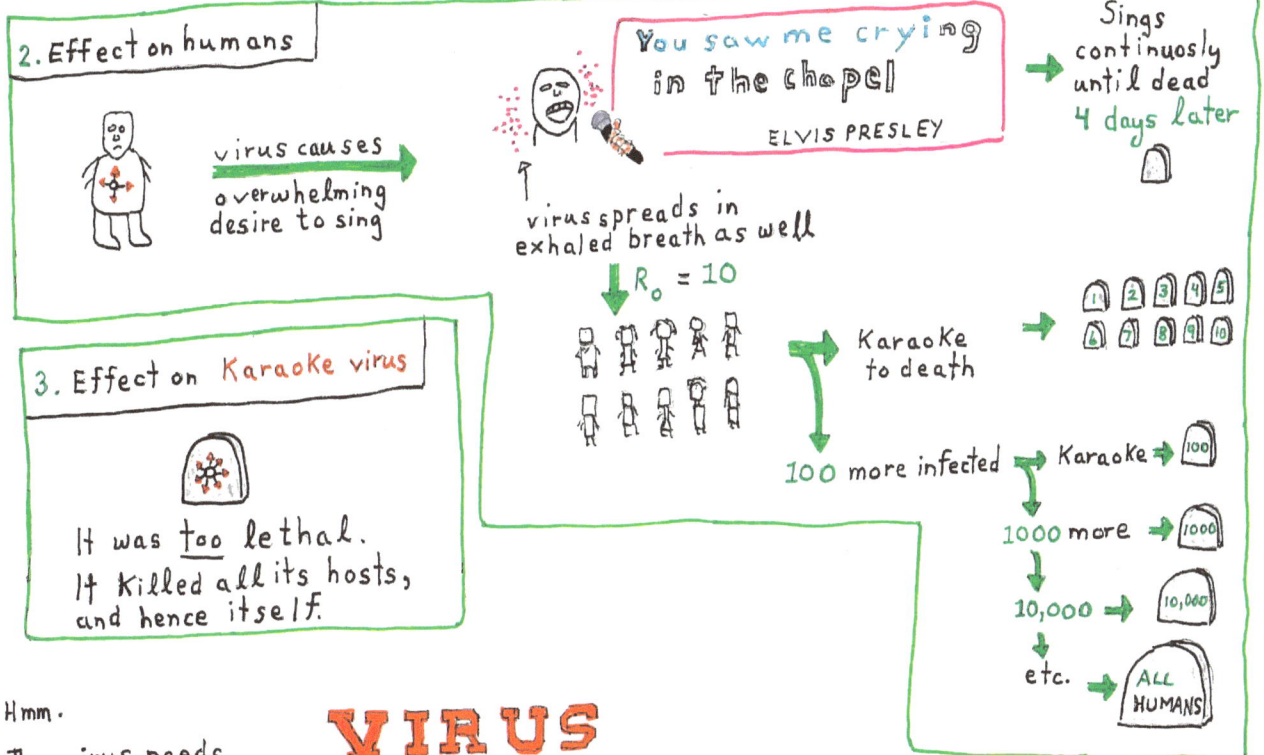

1. Spread

Karaoke virus

Spreads globally in clouds

← cloud

Plus, spread by:

mosquito + louse + flea + water + chocolate cake

2. Effect on humans

virus causes overwhelming desire to sing

You saw me crying in the chapel
ELVIS PRESLEY

Sings continuosly until dead 4 days later

↑ virus spreads in exhaled breath as well

$R_0 = 10$

Karaoke to death

100 more infected → Karaoke → 100

1000 more → 1000

10,000 → 10,000

etc. → ALL HUMANS

3. Effect on Karaoke virus

It was <u>too</u> lethal. It killed all its hosts, and hence itself.

- Hmm.
- The virus needs some rules.

VIRUS PLAYBOOK

1. Do not kill host until it has already had children who can fend for themselves. This assures an ongoing supply of hosts.

2. Diversify: Infect multiple hosts like Influenza virus or Coronavirus. ⌐bat ⌐human
└pig/chicken/human

3. Mutate to evade immune system and anti-viral drugs.

- This was a simple thought experiment - part fact, part silly. We'll return to it later, more seriously.

For now, let's ask: What kills us on a routine basis?

— Whatever is born, dies. Eventually. Or suddenly. Or prematurely.

Births + Deaths in 2017

↓ ZOOM

BIRTHS in ☀ 2017

140,950,000 = 16,090 births/hour

DEATHS in 2017

R.I.P. 58,000,000

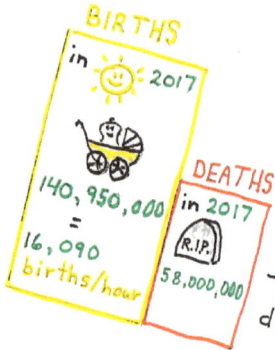

ZOOM on deaths →

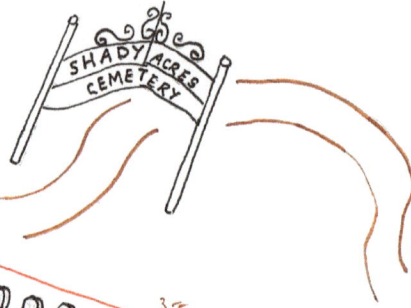

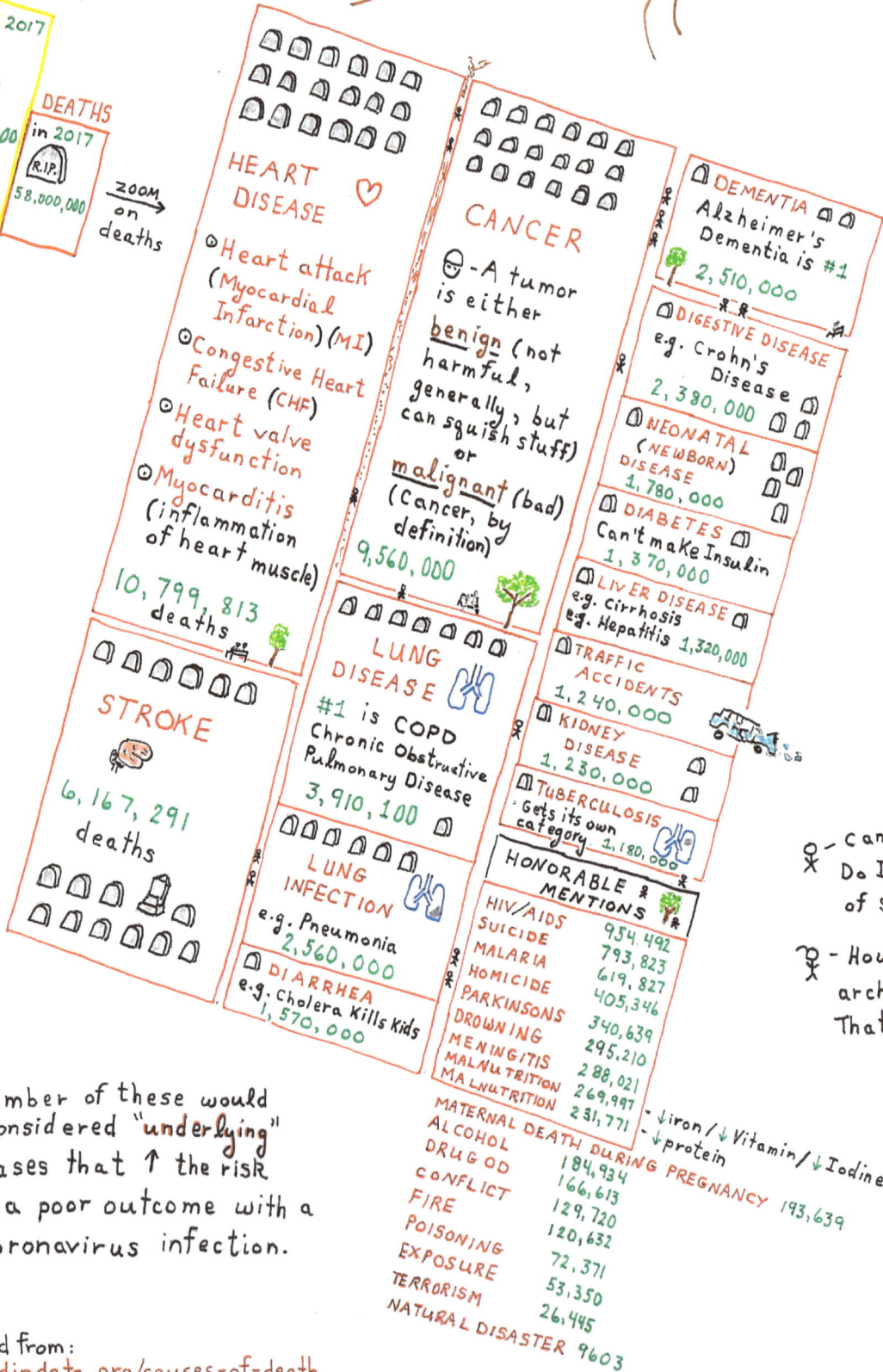

SHADY ACRES CEMETERY

HEART DISEASE ♡

- ⊙ Heart attack (Myocardial Infarction) (MI)
- ⊙ Congestive Heart Failure (CHF)
- ⊙ Heart valve dysfunction
- ⊙ Myocarditis (inflammation of heart muscle)

10,799,813 deaths

STROKE

6,167,291 deaths

CANCER

— A tumor is either benign (not harmful, generally, but can squish stuff) or malignant (bad) (Cancer, by definition)

9,560,000

LUNG DISEASE 🫁

#1 is COPD Chronic Obstructive Pulmonary Disease

3,910,100

LUNG INFECTION 🫁

e.g. Pneumonia

2,560,000

DIARRHEA

e.g. Cholera kills kids

1,570,000

DEMENTIA

Alzheimer's Dementia is #1

2,510,000

DIGESTIVE DISEASE

e.g. Crohn's Disease

2,380,000

NEONATAL (NEWBORN) DISEASE

1,780,000

DIABETES

Can't make Insulin

1,370,000

LIVER DISEASE

e.g. Cirrhosis
e.g. Hepatitis   1,320,000

TRAFFIC ACCIDENTS

1,240,000

KIDNEY DISEASE

1,230,000

TUBERCULOSIS

Gets its own category   1,180,000

HONORABLE MENTIONS

HIV/AIDS	954,492
SUICIDE	793,823
MALARIA	619,827
HOMICIDE	405,346
PARKINSONS	340,639
DROWNING	295,210
MENINGITIS	288,021
MALNUTRITION	269,997
MALNUTRITION	231,771

↓ iron / ↓ Vitamin / ↓ Iodine
↓ protein

MATERNAL DEATH DURING PREGNANCY   193,639

ALCOHOL	184,934
DRUG OD	166,613
CONFLICT	129,720
FIRE	120,632
POISONING	72,371
EXPOSURE	53,350
TERRORISM	26,445
NATURAL DISASTER	9603

— Can't I just die? Do I have to die of something?

— How about an archery accident? That's original.

A number of these would be considered "underlying" diseases that ↑ the risk for a poor outcome with a coronavirus infection.

Data adapted from:
ourworldindata.org/causes-of-death
There are 25 interactive graphs you can have deathly fun with. They put ♡ + Stroke in 1 category.

😐 - But a simple graveyard with numbers does not tell the full story.

R.I.P. — age, gender, location, risk factors (including occupational hazards)

The subtleties are buried in each tombstone.

65 65 65 65

20-40 20-40 20-40 20-40

5 5 5 5

↑
1918 Influenza Pandemic cemetery

😐 - Let's say tombstone height is age. OLD young
~And that tombstone color is gender.

♂ ♀

• ♂ and ♀ were killed in equal numbers globally.

• 3 distinct age groups died < 65 years or older
20-40 years
5 years or younger

↳ In statistics, this is called a tri-modal distribution

Amazon Africa is #1 India SE Asia

↑
Malaria cemetery

→ 57% of Malaria deaths (619,827 in total in 2017) are in children less than 5 years old

→ What's almost more telling about this map is where Malaria is **not** occurring.

😐 - As a broad generality, people in developed nations die of diseases of excess, and people in non-developed countries die of diseases of deficiency (like mal-nutrition).

How I Died Today

Natural causes
• Vast majority of deaths
• This includes infections

Non-natural (un-natural) causes

Accident   Suicide   Homicide

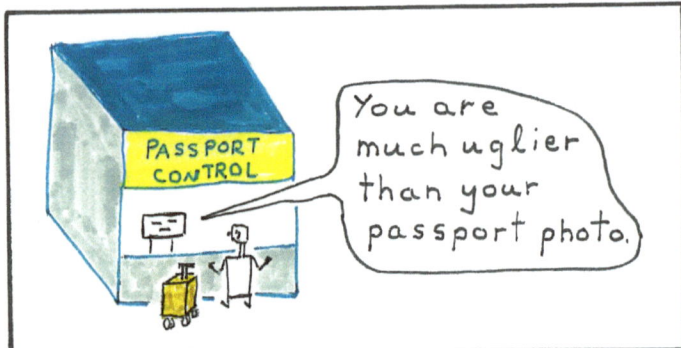

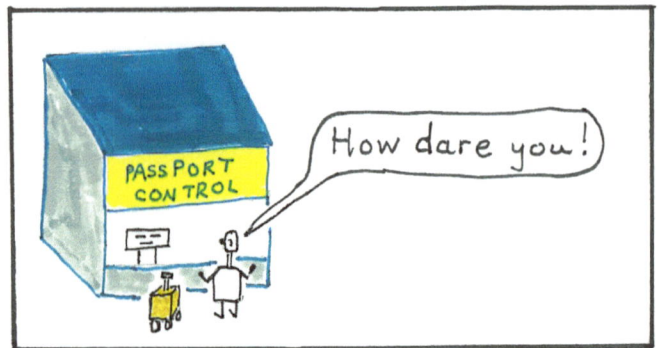

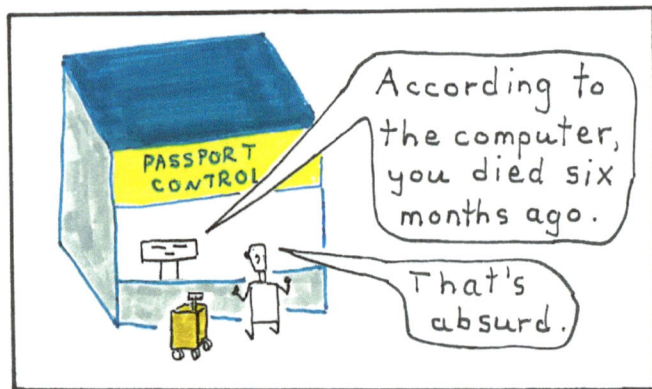

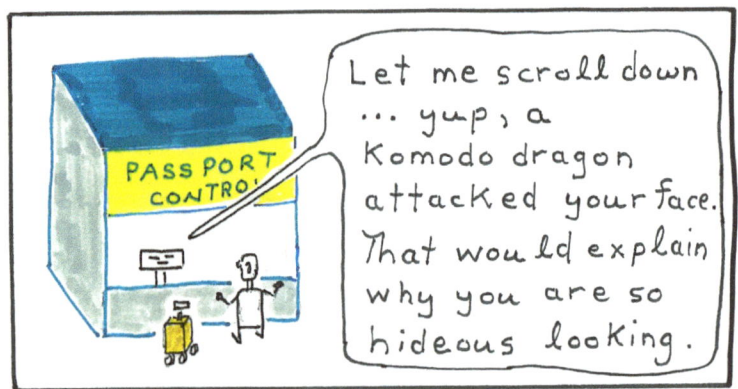

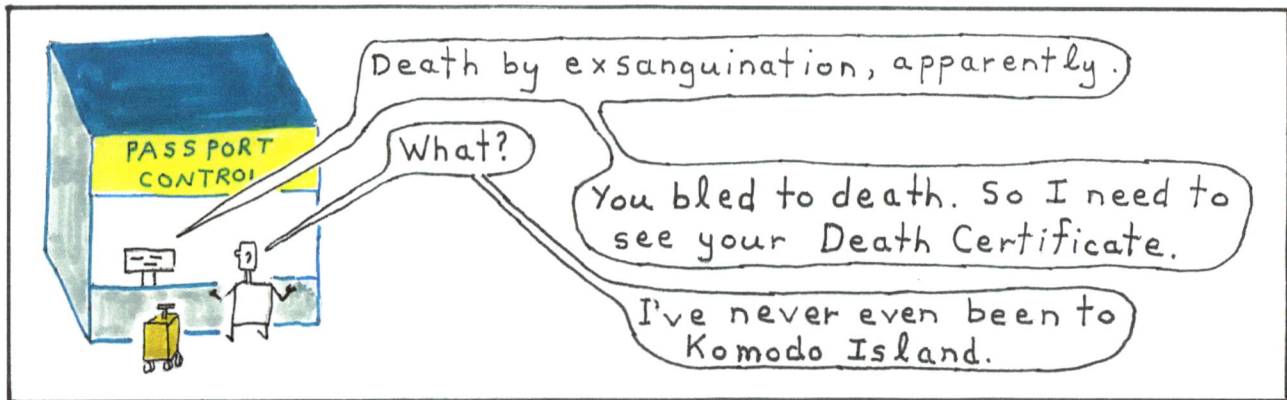

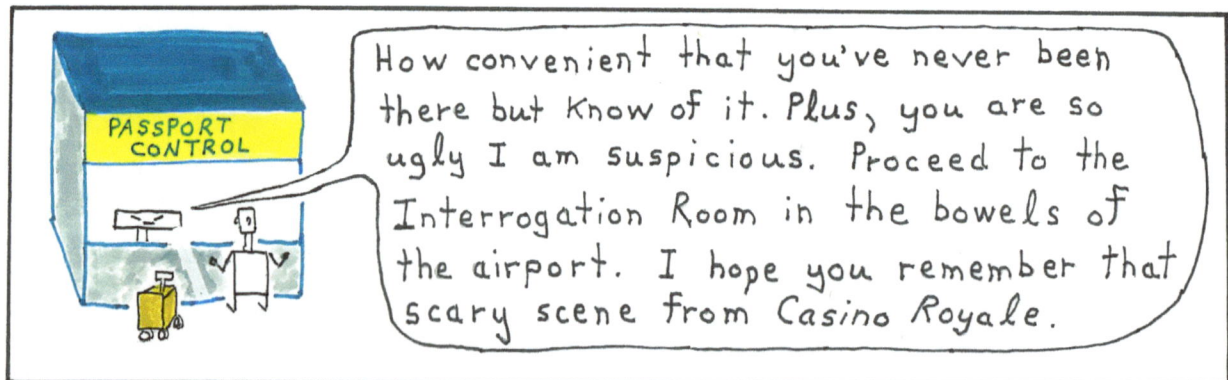

♀ - What's the purpose of a death certificate?

♀ - Besides the legal stuff like your Last Will and Testament,
   the medical purpose is to collect data on what kills people.

Certificate of Death

Decedent Name: JOHN DOE
Gender: MALE
Date of Birth (DOB): 1 MARCH 1950
Date of Death (DOD): 1 JULY 2020

Part I
   IMMEDIATE CAUSE OF DEATH: ACUTE RESPIRATORY DISTRESS SYNDROME
   UNDERLYING CAUSES OF DEATH: PNEUMONIA
                               COVID-19

Part II
   CONTRIBUTING CONDITIONS:

MANNER OF DEATH

   ■ NATURAL
   □ ACCIDENT
   □ SUICIDE
   □ HOMICIDE
   □ PENDING INVESTIGATION
   □ COULD NOT BE DETERMINED

I hereby certify this to be true.   1 JULY 2020

                                     Emma Smith, M.D.

😐 - That's the basic layout.
   ' The coroner/medical examiner has to be notified
     in cases of accident or suicide or homicide.

   ' 'Decedent' is a fancy way of saying 'deceased person.'

😐 - "da see dent"   ' Don't confuse this with the death certificate from
SOMPOO   a funeral home, which is a bit different.
SAYS

- Let's explore some death certificates to get you thinking about the <u>sequence</u> of events leading up to death.

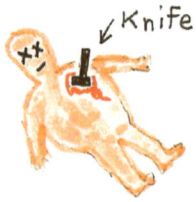

Knife

IMMEDIATE CAUSE OF DEATH: HEMORRHAGIC SHOCK

(final disease or condition resulting in death)

UNDERLYING CAUSES OF DEATH: STAB WOUND OF HEART

(diseases or injury that initiated the events resulting in death)

MANNER OF DEATH: ■ HOMICIDE

"hee mow raj ick"

"x sang gwin nation"

SOMPOO SAYS

- Fancy way of saying you bled to death
- A suitable synonym is EXSANGUINATION, probably something Sherlock Holmes would say.

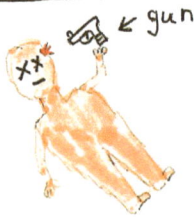

---

gun

IMMEDIATE CAUSE OF DEATH: PENETRATING INJURY OF BRAIN

UNDERLYING CAUSES OF DEATH: GUNSHOT WOUND (GSW) TO HEAD

MANNER OF DEATH: ■ SUICIDE

(Lost the will to live)

CONTRIBUTING CONDITION: INOPERABLE CANCER

(A medical condition that <u>contributed</u> to the death but was not a <u>direct cause</u>)

- Notice how the data is recorded as a probable chain of events, from bottom to top?

- Let's assume the coroner and police determined it was not a murder meant to look like a suicide.

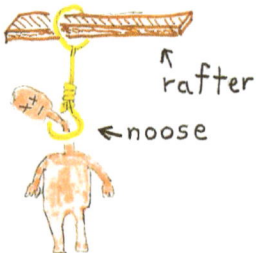

---

rafter

noose

IMMEDIATE CAUSE OF DEATH: ASPHYXIA

UNDERLYING CAUSES OF DEATH: HANGING

MANNER OF DEATH: ■ SUICIDE

- Hanging is a type of Asphyxia

"Ass fix ee ah"

SOMPOO SAYS

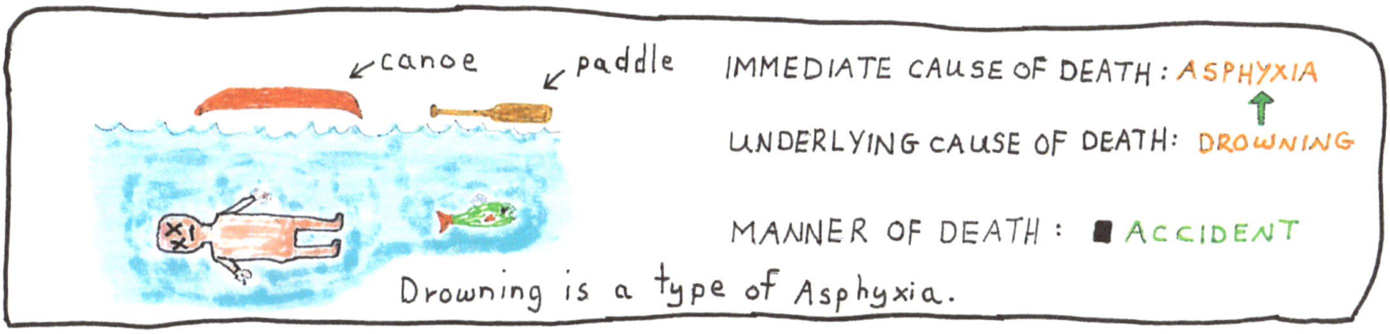

← canoe   ← paddle

IMMEDIATE CAUSE OF DEATH : ASPHYXIA ↑

UNDERLYING CAUSE OF DEATH: DROWNING

MANNER OF DEATH : ■ ACCIDENT

Drowning is a type of Asphyxia.

☻ – Asphyxia is an umbrella term for a bunch of bad things that interfere with breathing.

＼ Let's explore Asphyxia, because the more you understand the lungs and breathing, the more you understand ☼ coronavirus.

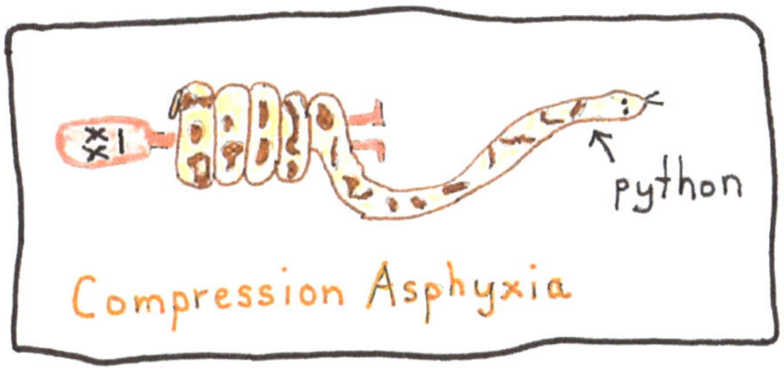

← python

Compression Asphyxia

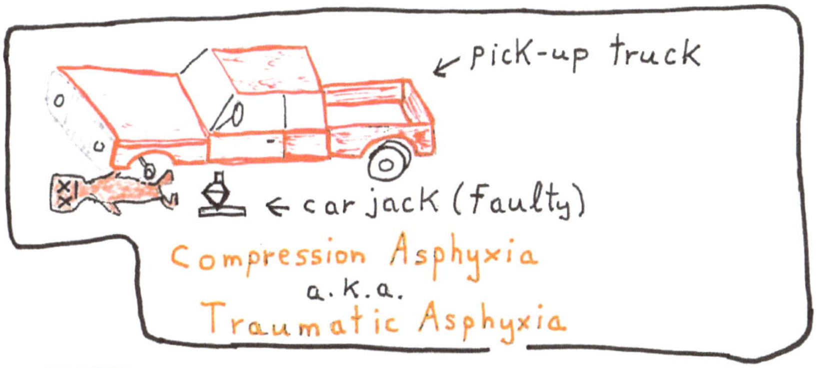

← pick-up truck

← car jack (faulty)

Compression Asphyxia
a.k.a.
Traumatic Asphyxia

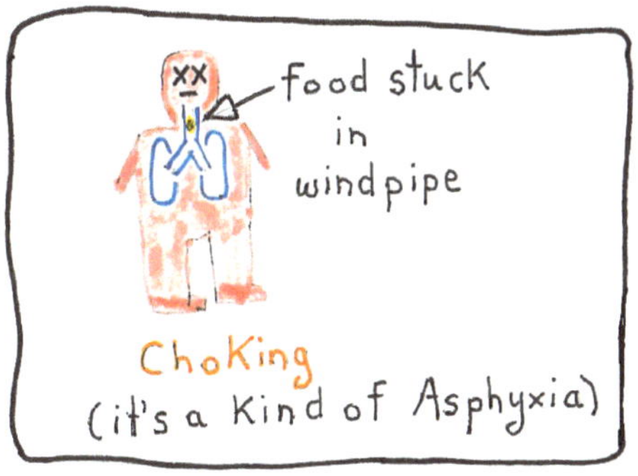

food stuck in windpipe

Choking
(it's a kind of Asphyxia)

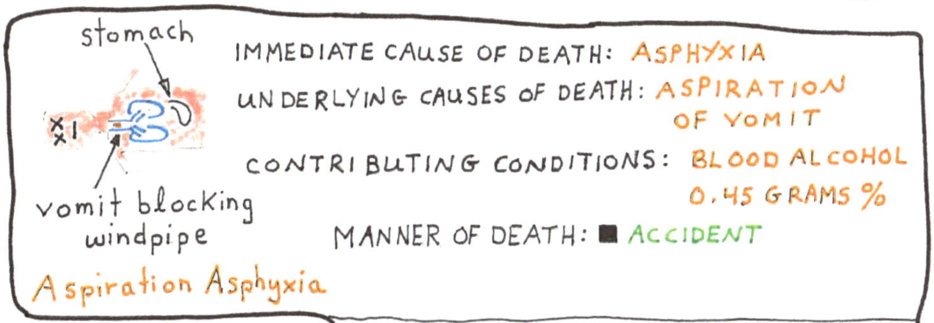

stomach

vomit blocking windpipe

Aspiration Asphyxia

IMMEDIATE CAUSE OF DEATH: ASPHYXIA
UNDERLYING CAUSES OF DEATH: ASPIRATION OF VOMIT
CONTRIBUTING CONDITIONS: BLOOD ALCOHOL 0.45 GRAMS %
MANNER OF DEATH: ■ ACCIDENT

☻ – Yes, he choked on his own vomit, but this is not considered Choking, per se. It is Aspiration Asphyxia.

Aspiration means he inhaled his own vomit.

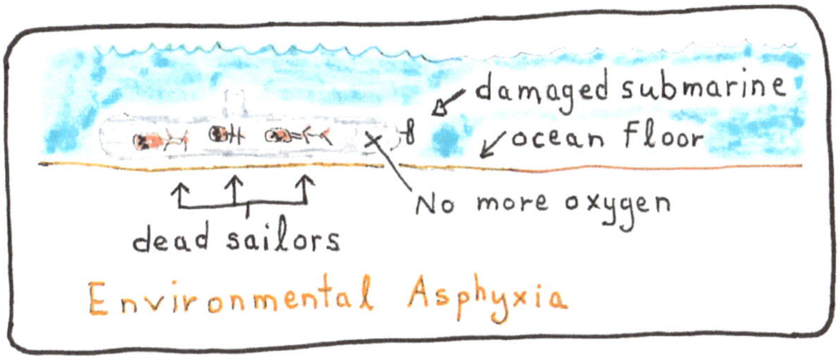

← damaged submarine
← ocean floor

No more oxygen

dead sailors

Environmental Asphyxia

pillow

←assailant

I have to be honest. I never liked you

←plastic bag

Smothering, also known as Suffocation, is a type of Asphyxia in which the mouth and nose are covered.

IMMEDIATE CAUSE OF DEATH: ASPHYXIA
UNDERLYING CAUSE OF DEATH: STRANGULATION
MANNER OF DEATH : ■ HOMICIDE

or

←electrical cord or rope

Strangulation is a type of Asphyxia.

☻ -The carotid arteries that supply the brain are squeezed shut.

☻ -In several examples (python, car on chest, hanging, strangling, smothering, choking), an External force or object physically interferes with breathing. This is called Mechanical Asphyxia. There is also Chemical Asphyxia.

CO gas inhaled

←water heater

Carbon monoxide (CO) gas (it's actually invisible)

natural gas flame to heat water

IMMEDIATE CAUSE OF DEATH: ASPHYXIA
UNDERLYING CAUSE OF DEATH: CARBON MONOXIDE POISONING
MANNER OF DEATH: ■ ACCIDENT

☻ - This is Chemical Asphyxia.
` Carbon monoxide (CO) gas is produced if natural gas (methane)(CH_4)($H-C-H$) is only partly burned.
` Carbon monoxide prevents our blood from transporting oxygen (O_2).

↗ cyanide tablet

Chemical Asphyxia

IMMEDIATE CAUSE OF DEATH: ASPHYXIA
UNDERLYING CAUSE OF DEATH: CYANIDE POISONING
MANNER OF DEATH : ■ SUICIDE
CONTRIBUTING CONDITIONS: ABANDONED ON MARS

☻ - Problems with breathing (as in, lungs expanding and contracting)? No.
 - Problems transporting oxygen? No.
 - Problems with cells producing energy? Yes.

Your lips turn a nice shade of blue called cyan ... hence cyanide

←heroin

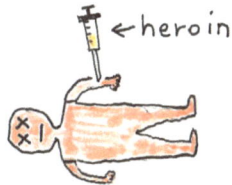

IMMEDIATE CAUSE OF DEATH: **RESPIRATORY ARREST**
UNDERLYING CAUSES OF DEATH: **HEROIN OVERDOSE**
: **OPIOID USE DISORDER**
(DRUG ADDICTION)

MANNER OF DEATH: ■ **ACCIDENT**

☺ - Heroin (and fentanyl and all the other opioids) turn off the brain's instructions to the lungs to expand/contract.

`Okay, it's not an actual ON ⊘ OFF switch

`More like a dial. 50 / 75 · 25 / 100 - ◯ - 0

`A big heroin overdose turns the dial to zero.

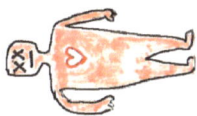

IMMEDIATE CAUSE OF DEATH : **MYOCARDIAL INFARCTION** (♡Attack)

muscle heart Cells die because blood supply is cut off

UNDERLYING CAUSE OF DEATH: **CORONARY ARTERY DISEASE (CAD)**
MANNER OF DEATH: ■ **NATURAL**

☺ - What does 'corona' mean?
- It means crown in Latin.

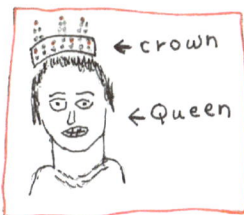

←crown
←Queen

←corona of Sun
• It's like a crown of hot gas
• 1,000,000 °C/F
• Becomes visible during solar eclipse

↙spikes
←Corona-virus
• The virus has a 'crown' of spikes (at least, in 2-D images)
(in 3-D, it's like a volleyball coated with peas)

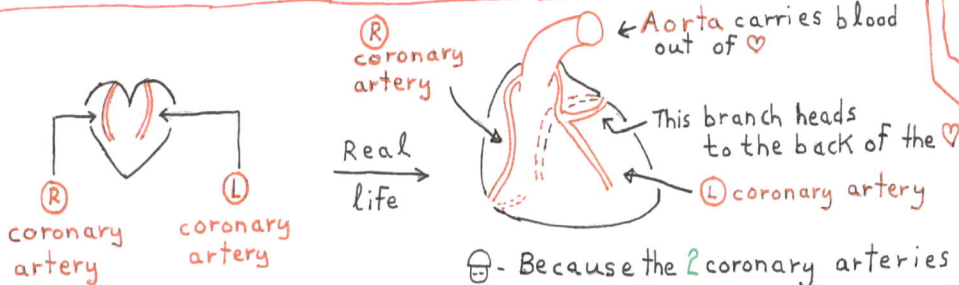

®coronary artery
←Aorta carries blood out of ♡
This branch heads to the back of the ♡
Ⓛ coronary artery

Real life

® coronary artery   Ⓛ coronary artery

These 2 arteries are the blood supply to the heart (which is a muscle, so it needs blood to beat non-stop)

☺ - Because the 2 coronary arteries have branches, a 'crown' of arteries encircles the heart.

`Guess what happens if the arteries get narrowed by fat deposits? Lack of blood to ♡ muscle, the worst-case scenario being a ♡Attack.

- Because there are multiple branches you can have a Quadruple Bypass operation.

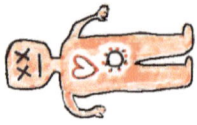

IMMEDIATE CAUSE OF DEATH: MYOCARDIAL INFARCTION (♡ ATTACK)

UNDERLYING CAUSES: CORONARY ARTERY DISEASE ⬆

PNEUMONIA ⬆

COVID-19 ☼

CONTRIBUTING CONDITIONS:

DIABETES
HIGH BLOOD PRESSURE
HIGH CHOLESTEROL
SMOKING
COPD ← Smoking causes COPD

↳ These 4 conditions make the narrowing of the coronary arteries worse

MANNER OF DEATH:
■ NATURAL

😐 - This is a complex patient.

- ☼ Coronavirus caused Pneumonia ... which made it hard to breath ... which makes the ♡ beat faster ... but the ♡ has a crappy blood supply (Coronary Artery Disease) because of Diabetes, High blood pressure, High cholesterol and Smoking ... and all of this made worse because the patient has very little lung 'reserve' because of COPD (Chronic Obstructive Lung Disease) ... and to get technical, Emphysema is a major component of COPD where lung tissue is destroyed (less air sacs) ... so the patient just can't get enough oxygen ... so the ♡ has to work even harder ... but it's not getting enough oxygen itself ... ♡ Attack.

\ Now, don't be a pessimist and assume, "He was gonna die anyway." Maybe he had another 10 years to live. Or 20.

\ Point is, ☼ coronavirus caused Pneumonia, and everything got worse from there.

😐 - Okay, so the point of (accurate) death certificates is to identify patterns and interrupt the sequence of events leading to death.

- And count deaths. If only 2 people per year are killed by Komodo dragons, the government does not need to spend $50 million on a Komodo Dragon Awareness Campaign.

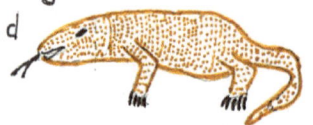

- p.s. You're not allowed to die of old age.

IMMEDIATE CAUSE OF DEATH: OLD AGE

100 years old

Autopsy incision (Y-shape)
• No specific findings
• Just normal aging of organs

That is not considered an acceptable answer.

But this is okay

IMMEDIATE CAUSE OF DEATH : UNDETERMINED NATURAL CAUSES
MANNER OF DEATH: ■ NATURAL

The vagueness is okay. This 100-year old man, without any offense to him, has an unremarkable tombstone, medically speaking.

- Why an autopsy on a 100-year old man?
- Maybe he's a billionaire found dead in a hotel room. The coroner would be contacted to rule out a suspicious death. Especially if his grandson just bought a Ferrari and was doing donuts in the parking lot.

A POTENTIALLY CONFUSING TOPIC

SYMPTOMS
= What the patient feels.

patient →
I feel weak

doctor measuring BP

Blood Pressure (BP) cuff

SIGNS
= What the doctor sees, hears, touches, measures.

My stomach hurts

doctor hand touching abdomen and seeing patient's reaction

This patient has involuntary guarding
↳ The muscles of the abdomen tighten involuntarily when the doctor's hand touches it.
• This is a sign of Appendicitis, potentially. Not a slam dunk.

- Low blood pressure is a sign.
`When in doubt, think of a Stop sign. You can see it. So it's a sign.
(Plus, stop signs don't talk about how they are feeling).

STOP

I'm having trouble breathing

There are decreased breath sounds in the Right Lower Lobe of the lungs
↳ This is a sign of Pneumonia, potentially

back
stetho-scope to hear lungs

I feel fine

I'm short of breath

corona-virus

Asymptomatic
• Feels nothing

Symptomatic
• Feels something

- What are Vital Signs?
- Blood Pressure, Heart Rate, Respiratory Rate, Temperature
   (BP)   (HR)   (RR)   (T)   → Vital Signs Stable

`If these are all normal, then in the patient's chart, "VSS" is written.

- Let's knock off a few more concepts of Epidemiology and then head back to infections.

Case Fatality Rate

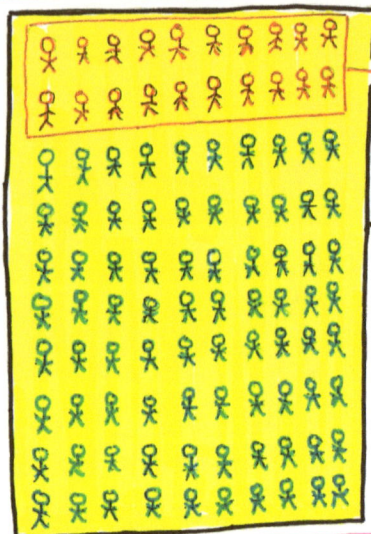

20 people died R.I.P.
―――――――――――――――――――
100 people infected

↑
Think, 100 cases in total

= 20% Case Fatality Rate (CFR)

Correlation

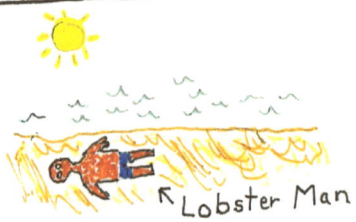

↑ sun → ↑ sunburn
(positive correlation)

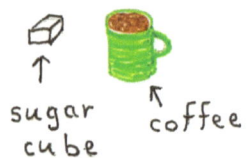

↑ Lobster Man

↑ sugar → ↑ sweetness
(positive correlation)

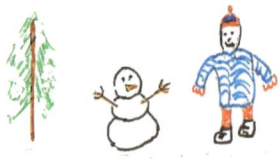

sugar cube   ↑ coffee

↓ Temperature → ↑ clothing
(negative correlation)

- Correlation is a fancy word to describe relationships.
- We notice these relationships practically our whole lives
- co-relation
  ⌐
  together

- But!, we can make errors when trying to connect 2 sets of correlations.

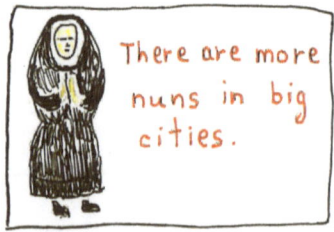

There are more nuns in big cities.

There are more murders in big cities

∴ therefore

Come Get Some
Nuns commit the most murders in big cities

Correlation #1
TRUE

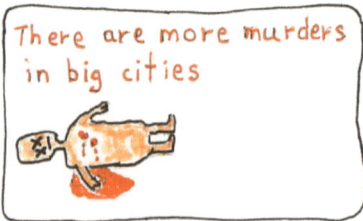

Correlation #2
TRUE

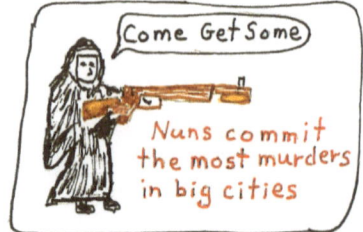

Probably not true

Risk Factors

Glub, glub glub

Why don't you just stay on land?

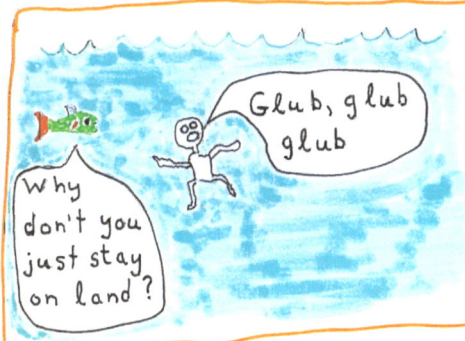

Risk Factors (RF) for drowning

#1 - Cannot swim
#2 - No Life Preserver
#3 - Alcohol
#4 - Rip current
etc.

😐 - Virtually every single illness has a set of Risk Factors

😐 - Doctors tend to stratify patients into ⟨ High Risk (HR)
Medium Risk (MR)
Low Risk (LR)

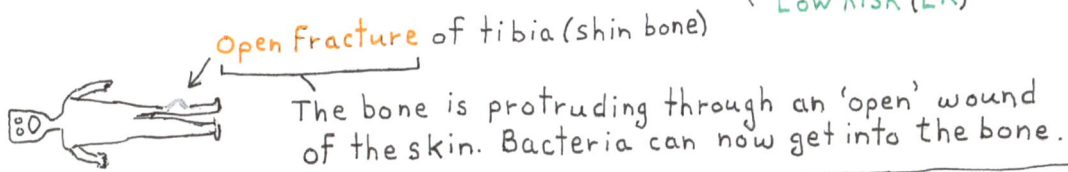

Open Fracture of tibia (shin bone)

The bone is protruding through an 'open' wound of the skin. Bacteria can now get into the bone.

This patient is high risk for a bone infection. We need to get him to the OR and clean up the bone within 6-8 hours. After we clean it, we'll put some plates and screws in it.

↑ bone (orthopedic) surgeon

Risk Factors (RF) for Bone Infection

- Open Fracture
- ↓ immunity
- IV injection of drugs (eg., heroin)
- several others

Risk Factors (RF) for ♡ Coronary Artery Disease ♡

D - iabetes
H - igh blood pressure
H - igh cholesterol
S - moking

[I remember this as DHHS]
There are apps to calculate risk.

Risk Factors (RF) for severe COVID-19

- ↓ immunity (we'll get into some examples later on)
- Cancer (you're already weak and vulnerable)
- COPD (Chronic Obstructive Pulmonary Disease) (= can't get enough oxygen)
- Coronary Artery Disease (♡ muscle not getting enough blood)
- Diabetes requiring insulin
- Sickle Cell Anemia (details later)
- Chronic Kidney Disease
  └ That means it's being going on for a long time.
- Obesity with Body Mass Index (BMI) 30 or higher.

5'5"
(65")
=
1.65 meters

240 LB = 109 KG

$BMI = \dfrac{weight}{height^2}$

$= \dfrac{240\ LB}{65" \times 65"} \times 703$

$= \dfrac{109\ KG}{1.65\ m \times 1.65\ m}$

$= BMI\ 40$

☻ - Greek is important

En-demic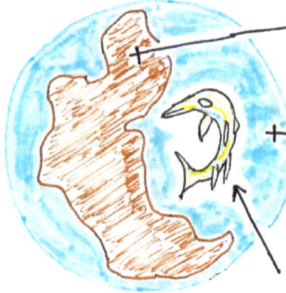
↑ ↑
'in' 'people'
(Greek 'demos' means
people hence democracy)

The disease is <u>in</u> the people,
continuously present.

Epi-demic ⊙
↑ ↑
'upon' 'people'

The disease is
<u>upon</u> the people,
temporarily.

Pan-demic ⊙
↑ ↑
'all' 'people'

The disease has spread
to <u>all</u> people.

Pan

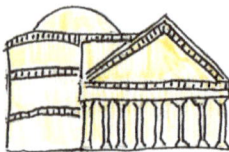

Pan-gea = <u>1</u> landmass (super-continent)
| |
all Earth   250 million years ago

Pan-thalassa = single large ocean
| | surrounding Pangea
all sea

Thalatto-saur = marine reptile that
| | swam in Panthalassa
sea lizard

☻ - 'Pan' is found in many medical words. Watch for it

Pan

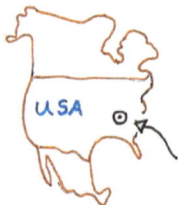 **Pan-theon** = Temple in Rome
| |
all gods

CDC

☻ - The CDC collects <u>vast</u> amounts of information on disease.

`If you intend on traveling anywhere in the world and want to know
what diseases you can catch there, Google this: CDC <u>name of country</u>

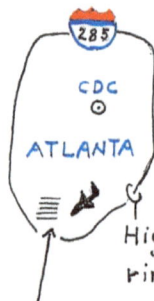

CDC
1600 Clifton Road
Atlanta, Georgia
30333

285
CDC
ⓞ
ATLANTA

Highway 285
ring road

Hartsfield-Jackson Atlanta Airport
• Code: ATL / KATL
• 5 parallel Runways
• World's busiest airport

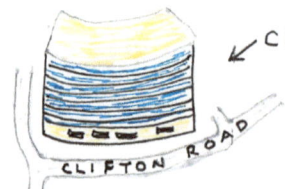 ← CDC

CLIFTON ROAD

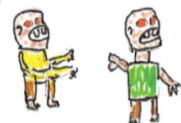 ← Zombies

Zombies always attack
the CDC. Somehow they
know the address.

USA ⊙

- Time for a sense of scale.

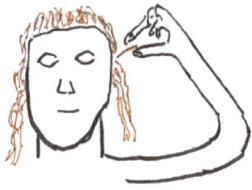

Pluck! a single hair

enlarge

flow

capillary
• smallest blood vessel
• 4 microns diameter

Red Blood Cell (RBC)
• It carries oxygen.
• It deforms in shape to travel through the capillary.
• 7 microns in diameter

7 microns (side view)

Yersinia pestis
• Bubonic Plague (Black Death)
• 0.5 × 2 microns
• rod shape
• can it travel (and multiply) in the blood? Yes! That's blood poisoning.

Vibrio cholera
• Cholera (death by diarrhea)
• 0.3 × 1.3 microns

100 microns
• Diameter of hair

• ← Coronavirus
• ← Influenza virus
• ← Smallpox virus
• ← Ebola virus (it's like string)

In fact, these dots are 5 times too big

Type 2 Pneumo-cyte
lung   cell
• Coronavirus infects this guy. Details later.
• 9 microns diameter

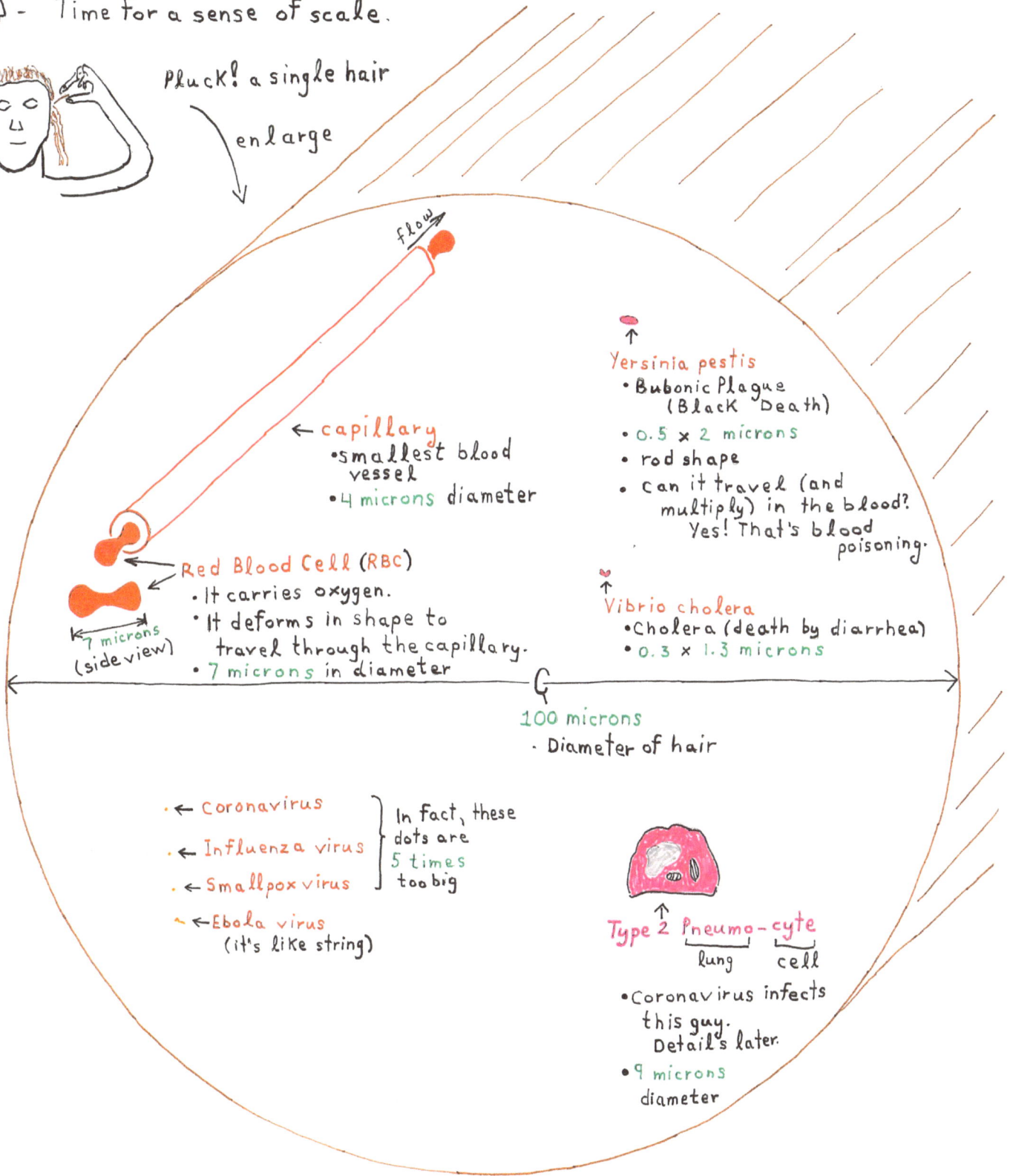

- Pretend the plucked hair is a tube

- I have no idea what a micron is

- Patience ...

Panel 1 (top left):

♀ -?

♂ - Chop the credit card edge into 762 slices. Each slice will be 1 micron thick

→ Japanese Knife

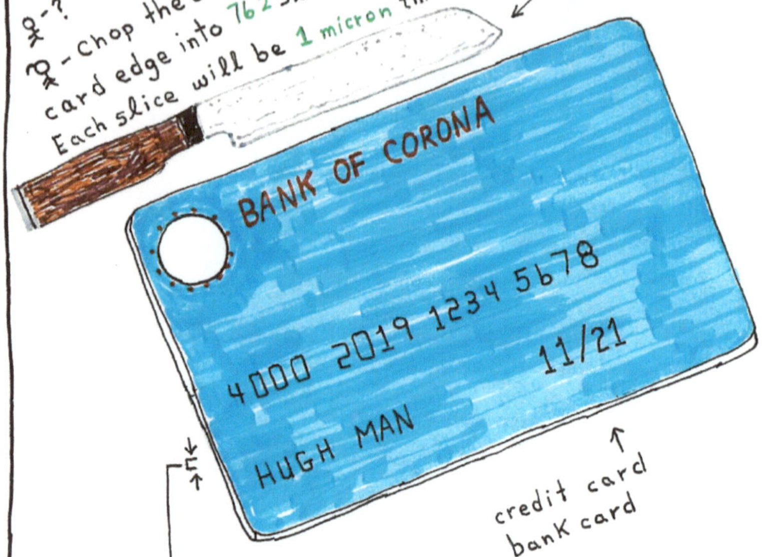

BANK OF CORONA

4000 2019 1234 5678

11/21

HUGH MAN

↑ credit card bank card

762 microns thick = 0.762 milli-meters (mm)
- Fits in ATM / bank machine / card reader.
- Global standard set by the International Organization for Standardization (ISO).

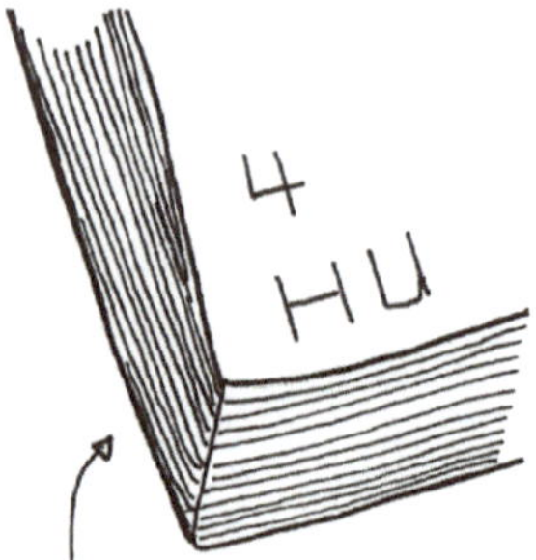

Panel 2 (middle left):

4
HU

Like this, but 762 slices

♀ - So each slice is 1 micron?

♂ - Correct. You'd need a steady hand and an exceedingly sharp blade.
1 micron is extremely small - smaller than the eye 👁 can see. Need a microscope. On the scale of microns we can see stuff like blood cells, and, just barely, bacteria.

Panel (bottom left):

♀ - What about viruses?
♂ - You'd have to slice that credit card 7620 times

Panel (middle column, green):

paper clip 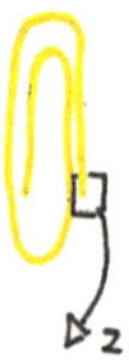
↓ zoom

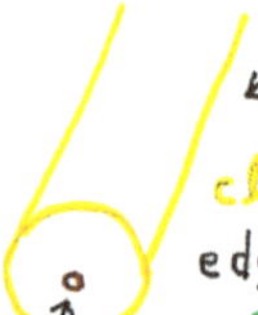

paper clip wire edge-on is 0.8 mm wide (800 microns)

hair (previous page) 0.1 mm wide (100 microns)

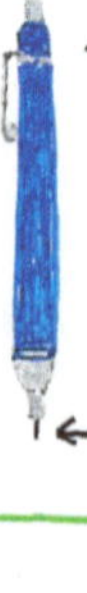

← mechanical pencil
- 0.5 mm lead (500 microns)

Panel (right column):

yardstick   meterstick

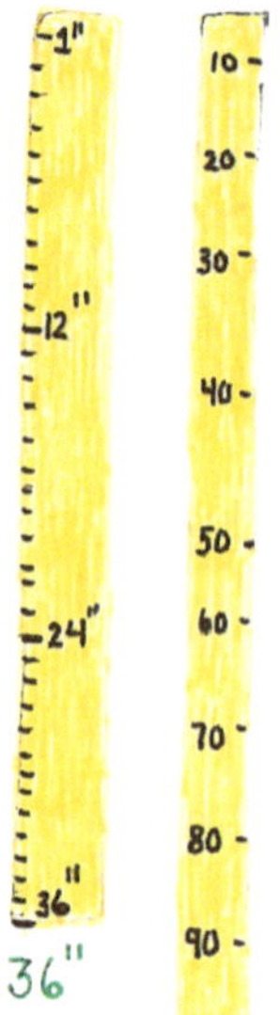

1"
12"
24"
36"
36"

10
20
30
40
50
60
70
80
90
100
39"

☻ - 1 micron is 1/25,400th of an inch

cm = 1000 mm = 1,000,000 microns

☻ - The Latin 'centuria' means 100 ... hence 21st Century ... hence a Roman Centurion who commanded 100 men (or so)

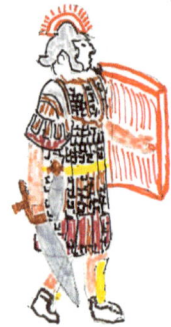

... hence 100 centi-meters in 1 meter

☻ - Milli means 1000 ... hence a milli-pede with 1000 legs Actually, 750 is the max. ... hence 1000 milli-meters in 1 meter

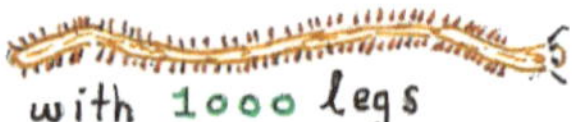

☻ - You guessed it, micro means 1,000,000. To be specific 1/1,000,000th ... hence 1,000,000 micro-meters (microns) in 1 meter

- Because I'm a slave to detail, I want you to understand the size of coronavirus in pictures you'll encounter.

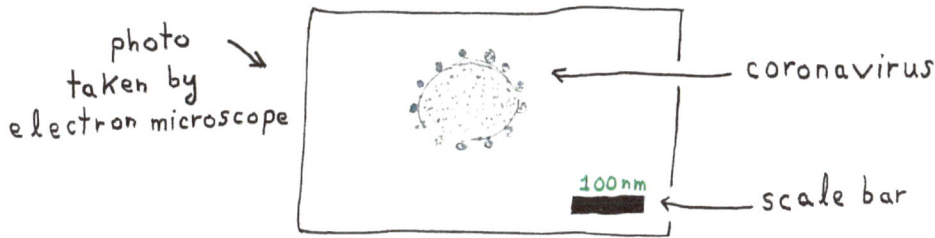

photo taken by electron microscope →

coronavirus →

100nm

scale bar →

- That scale bar uses the metric system, which is based on the number 10. You probably already use half of these terms.

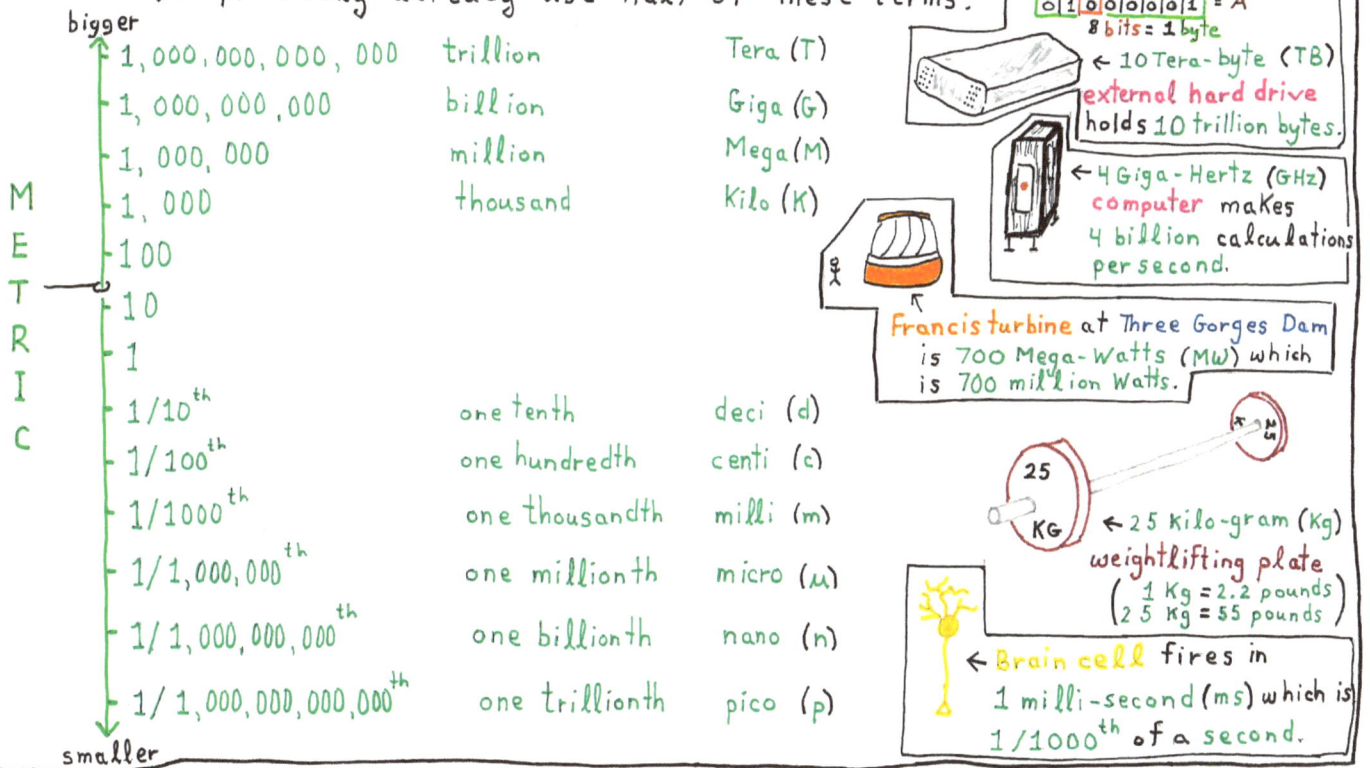

bigger

M E T R I C

1,000,000,000,000	trillion	Tera (T)
1,000,000,000	billion	Giga (G)
1,000,000	million	Mega (M)
1,000	thousand	Kilo (K)
100		
10		
1		
$1/10^{th}$	one tenth	deci (d)
$1/100^{th}$	one hundredth	centi (c)
$1/1000^{th}$	one thousandth	milli (m)
$1/1,000,000^{th}$	one millionth	micro (μ)
$1/1,000,000,000^{th}$	one billionth	nano (n)
$1/1,000,000,000,000^{th}$	one trillionth	pico (p)

smaller

↰ bit
| 0 | 1 | 0 | 0 | 0 | 0 | 0 | 1 | = 'A'
8 bits = 1 byte

← 10 Tera-byte (TB) external hard drive holds 10 trillion bytes.

← 4 Giga-Hertz (GHz) computer makes 4 billion calculations per second.

Francis turbine at Three Gorges Dam is 700 Mega-Watts (MW) which is 700 million Watts.

25 KG

← 25 kilo-gram (Kg) weightlifting plate
(1 Kg = 2.2 pounds)
(25 Kg = 55 pounds)

← Brain cell fires in 1 milli-second (ms) which is $1/1000^{th}$ of a second.

100 nm

← Coronavirus diameter

↘ 0.1 micro-meters (μm) (microns)
↗ 100 nano-meters (nm)

"Zero point one microns"
"one hundred billionths of a meter"

CREDIT CARD 4000 2019

$1/7620^{th}$ of a credit card thickness (Yes, $1/10^{th}$ of a micron)

- These are <u>exactly</u> the same.
- But nano-meters (nm) is what you'll usually read.
- The actual range in size of Coronavirus is 50 to 200 nm.
- If you say, "The Coronavirus diameter is one tenth of a micron," you're right on the money.

0.1 μm

You might see this

μ
↖ That's the Greek letter mu
Hence 0.1 μm diameter.

- How about I just say that coronavirus is insanely small?

- No problemo

☺ —We were never properly introduced. This is my family tree.

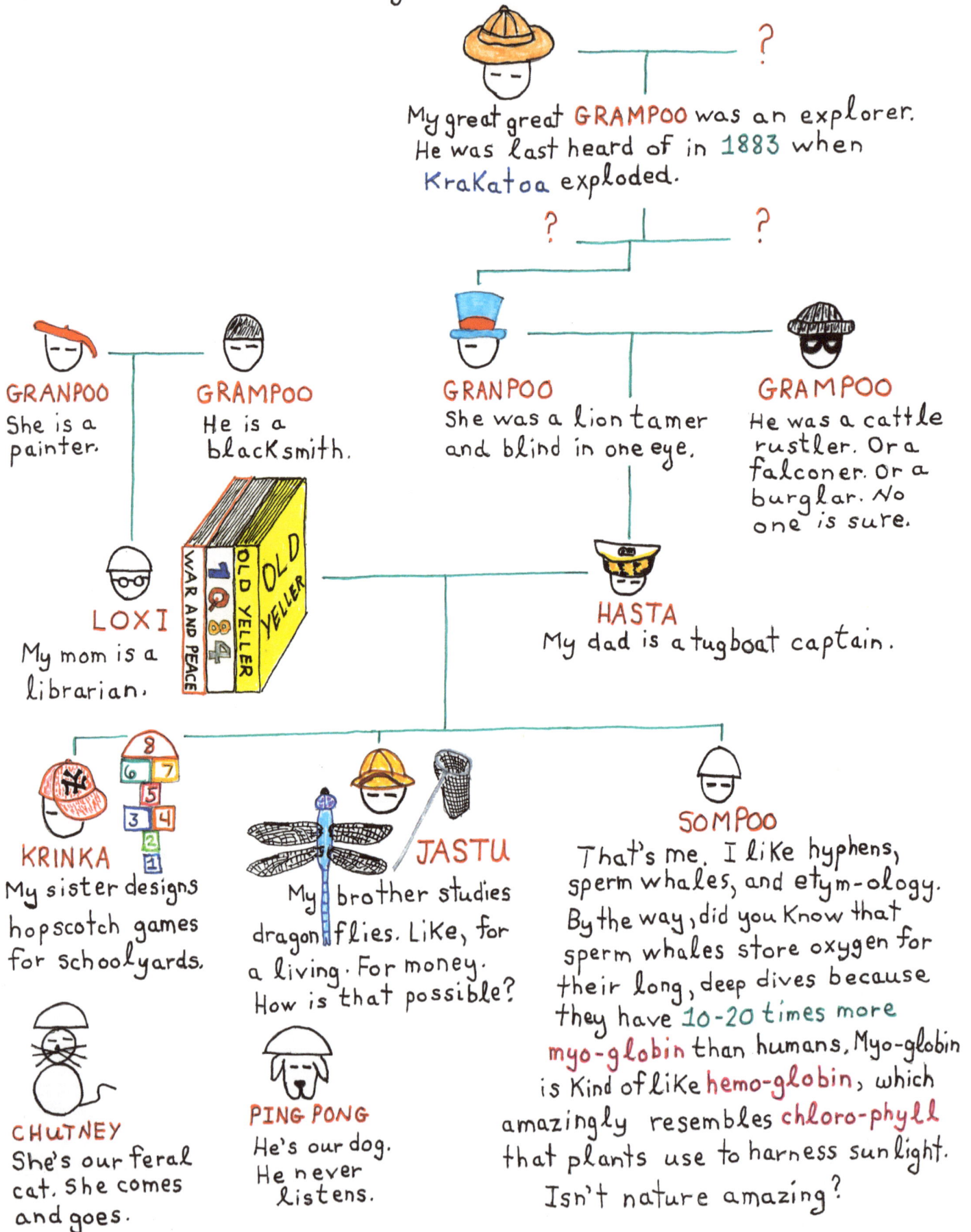

?

My great great **GRAMPOO** was an explorer.
He was *last heard of* in 1883 when
KraKatoa exploded.

?   ?

GRANPOO
She is a
painter.

GRAMPOO
He is a
blacksmith.

GRANPOO
She was a lion tamer
and blind in one eye.

GRAMPOO
He was a cattle
rustler. Or a
falconer. Or a
burglar. No
one is sure.

WAR AND PEACE 1984 OLD YELLER

LOXI
My mom is a
librarian.

HASTA
My dad is a tugboat captain.

KRINKA
My sister designs
hopscotch games
for schoolyards.

JASTU
My brother studies
dragonflies. Like, for
a living. For money.
How is that possible?

SOMPOO
That's me. I like hyphens,
sperm whales, and etym-ology.
By the way, did you Know that
sperm whales store oxygen for
their long, deep dives because
they have 10-20 times more
myo-globin than humans. Myo-globin
is Kind of like hemo-globin, which
amazingly resembles chloro-phyll
that plants use to harness sunlight.
Isn't nature amazing?

CHUTNEY
She's our feral
cat. She comes
and goes.

PING PONG
He's our dog.
He never
listens.

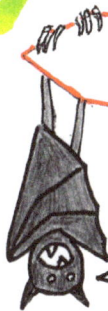

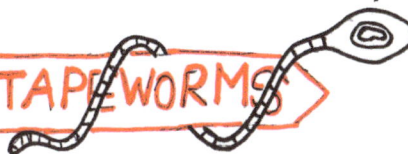

WHO LIVES ON EARTH?

← Earth from 30,000 miles
(Google Earth maximum altitude)

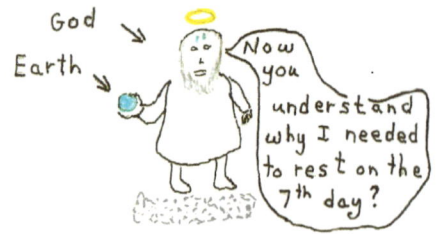

God →
Earth →
Now you understand why I needed to rest on the 7th day?

☺ - All life can be divided into 5 Kingdoms.

Life

Kingdom of Bacteria	Kingdom of Amoebas	Kingdom of Fungi	Kingdom of Plants	Kingdom of Animals

Kingdom of Bacteria

bacteria
(It's a single cell)
This one is a rod

← round bacteria

← corkscrew bacteria

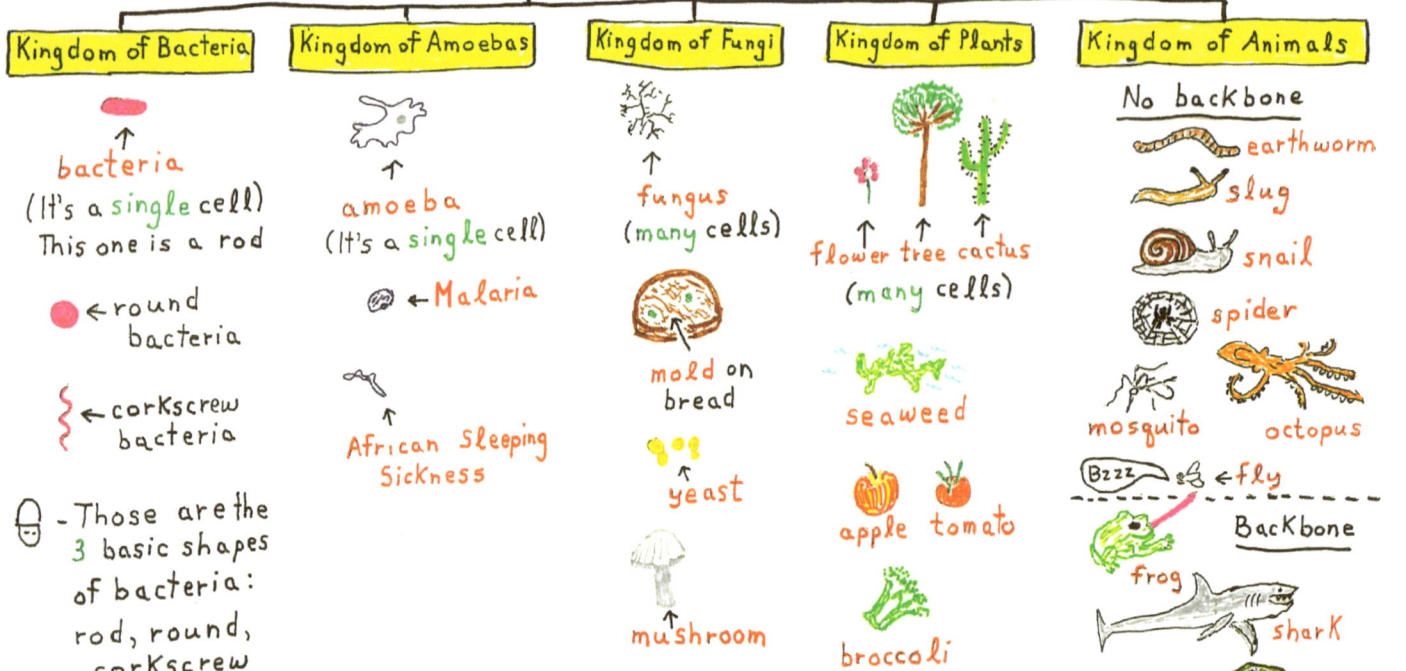

☺ - Those are the 3 basic shapes of bacteria: rod, round, corkscrew

Kingdom of Amoebas

amoeba
(It's a single cell)

← Malaria

African Sleeping Sickness

Kingdom of Fungi

fungus
(many cells)

mold on bread

yeast

mushroom

Kingdom of Plants

flower tree cactus
(many cells)

seaweed

apple tomato

broccoli

Kingdom of Animals

No backbone

earthworm
slug
snail
spider
mosquito octopus

Bzzz ← fly
_____
Backbone

frog

shark

T. rex (extinct reptile)

← finger bones are 'frame' of wing

ptero-dactyl
wing finger
(extinct flying reptile)

crocodile

← black mamba

← eagle

← finger bones? yes

bat (extant flying mammal)
The opposite of extinct

← giraffe
230 feet of intestines

That was his signature. Hard to forge?

Robert Harding Whittaker

○ 1920 - 1980
○ Plant ecologist (study of plant communities)
○ He came up with the 5 Kingdoms

Human →
(many cells)

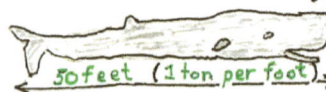

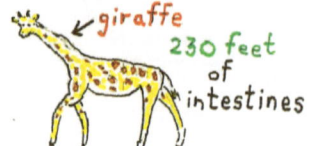

Lion

sperm whale
50 feet (1 ton per foot)

giraffe

- What about viruses? Are they *Life*?

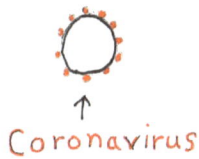

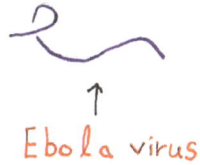

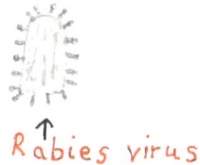

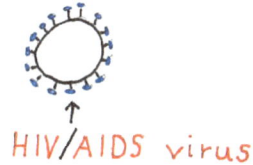

Coronavirus   Ebola virus   Rabies virus   HIV/AIDS virus

- What is *Life*?

- Strictly speaking, *Life* can reproduce.
  It can make a copy of itself without help.

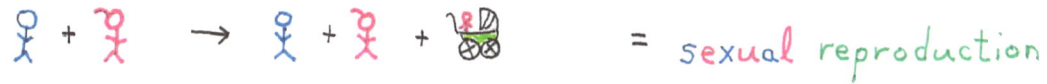

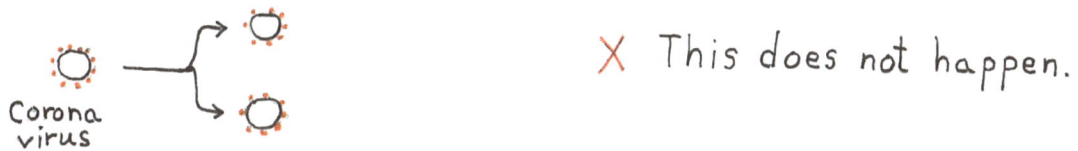

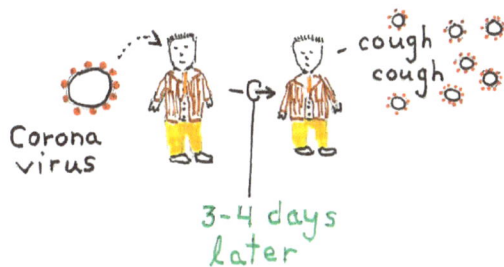

♀ + ♂ → ♀ + ♂ + 👶   = sexual reproduction

1
rod bacteria   2
rod bacteria   = asexual reproduction

X This does not happen.

X This does not happen.

Corona
virus

= This happens.

⊙ The only way a virus can
reproduce is to hijack
a cell (details later)
from 1 of the 5 Kingdoms.

Corona
virus   cough
cough

3-4 days
later

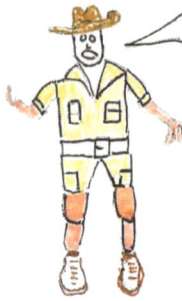

Nasty = **Typhoid Fever**   ⊖ - Do NOT confuse with Typhus. Totally different.

hence

Spread is person-to-person (by feces) (or urine)

Salmonella enterica sub-type Typhi

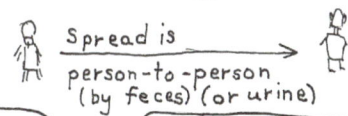

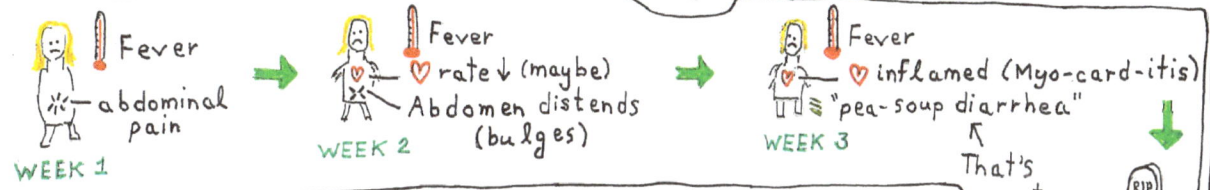

WEEK 1
Fever
—abdominal pain

WEEK 2
Fever
♡ rate ↓ (maybe)
Abdomen distends (bulges)

WEEK 3
Fever
♡ inflamed (Myo-card-itis)
≡ "pea-soup diarrhea"

That's nasty. So's that.

(maybe) RIP

⊖ - But(!) some people are ' asymptomatic carriers '
They feel normal ... but are still infected

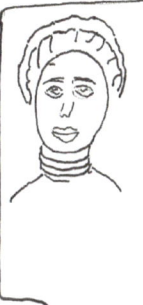

← Typhoid Mary a.k.a. Mary Mallon
- ⊙ She's a <u>cook</u> in Manhattan from 1900-1907 → 53 people infected → 3 deaths
- ⊙ She refuses to wash her hands
- ⊙ She changes her name.
- ⊙ She is tracked down.
- ⊙ She is quarantined ...

⊖ - Let's be blunt.
- Mary's Salmonella-infected feces end up in your mouth.
  \Or her urine (less common).

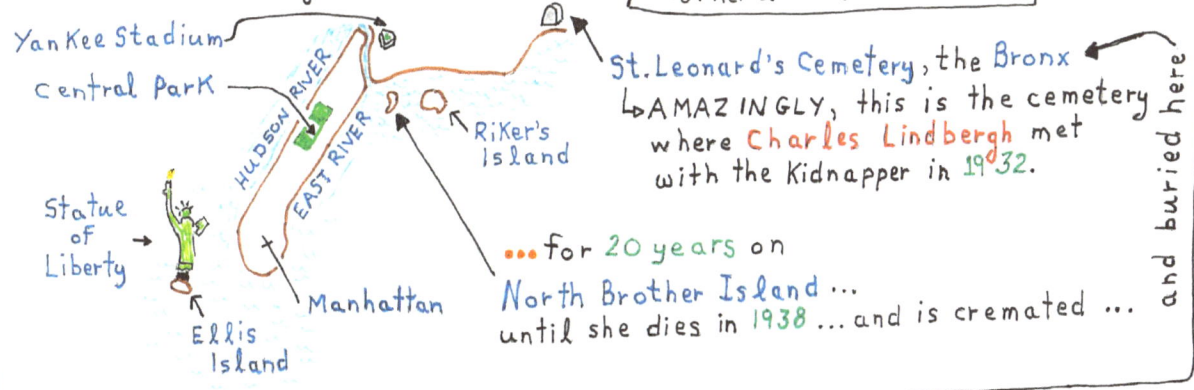

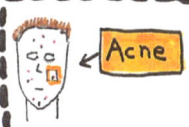

Yankee Stadium
Central Park
HUDSON RIVER
EAST RIVER
Riker's Island
Statue of Liberty
Manhattan
Ellis Island

St. Leonard's Cemetery, the Bronx
↳ AMAZINGLY, this is the cemetery where Charles Lindbergh met with the kidnapper in 1932.

and buried here

... for 20 years on North Brother Island ... until she dies in 1938 ... and is cremated ...

Acne   Genus   species
Propioni-bacterium acnes

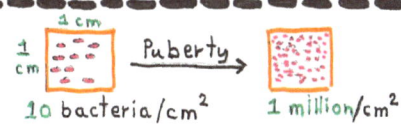

1 cm / 1 cm   10 bacteria/cm² → Puberty → 1 million/cm²

⊖ SOMPOO SAYS - "Pro pie on ih back teer ee um ack knees"

Urinary Tract Infection (UTI)

E. coli

⊖ - E. coli is the short name.
- Escherichia coli is the long name.

↑ sugar cube of human feces contains 5 billion E. coli. Yay.

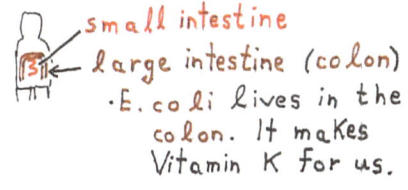

small intestine
large intestine (colon)
· E. coli lives in the colon. It makes Vitamin K for us.

85% of UTIs are caused by E. coli. That's why little girls are taught to wipe front to back.

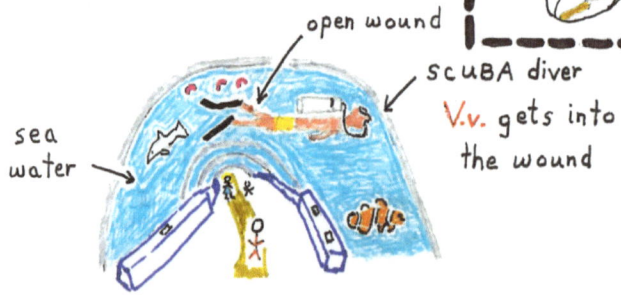

Mommy, can we take a rest?

Only if you can spell Escherichia

Cholera

←rice-water stool

▬ rod

↓

◗ curved (sometimes described as a comma)

☻ -Interestingly, Vibrio cholera changes to a curved shape when it infects us. This is thought to allow it to better penetrate the mucous lining of the small intestine.

Sahara Desert

Sub-Saharan Africa (SSA)

AFRICA

· Cholera persists in SSA and kills children.

Scenario #1

TB growing in the lungs

⊙ This is called a 'Ghon lesion' and is characteristic of TB.

Scenario #2

TB
HIV/AIDS virus

} This is called a co-infection

☻ -The HIV/AIDS virus ✳ destroys our immune system

↓

20 times more likely to get infected by TB ▬

↓

⅓ of HIV/AIDS deaths are due to TB.
⊙ This is called

HIV-Associated TB

↓

251,000 deaths in 2018

↓

84% of these deaths were in

AFRICA

Tuberculosis (TB)

↑
Myco-bacterium tuberculosis

☻ - Remember where Ebola outbreaks occur? In the Democratic Republic of the Congo. It's in SSA.

· So Ebola + Cholera is a double-whammy.

WATCH YOUR STEP

☻ - Who is on top of these statistics like white on rice?

· World Health Organization (WHO)
· Centers for Disease Control (CDC)

- Tuberculosis is endemic in parts of Africa, meaning it is always there.

Nasty infection in SCUBA divers

⟨ ← Vibrio vulnificus

open wound

sea water

SCUBA diver

V.v. gets into the wound

Nasty skin infection a.k.a. Necrotizing skin infection
└Fancy word for dead tissue

☻ - "Nasty" is not far off the mark because the technical term is Necrotizing Soft Tissue Infection (NSTI).

- Skin is soft tissue.   Bone is hard tissue.

SPECIAL EXHIBITION
★ THE NASTY COUSINS ★

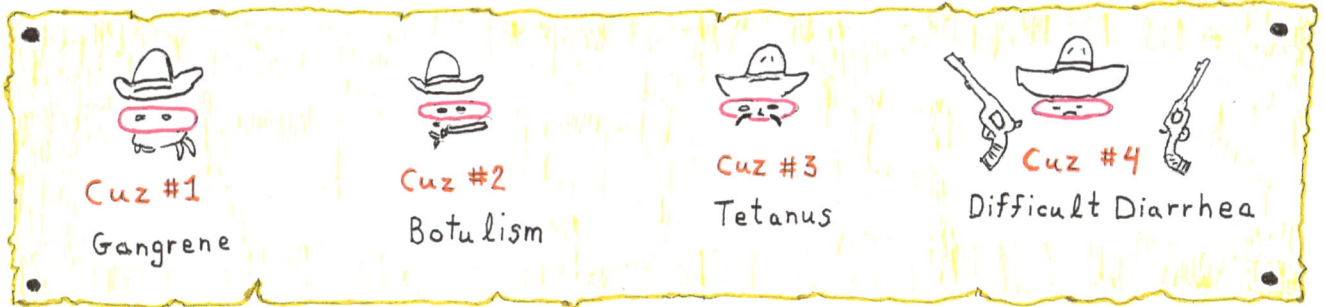

Cuz #1
Gangrene

Cuz #2
Botulism

Cuz #3
Tetanus

Cuz #4
Difficult Diarrhea

- Some background:
  - The cousins die in the presence of 21% oxygen (what we humans breathe).
    - Therefore they are called 'obligate anaerobes.'

      They are obligated to live without oxygen

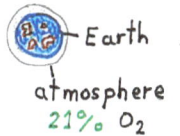

      Earth atmosphere 21% O_2

  - They live in the soil.
  - They are protected by a heat-resistant and dehydration-resistant coat called a spore (not the same as a fungus spore).

Gangrene

Cuz #1

Clostridium perfringens
- Likes to infect wounds
- Produces gas
  → 'Gas Gangrene'

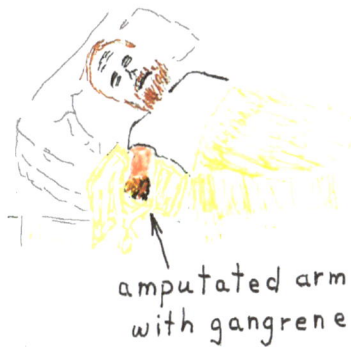

Forlorn U.S. Civil War soldier wounded by a musket bullet

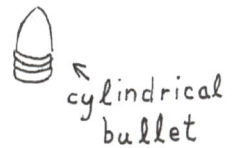

cylindrical bullet

amputated arm with gangrene
(Painting by Edward Stauch, 1863)
(Wikipedia - Gangrene)

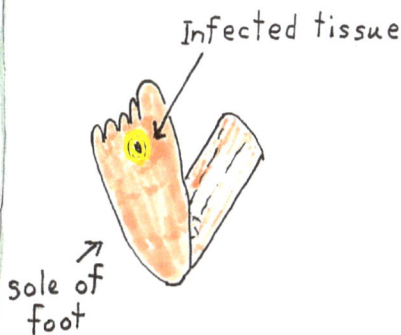

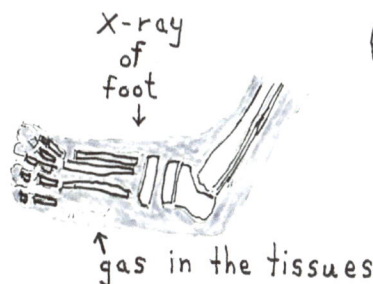

Infected tissue

sole of foot

X-ray of foot
↓

gas in the tissues

- A modern scenario is the 'Diabetic Foot', which is a breakdown of the tissue. Cuz #1 gets in there and makes it worse.

Gangrene (continued)

- When you see the word 'gangrene', think rotting, dead flesh.
- Other bacteria can cause it also... and the tissues look moist... so it's called **Wet Gangrene**. I know, not very appetizing.

` By contrast, **Dry Gangrene** can occur in the absence of bacteria (or at least not the direct cause). For example:

① **Earlier stages of Diabetic Foot**

← dry, dead toe

It can actually just die and fall off, which is called **auto-amputation**.

All About Wet Gangrene

↑ You would not want that as your in-flight movie

② **Septicemic Plague**

black hand of Black Death

If you recall, in this *Horrible Menu* choice, *Yersinia pestis* is in the blood.

↓ Blood clots form ↓ Block arteries to fingers

③ **Frostbite**

- This is rather fascinating.
◇ In response to cold, the arteries in the fingers alternate between constricting and dilating.
  'vaso-constriction'   'vaso-dilation'

← Mount Everest 29,035 FT (8850 m)

This is called the Hunting reaction.

◇ When it gets too cold, the Hunting reaction stops → sustained constriction of the arteries → no blood to fingers (or toes)
→ black, dead tissue (Dry Gangrene)

Ⓛ palm view   Ⓛ pinky

→ digital arteries (supply fingers)

← ulnar artery

radial artery

↻ This is the pulse you can feel in your wrist

The blood supply is more complex than this but it's close enough

Botulism

Cuz #2
Clostridium botulinum

- It likes to infect improperly canned food.
- This is called **Food-Borne Botulism.**

Fresh food

← Cuz #2
← fresh food

♀ - Can Cuz #2 grow on fresh food?

♂ - No. Fresh food is exposed to the air. Cuz #2 can only grow in the absence of oxygen.

Home canning

home-canned food   Cuz #2

Ideal conditions for Cuz #2 to grow are:

← Less than **2%** oxygen
← Temperature **40°-120°F (4°-49°C)**
← moist, low-acid food
  eg. green beans
     beets
     fish
     meat

☺ - To do it safely, Google this:
  USDA complete guide to home canning
  United States Department of Agriculture
  It's super detailed.

☺ - Cuz #2 secretes **Botulinum Toxin (BTX)** which begins to accumulate in the (improperly) canned food.

Cuz #2 → ⟿ BTX   ⟿ ← beet

SYMPTOMS

- Double vision ÅÅ
- Difficulty swallowing
- Difficulty breathing → **Respiratory Paralysis** → [RIP] **5-10%** Fatality rate
  └ In some people

↑
Botulism
- This starts about **18-36 hours** after eating the contaminated food.

☺ - What's happening? | The toxin interferes with nerve talking to muscle ← eye muscles / throat muscles / breathing muscles.

nerve   muscle →   ZOOM   BTX↓   ☺ - The toxin prevents the release of neuro-transmitters.

A **neuro-transmitter** called **acetyl-choline** is stored in here. It excites muscle.

★ - If the affected muscle controls the <u>lungs</u> (expand/contract) ... you die. 🪦. Maybe.

☺ - You will learn later that the muscle called the diaphragm controls the lungs.

Botox
wrinkles

Cuz #2 ⟿ ⟿ BTX
collect this + put it in a syringe

Botox = Botulinum toxin = **$500**

★ - If this is the <u>muscle</u> controlling the <u>forehead</u>, your wrinkles go away because the muscle is paralysed.

Infant Botulism

Cuz #2 can grow in honey ... and for unknown reasons can cause Botulism in babies less than **1-year old.**

↑ honey   ↑ baby   Cuz #2

Tetanus

Cuz #3
Clostridium tetani

Hence the species name

- It likes to cause muscle spasms.
- A muscle in continuous spasm is said to be in tetany.

θ - A plain ol' muscle spasm is not Tetanus, however.

SYMPTOMS

← spasm of jaw muscles = "Lockjaw"
← spasm of body muscles can break your bones. Ouch.
← spasm of breathing muscles → death 🪦. Maybe.

What is going on?

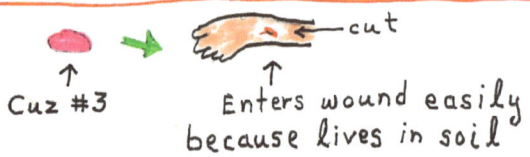

Cuz #3 → cut
Enters wound easily because lives in soil

→ Infection of the wound is not the problem

This is the problem

Tetanus NeuroToxin
a.k.a.
Spasmo-genic Toxin

nerve to jaw
bone → nerve to arm
CRACK! muscle
nerve to diaphragm

← Toxin does not enter brain

← Toxin causes spinal cord to continuously excite muscles

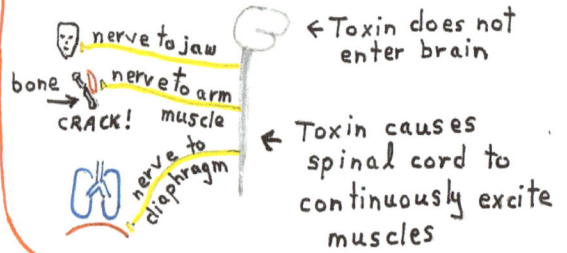

Difficult Diarrhea

Cuz #4
Clostridium difficile
"c. diff" for short.

- Diarrhea is its thing.

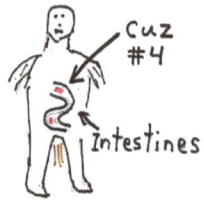

Cuz #4
Intestines

Doctor's Dilemma
(and yours)

I will give you this anti-biotic for your pneumonia, which is good because it will kill the bacteria causing the pneumonia ... but it can also kill some of the bacteria in your intestines ... allowing c. diff to multiply ... causing **C.diff Diarrhea**.

θ - "Closs trid ee um"

SOMPOO SAYS

"per fringe ens"   Cuz #1   Gangrene
"botch you line um"   Cuz #2   "Botch you lizm"
"tet an eye"   Cuz #3   Tetanus
"diff ih seal"   Cuz #4   C. diff Diarrhea

EXIT →

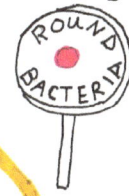
ROUND BACTERIA

Staphylo-coccus aureus

Staphylo- ← Latin
coccus ← Latin
aureus ← Latin

cluster | berry | golden ← English

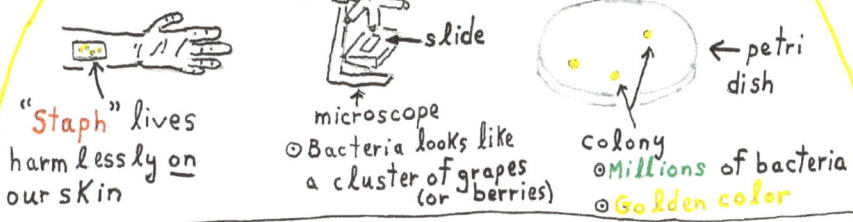

← slide
← petri dish

"Staph" lives harmlessly on our skin

microscope
⊙ Bacteria looks like a cluster of grapes (or berries)

colony
⊙ Millions of bacteria
⊙ Golden color

⊖ - Round bacteria are known as:
coccus = 1 ●
cocci = 2 or more
●●●

⊖ -If staph gets under our skin or inside us, it can harm us.

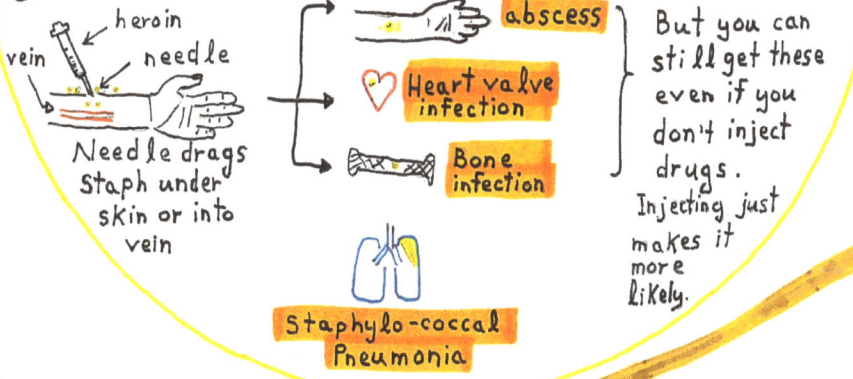

heroin
needle
vein

Needle drags Staph under skin or into vein

abscess
Heart valve infection
Bone infection

But you can still get these even if you don't inject drugs. Injecting just makes it more likely.

Billy, liquified seaweed is used to make the agar growth medium in a petri dish

Mom, I'm only in Grade One

Staphylo-coccal Pneumonia

⊖ - "Staff low cock us"
"or ee us"
SOMPOO SAYS
"Staff low cock ul"

Strepto-coccus
●●●●●

⊖ -These tend to grow in chains.

⊖ - Strep names are a challenge to memorize.

⊖ -The shortest chain is 2.
●●
Strepto-coccus pneumoniae
a.k.a.
Pneumo-coccus (PC)

⊖ - "strep toe cock us"
"new moan ee a"
SOMPOO SAYS
rhymes with day

Strepto-coccal Pneumonia
a.k.a.
Pneumo-coccal Pneumonia

⊖ - This guy normally lives peacefully in the back of our throat.
- But it can cause: Pneumonia
Ear infections
Sinus infections (↑risk if smoke)

⊖ - At the end of the day, if you remember that Staph and Strep are round, you're in good shape.

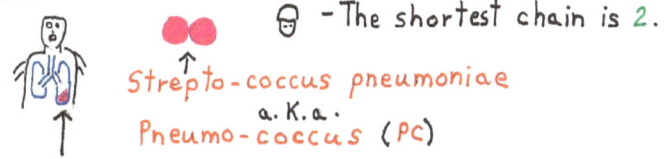
⊖ -Why stop here?
There are also:
Group A Strep
Group B Strep
Group C Strep
Group D Strep
Group F Strep
Group G Strep
We'll limit your mental torture to just these 2.

⚥- What about E?
⚥ -Strangely absent

😐 - In the 1918 Influenza Pandemic, guess which bacteria caused the super-infection in the lungs?

Staph aureus
Strep pneumoniae
Group A Strep

← The chain does not have to be straight

Group A Strep (GAS)

😐 - However, you might be an asymptomatic carrier.

"Mummy, my throat hurts"

Strep Throat

⊙ GAS causes Strep Throat, usually in children
⊙ Usually there is no cough.   4-7y old.

FLESH-EATING DISEASE a.k.a. Necrotizing Fasciitis

😐 - The key to understanding this is knowing what fascia is.

←fascia

muscle

⊙ It's like biological Saran wrap that wraps individual muscles. } This is thought to ↓ friction to allow muscles to slide past each other.

😐 - Fascia also wraps groups of muscles, creating what are called compartments.

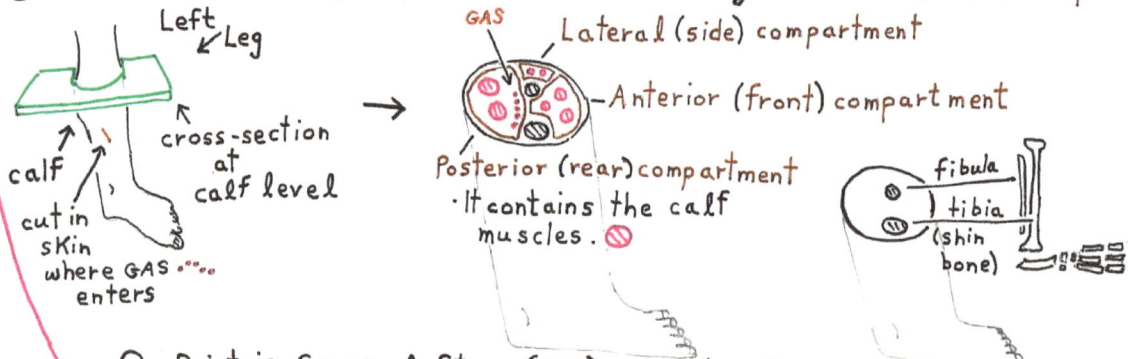

Left Leg

cross-section at calf level

calf

cut in skin where GAS enters

GAS

Lateral (side) compartment

- Anterior (front) compartment

Posterior (rear) compartment
· It contains the calf muscles.

fibula
tibia
(shin bone)

😐 - Point is Group A Strep (GAS) spreads along 'fascial planes'.
It destroys the fascia.

Necrotizing   Fasciitis

Dead/dying tissue   Inflamed fascia

2/3 of cases involve the leg.

😐 - In a totally different scenario, severe burns can cause swelling within a compartment. That's called a Compartment Syndrome

A surgeon will slice the fascia to relieve the swelling.

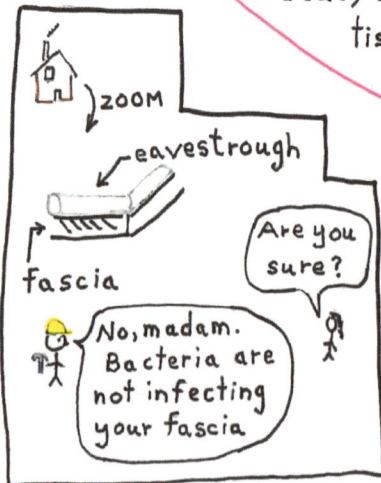

ZOOM

house → eavestrough

fascia

Are you sure?

No, madam. Bacteria are not infecting your fascia

"fah shah"
😐 - "Neck row tie zing"
SOMPOO SAYS   "fash ee eye t iss"

♀ - If I have Strep Throat, will I get Flesh-Eating Disease?

♀ - This happens once per million cases. It affects fascia in the throat.

That's less likely than being struck by lightning (1/700,000).

♀ - What can you tell me about the fetus?

♂ - The fetus is surrounded by 2 membranes - the amnion and the chorion.
They protect the fetus from the outside world.
When it is time to be born, they rupture (the dramatic scene in a Hollywood movie
when a pregnant woman gasps, "My water broke!"). This is called the
Rupture Of Membranes (ROM). And the 'water' is amniotic fluid. So far so good.

♀ - What's not good?

♂ - Premature ROM
a.k.a.
PROM
The membranes
rupture
too soon.
...

← magnified 900 x

Group B Strep (GBS)

♂ ... but may be not
an outright rupture.
Maybe a small
leak.
Nevertheless,
a security
breach.

← Pregnant
← uterus

muscular wall
of uterus

amniotic
fluid

SEQUENCE OF PROBLEMS:

1. GBS present in vagina
ascend into uterus. This
is called an 'ascending
infection.'

2. GBS infect chorion

3. GBS infect amnion

4. GBS infect fetus

← uterus
(womb)

amnion
·inner
membrane

chorion
·outer membrane

← vagina

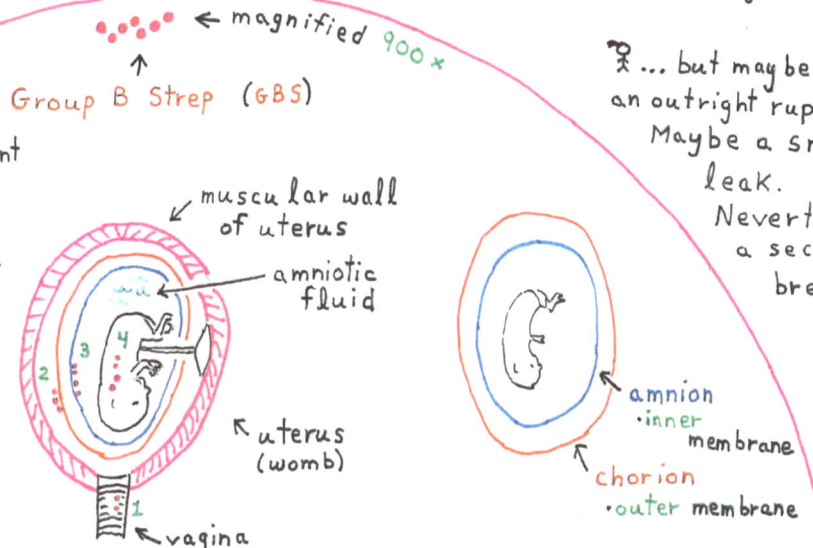

·GBS are found normally in 10-30% of
pregnant females (in the vagina).

PROM makes it more likely for GBS to ascend (by multiplying) and infect the 2
membranes. The infection is called Chorio-amnion-itis. Yes, doctors use anti-biotics. ⊗

AMAZING ZOOLOGY STORY

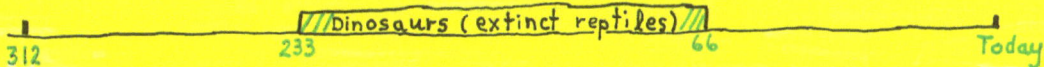

Dinosaurs (extinct reptiles)

| 312 | 233 | 66 | Today |

312 million years ago, reptiles evolve a H_2O-proof egg.
The amnion makes it H_2O-proof. (Think, Keep H_2O inside the egg.)

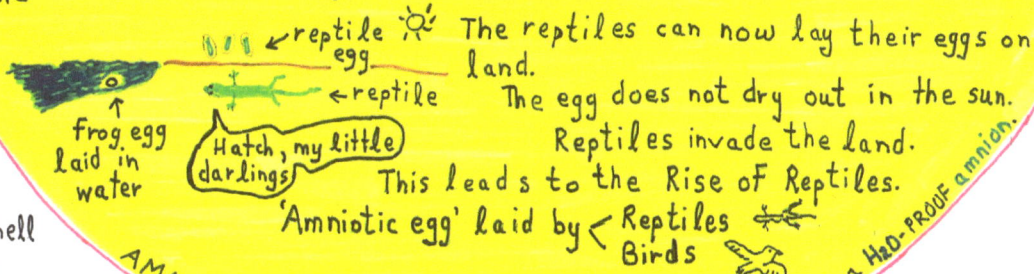

← reptile
egg

The reptiles can now lay their eggs on
land.
The egg does not dry out in the sun.
Reptiles invade the land.
This leads to the Rise of Reptiles.

← reptile

frog egg
laid in
water

Hatch, my little
darlings

'Amniotic egg' laid by < Reptiles
Birds

chorion

amnion

←shell

reptile egg

chorion

shell

amnion

chicken
egg

AMAZINGLY, 312,000,000 years later, humans still have a H_2O-PROOF amnion.

⊗ The American College of Obstetricians and Gynecologists (ACOG) has rather detailed
                          deliver babies   ♀ reproductive parts

'decision trees' (fancy flowcharts) depending on when the Premature Rupture of Membranes occurs.

PROM

PPROM: That means Pre-term Premature Rupture of Membranes.
Before 37 weeks of the 40-week pregnancy.

SOMPOO
SAYS
- "P,rom"
"P,P,rom"

Mommy, my head is exploding with all these doctor words

Billy, you are going to learn all of them, then become an Infectious Disease doctor so you can save me from Coronavirus

But I want to be a professional gamer

Meningitis

← Looks like 2 balls squished together

Meningo-coccus

It infects the membranes (meninges) of the brain

3 layers of brain membranes

brain

ZOOM →

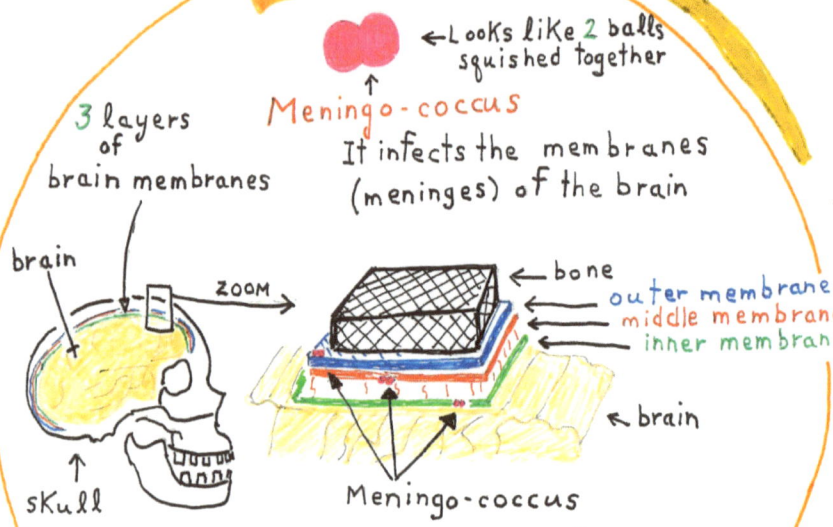

bone
outer membrane
middle membrane
inner membrane
brain

skull

Meningo-coccus

☺ - In Meningitis, the 3 layers of membranes (meninges) that surround and protect the brain are invaded by bacteria.
- That's **Bacterial Meningitis**.
Many other bacteria can cause Meningitis. Plus fungi, viruses, and amoebas

☺ - "menin jeez"
SOMPOO SAYS   "men in jy tiss"
    rhymes with sky

☺ - The outermost membrane is the 'tough mother'

As in durable   Latin for 'mother'

Dura mater } meninges

"der ah" "mah ter" - ☺
SOMPOO SAYS

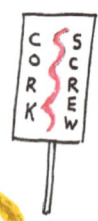

The reason for the stiffneck is that the meninges also surround the spinal cord.

Lyme disease

corkscrew shape ↘

5-20 microns (μm) long

0.3 μm

Borrelia burgdorferi

forest

you

deer tick

Borrelia ·Lives in mid-gut

mid-gut

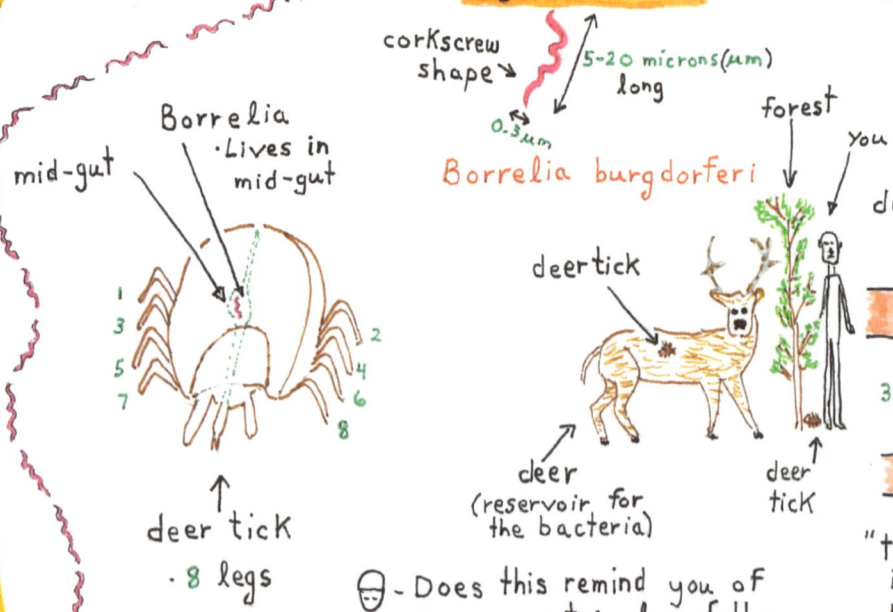

1 3 5 7   2 4 6 8

deer tick
· 8 legs

deertick

deer (reservoir for the bacteria)

deer tick

deer tick

3-32 days later

"target lesion" is characteristic red skin rash

☺ -Does this remind you of the pro-ventriculus of the flea in Bubonic Plague?

☺ - Lots of weird manifestations:
⊙ **Arthritis** (even after B.b. is long gone)
⊙ ♡ **muscle inflammation** (☼ coronavirus also does this)
⊙ **Meningitis**

☺ - There are a gazillion more bacteria that cause infections but let's move on to the next Kingdom.

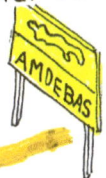

AMOEBAS

☺ - Amoebas, like bacteria, are a single-celled organism.

MALARIA in 11 easy steps

☺ - Malaria showcases the complexity that even a single cell possesses.

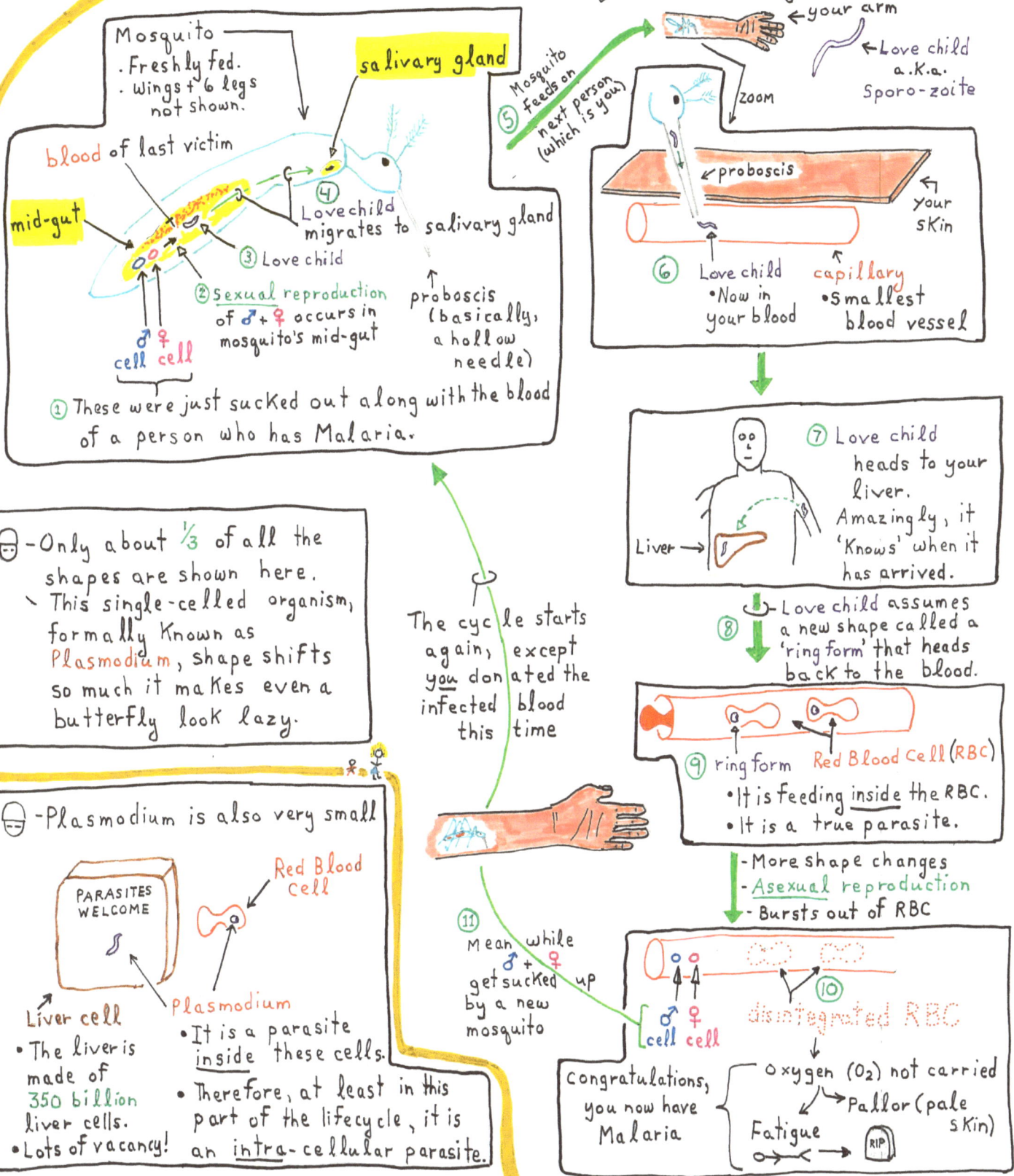

Mosquito
. Freshly fed.
. Wings + 6 legs not shown.

salivary gland

blood of last victim

mid-gut

④ Lovechild migrates to salivary gland

③ Love child

② Sexual reproduction of ♂ + ♀ occurs in mosquito's mid-gut

proboscis (basically, a hollow needle)

♂ cell ♀ cell

① These were just sucked out along with the blood of a person who has Malaria.

Mosquito feeds on next person (which is you) ⑤

← your arm

← Love child a.k.a. Sporo-zoite

zoom

← proboscis

your skin

⑥ Love child • Now in your blood

capillary • Smallest blood vessel

⑦ Love child heads to your liver. Amazingly, it 'Knows' when it has arrived.

Liver →

☺ - Only about ⅓ of all the shapes are shown here.
This single-celled organism, formally known as Plasmodium, shape shifts so much it makes even a butterfly look lazy.

⑧ Love child assumes a new shape called a 'ring form' that heads back to the blood.

The cycle starts again, except you donated the infected blood this time

⑨ ring form   Red Blood Cell (RBC)
• It is feeding inside the RBC.
• It is a true parasite.

- More shape changes
- Asexual reproduction
- Bursts out of RBC

☺ - Plasmodium is also very small

PARASITES WELCOME

Red Blood Cell

Liver cell
• The liver is made of 350 billion liver cells.
• Lots of vacancy!

Plasmodium
• It is a parasite inside these cells.
• Therefore, at least in this part of the lifecycle, it is an intra-cellular parasite.

⑪ Meanwhile ♂ + ♀ get sucked up by a new mosquito

♂ cell ♀ cell

disintegrated RBC ⑩

Oxygen (O₂) not carried
→ Pallor (pale skin)
Fatigue →← → RIP

congratulations, you now have Malaria

Treating / Preventing Malaria

- As a broad generality, we try to kill the Plasmodium:

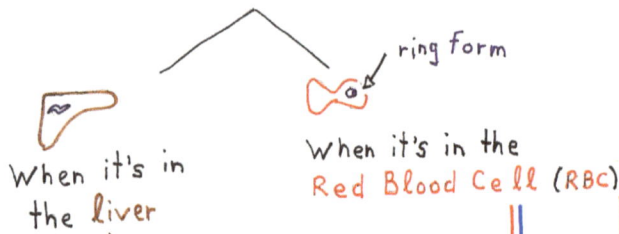

ring form

When it's in the liver

When it's in the Red Blood Cell (RBC)

Billy OD'ed on information!

Don't worry, Ma'am, we'll take him to the infirmary

SCUBA... seaweed... corkscrew

← pill

PRIMAQUINE
- It prevents the Plasmodium from creating energy to live. (Technically, it inhibits the mitochondria that powers the Plasmodium)

cinchona tree / bark of tree → **quinine**
- Extract from bark
- Used for centuries

chomp, chomp

sugar (glucose)

- It prevents the ring form from being able to use sugar.
- [I got intra-venous quinine when I got Malaria in Uganda. It was the nasty version known as Plasmodium falciparum]

sweet wormwood leaves

Artemisinin Combination Therapy

This is better

Artemisinin is never given alone! **ASK your doctor.**

HMM, WHAT IF THE RED BLOOD CELL HAS A WEIRD SHAPE?

concave / concave → "bi-concave disk" $r = 2$
- This is the normal shape of an RBC (viewed from the side)

← sickle

← sickle shape RBC

← Grim Reaper

- In the blood disease called **Sickle Cell Anemia**, the sickle shape screws up the ability of the Plasmodium to carry out its life cycle.
- The disease probably evolved as protection against Malaria.

↑ pill

Chloro-Quine (CQ)
- Synthetic (man-made).
- Similar to quinine.

↑ pill

Hydroxy-Chloro-Quine (HCQ)
- Synthetic.
- Made from CQ in 1946.
- It's not precisely known how it kills the ring form.

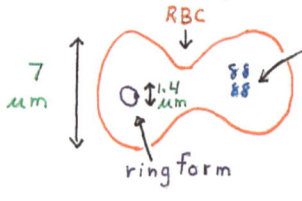

RBC

7 um   1.4 um

ring form

Hemoglobin (not to scale) (it's invisible)

- Getting downright technical, Hemoglobin is a large protein that carries oxygen.
- 250,000 Hemoglobins in every RBC !!
- It's made of Heme (contains iron) plus globin (the protein).
- The Heme may accumulate in the Plasmodium, killing it. That's maybe how Hydroxychloroquine works to treat Malaria.
- HCQ is not used much.

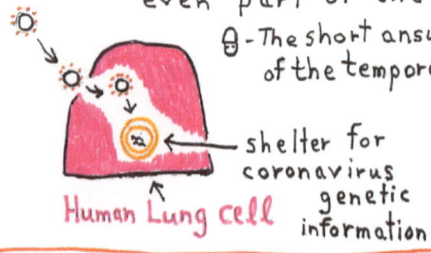

- The obvious question is: How does Hydroxychloroquine (HCQ) which isn't even part of the 5 Kingdoms of Life theoretically work against Coronavirus ?
- The short answer is that HCQ screws up the pH (acidity) of the temporary shelter the virus needs.
  ★ At least, this is what happens in a glass petri dish. ★
  ★ But what happens in a petri dish (or an animal model) may not translate to what happens in a human! ★

shelter for coronavirus genetic information

Human Lung cell

Amoebic Dysentery
(sicker than a dog)

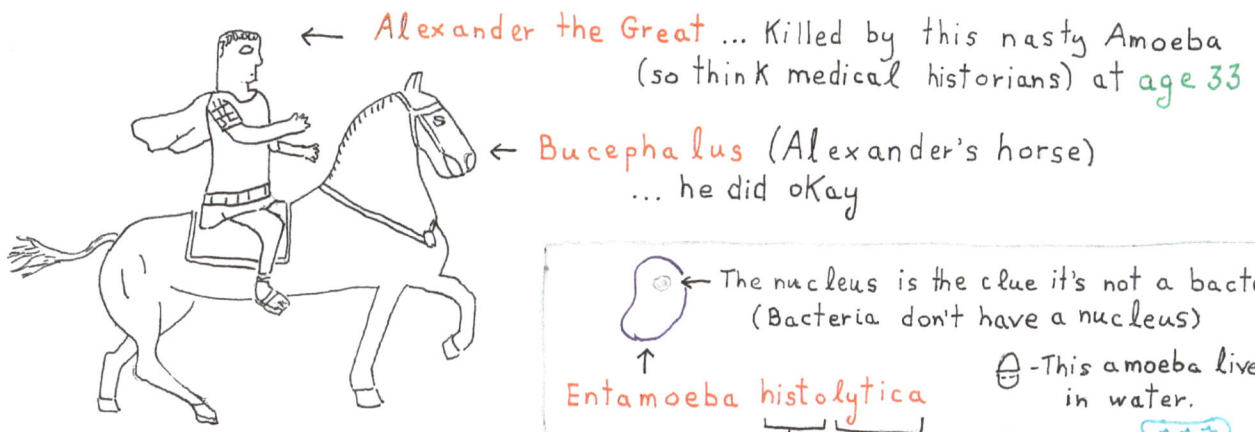

Alexander the Great ... Killed by this nasty Amoeba (so think medical historians) at age 33

Bucephalus (Alexander's horse) ... he did okay

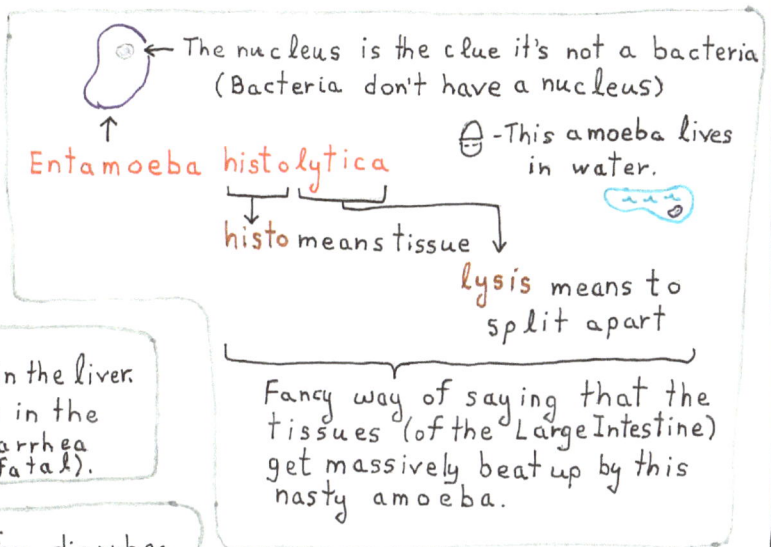

← The nucleus is the clue it's not a bacteria (Bacteria don't have a nucleus)

Entamoeba histolytica

-This amoeba lives in water.

histo means tissue

lysis means to split apart

Fancy way of saying that the tissues (of the Large Intestine) get massively beat up by this nasty amoeba.

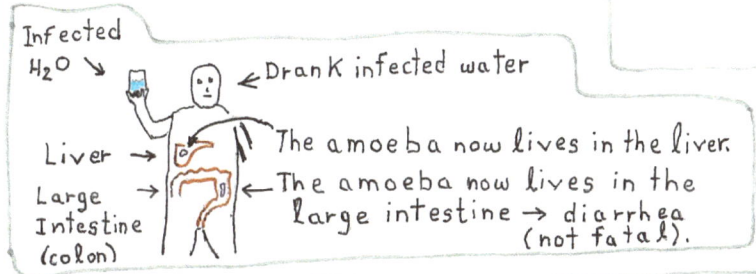

Infected H₂O ↘

→ Drank infected water

Liver →
Large Intestine (colon) →

The amoeba now lives in the liver.
← The amoeba now lives in the large intestine → diarrhea (not fatal).

dys-entery is an old term for diarrhea

enteron is the Greek word for intestines } = bad intestines

dys means bad, like a dys-functional family

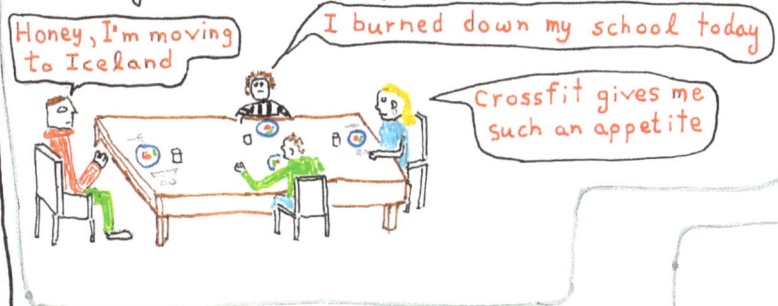

Honey, I'm moving to Iceland

I burned down my school today

Crossfit gives me such an appetite

"am ee bik"
"diss en terry"   SOMPOO SAYS

"ent am ee ba"
"hiss toe lit ick ah"

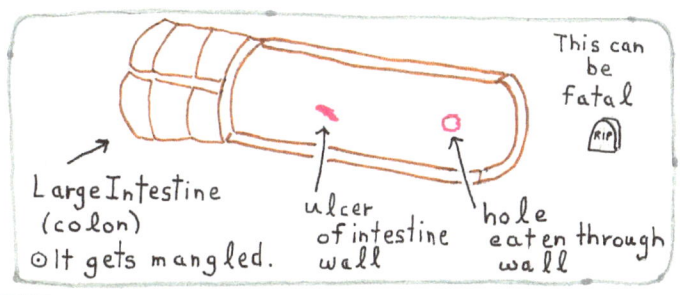

This can be fatal

Large Intestine (colon)
⊙ It gets mangled.

ulcer of intestine wall

hole eaten through wall

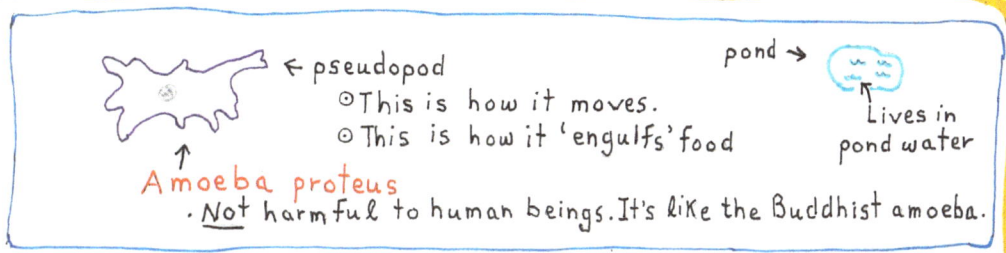

← pseudopod
⊙ This is how it moves.
⊙ This is how it 'engulfs' food

pond →

Lives in pond water

Amoeba proteus
· Not harmful to human beings. It's like the Buddhist amoeba.

Okay, we're done with Amoebas

- I lied. For all you cat lovers, here's a bonus page with 2 bacteria and 1 amoeba.

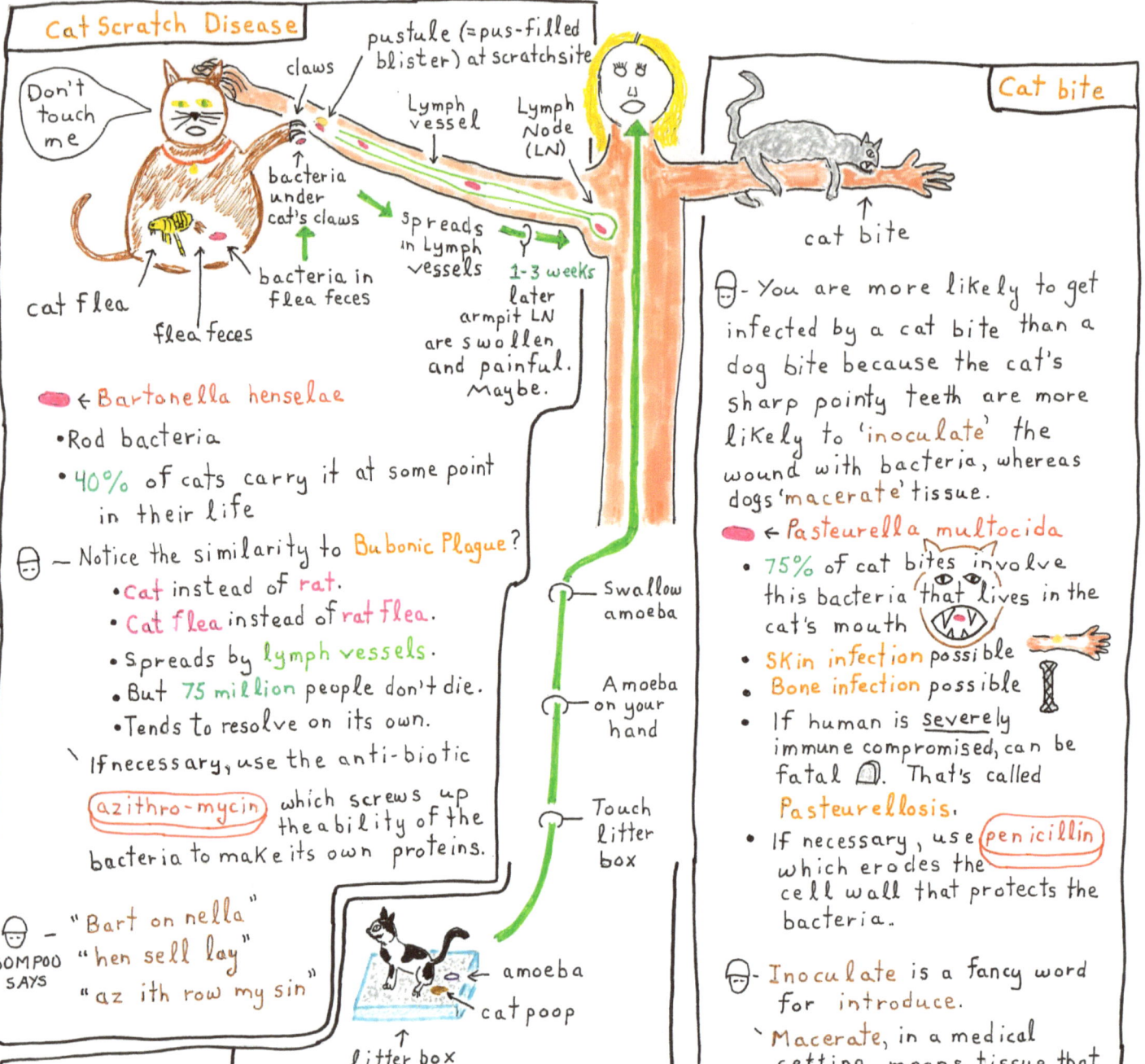

Cat Scratch Disease

"Don't touch me"

claws

pustule (=pus-filled blister) at scratchsite

Lymph vessel

Lymph Node (LN)

bacteria under cat's claws

Spreads in Lymph vessels

1-3 weeks later armpit LN are swollen and painful. Maybe.

cat flea

flea feces

bacteria in flea feces

← Bartonella henselae
- Rod bacteria
- 40% of cats carry it at some point in their life

- Notice the similarity to Bubonic Plague?
  - cat instead of rat.
  - Cat flea instead of rat flea.
  - Spreads by lymph vessels.
  - But 75 million people don't die.
  - Tends to resolve on its own.
  - If necessary, use the anti-biotic
  (azithro-mycin) which screws up the ability of the bacteria to make its own proteins.

SOMPOO SAYS - "Bart on nella" "hen sell lay" "az ith row my sin"

Swallow amoeba

Amoeba on your hand

Touch litter box

amoeba

cat poop

litter box

Cat bite

cat bite

- You are more likely to get infected by a cat bite than a dog bite because the cat's sharp pointy teeth are more likely to 'inoculate' the wound with bacteria, whereas dogs 'macerate' tissue.

← Pasteurella multocida
- 75% of cat bites involve this bacteria that lives in the cat's mouth
- Skin infection possible
- Bone infection possible
- If human is severely immune compromised, can be fatal. That's called Pasteurellosis.
- If necessary, use (penicillin) which erodes the cell wall that protects the bacteria.

- Inoculate is a fancy word for introduce.
- Macerate, in a medical setting, means tissue that looks beat up.

- Okay, now we're officially done with single cells - bacteria and amoebas. Everything else that infects us is made of many cells a.k.a. multi-cellular.

Toxoplasmosis

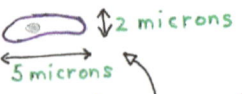

↕ 2 microns
← 5 microns →

Toxoplasma gondii
- It's an amoeba cousin
- The 'swamp' it lives in is a cell. As in, inside the cell of a cat or human.
- If you become infected, that's called Toxoplasmosis.

- If a pregnant woman touches cat litter and swallows the amoeba, it can infect the unborn baby (fetus). This mother-to-baby route is called: VERTICAL TRANSMISSION

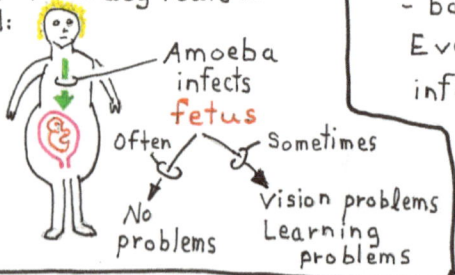

Amoeba infects fetus

Often → No problems

Sometimes → Vision problems Learning problems

FUNGAL SKIN INFECTIONS

Athlete's Foot

scaly, red skin

↑ stinky

Trichophyton rubrum

S
K
I
N
- epidermis →
- dermis →
- hair follicle →

fungus
· Growing downwards into epidermis

free nerve ending
⊙Fungus activates it
→ itchy feeling

Ringworm

· Not caused by a worm
· Caused by Trichophyton

FUNGI

☺ -Fungi live by absorbing

plant and animal matter.

☣ BIOHAZARD STINKY FEET STAY BACK 50 FEET

Rare scenario

LeuKemia (blood cancer)
· ↓ White Blood Cells (WBCs) to fight infections

↓ immunity
a.k.a.
immuno-compromised

epidermis

dermis

This is very rare

dermal invasion by Trichophyton

☺ - Remember the Disease Triangle?

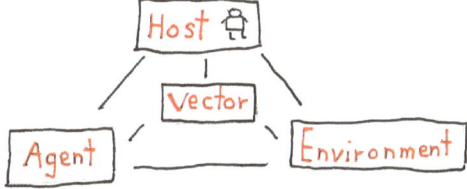

Host 🧍
|
Vector
Agent ———— Environment

In this scenario, the Host has ↓ immunity.
· The Agent (a pretty run-of-the-mill fungus) gets ↑ access to the Host's body

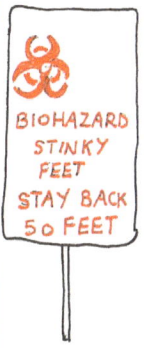

♀ - Who Knew stinky feet could be so interesting?

♂ - I agree although I'm not encouraging it

fingerprint
is created by
dermal ridges

☺ - "Epi" means upon (think, on top of)
→ Epi - dermis = It's on top of the dermis
   upon dermis

→ Epi - demic = It's on top of the people
   upon people

NASTY FUNGUS ... some of the time 🕘

Aspergillus fumigatus
· What a great name

SOMPOO SAYS - "Ass per jill us"

- Aspergillus is the perfect example of how an "underlying illness" can markedly alter what happens next.

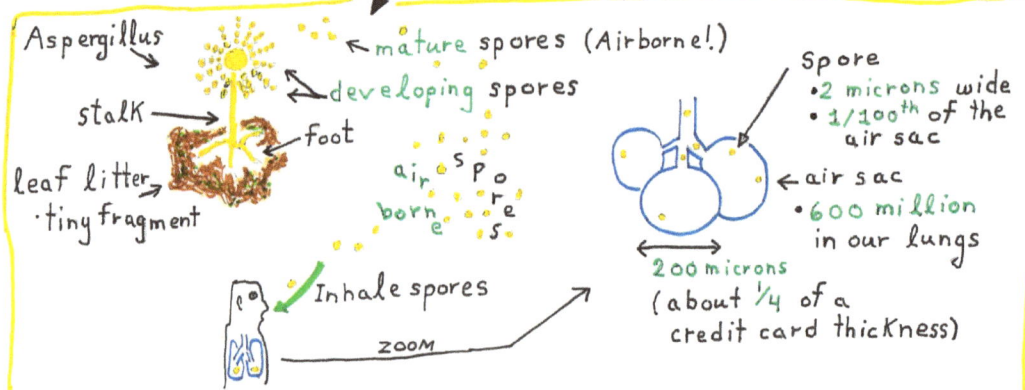

- There are 3 basic scenarios:
  Good, Bad, Ugly

- Aspergillus is everywhere.

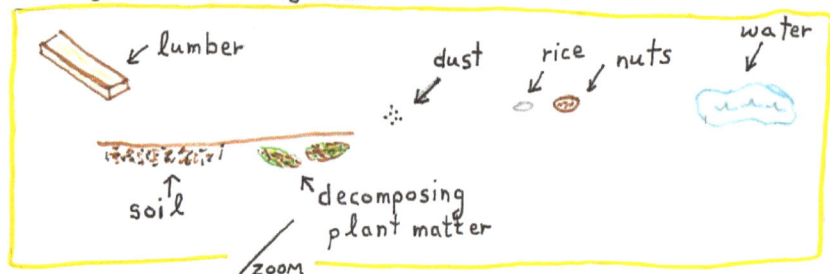

← lumber
dust   rice   nuts   water
soil   ← decomposing plant matter

ZOOM

Aspergillus
stalk
leaf litter
· tiny fragment
foot
← mature spores (Airborne!)
← developing spores
air borne spores

Inhale spores

ZOOM

Spore
· 2 microns wide
· 1/100th of the air sac
← air sac
· 600 million in our lungs

200 microns
(about 1/4 of a credit card thickness)

- The moral of the story is that Aspergillus fungal spores are so small they travel deep into your lungs.
- This happens every day ... obviously you survive this.

Good
←Joe

Joe is healthy
He inhales the spores
Nothing happens
It's all good

Bad
← Margaret
← pre-existing cavity in lung   ... due to

- Clearly, an abnormal starting point

TB (Tuberculosis) ← bacteria
· It can create cavities in lung tissue.

Emphysema
· Basically, 20 years of smoking a pack a day.
· The smoke particles destroy lung tissue.

SOMPOO SAYS - "Ass per jill oh ma"
↘ I love ♡ this word

cavity
Aspergillus
· Grows in the cavity.
· Kinda looks like a ball.
· This is called an :
  Aspergilloma
  or
  Aspergillus Intra-Cavitary Fungus Ball

← At first, only a mild cough
But later, in some people

R.I.P.
Possible.

Margaret coughs up blood
· Can be severe

Ugly

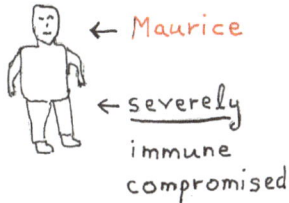

← Maurice

← severely immune compromised

- As a broad generality, patients are:

Immuno-competent
- That means an intact, functioning immune system.
- A normal number of White Blood Cells (WBC).

Immuno-compromised
- Not enough White Blood Cells.

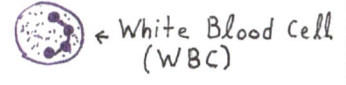

← White Blood Cell (WBC)

- "Not enough" is pretty vague.

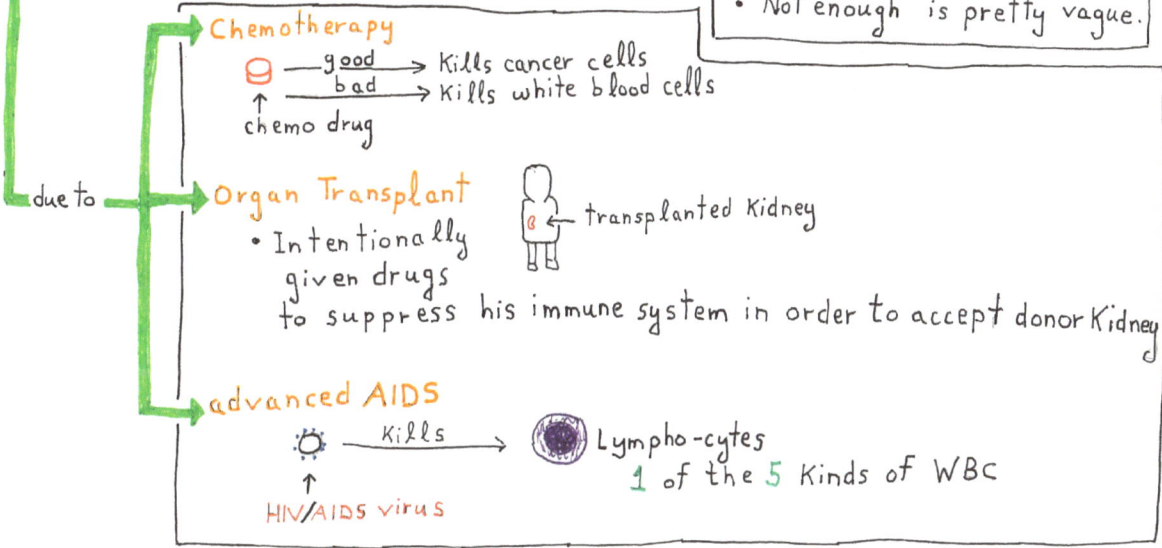

Chemotherapy

good → Kills cancer cells
bad → Kills white blood cells

↑ chemo drug

due to

Organ Transplant
- Intentionally given drugs to suppress his immune system in order to accept donor kidney

← transplanted kidney

advanced AIDS

Kills → Lympho-cytes
1 of the 5 kinds of WBC

↑ HIV/AIDS virus

- The underlying illnesses above are risk factors for progression to...

This is rare, fortunately.
This is called
Invasive Aspergillosis

Aspergillus in brain
- 100% fatal

Aspergillus growing on ♡ valve
- 100% fatal without surgery

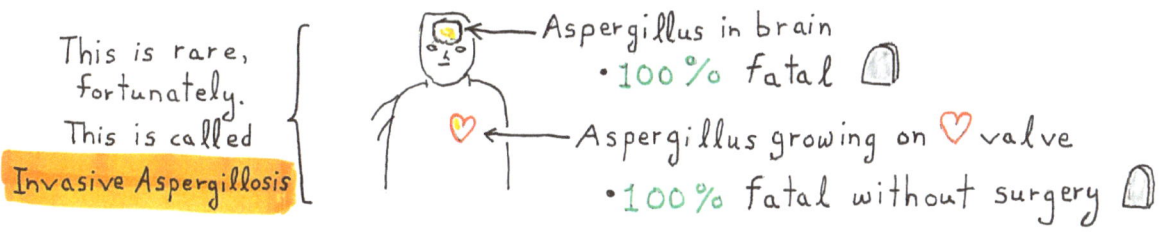

Random Violation of Intuition

← 74-year-old man with Coronavirus
- Intensive Care Unit (ICU) → ventilator
→ dies of Aspergillus despite having an intact immune system
- This is an Aspergillus super-infection.

Fatal Invasive Aspergillosis and Coronavirus Disease in an Immunocompetent Host
Emerging Infectious Disease, July 2020
↖ The CDC publishes this journal

Maurice, nothing personal.
I like to grow wherever I can

- Aspergillus looks like a miniature tree.

- True, but it's not a plant.
`Plants contain chlorophyll to harness sunlight.
`Fungi don't have chlorophyll

PLANTS

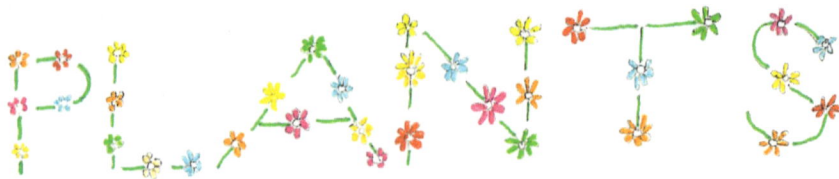

☺ – Plants do not infect humans.
Restated, plants do not invade and reproduce on us or in us.

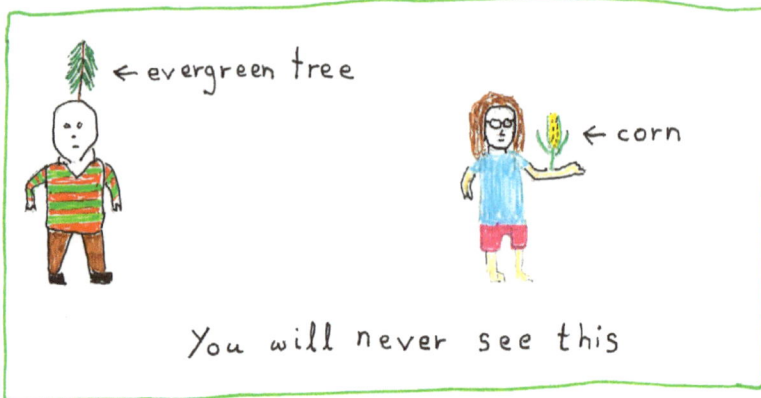

← evergreen tree

← corn

You will never see this

Pollen

Call the minister. Cancel my wedding

100* microns

itchy eyes
runny nose

☺ – Plant pollen can cause Allergies.
↘ Yes, White blood cells are responsible.
↘ But that's not an infection.

pollen

↑ Allergy sufferer

* Much larger than fungal spore (2 microns)

air-filled sac →

← air-filled sac

↑ pollen (of a pine tree)

↑ pine tree

~75 FEET
25 meters

☺ – Some pollen grains have air-filled sacs
↓
increased dispersal distance

Poison Ivy

←poison ivy →

↑ North America

"Leaves of 3
Let it be"

(Don't touch it)

←blister

☺ – Poison ivy contains a toxin called urushiol.
↘ The reaction of the skin is Allergic Contact Dermatitis.
↘ White blood cells involved? Yes. Infection? No.

Rose Handler's Disease

←rose
←fungus lives on rose bush

cut
⦿Fungus gets in cut

1-12 weeks later

bump on skin a.k.a. nodule (oozes pus)

fungus spreads by lymph vessels

another bump

☺ –Did the rose infect you? No. It was the fungus (Sporothrix).

(Remember Bubonic Plague?)

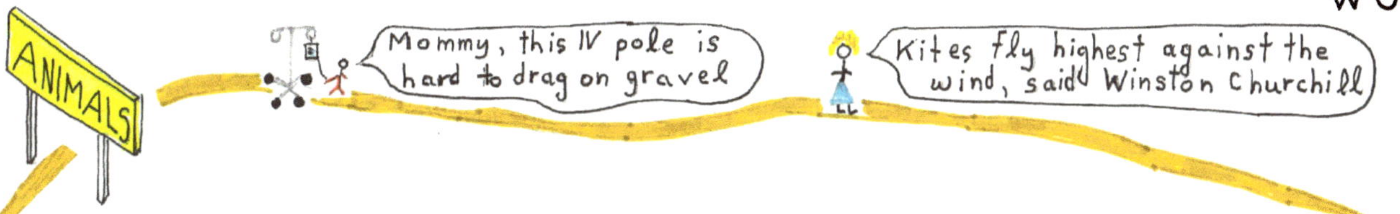

ANIMALS

Mommy, this IV pole is hard to drag on gravel

Kites fly highest against the wind, said Winston Churchill

Within the colossal Kingdom of Animals, parasitic worms tunnel their way through, causing much grief.

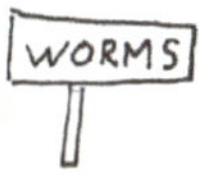

WORMS

RIVER BLINDNESS

– a short play –

☆ Starring ☆
◉ Detective Ling
◉ Understudy Kip

ACT I

KIP

Sir, men are going blind.

DETECTIVE LING

Only men?

KIP

No, men and women.

DETECTIVE LING

What do they have in common?

KIP

They live near a river.

DETECTIVE LING

I need a microscope.

KIP

A microscope?

DETECTIVE LING

Yes. And the eye of a blind man. Or woman.

KIP

Coming right away, Sir.

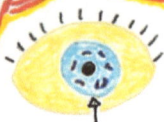

dead worms

live worm

← Oncho-cerca volvulus
- ⊙ It's a worm
- ⊙ Made of millions of cells.

SOMPOO SAYS

 - That's a mouthful
"Ong Kow sir Ka"
⌐rhymes with row
"vol view luss"

 - What's going on here?
 - Dead worms in the eye?

ACT II

DETECTIVE LING
Where are we?

KIP
Africa, Sir.

DETECTIVE LING
What is that infernal buzzing sound, Kip?

KIP
Sir, I believe those are black flies.

DETECTIVE LING (brows furrow, then relax)
I have solved the mystery.

KIP
Sir?

DETECTIVE LING
The flies, Kip. The flies! The flies breed near rivers.
The worms live in the flies.
The flies feed on human blood.
The worms are transmitted during feeding.
The female worms live under the skin of the infected human.
The male worms live close by.
They live for 10-15 years.
The female produces 1000s of baby worms every day.
The baby worms are tiny.
There can be 200,000,000 baby worms in 1 person.
The babies spread via the lymph vessels that are
 essentially invisible but found throughout the body.
Some baby worms end up in the eye, specifically
 the cornea, and die there, causing it to become cloudy.

KIP
As usual, Sir, your brilliance astounds. I shall book our return
flight to Macau.

River Blindness — AFTER PARTY

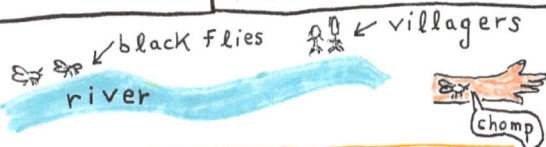

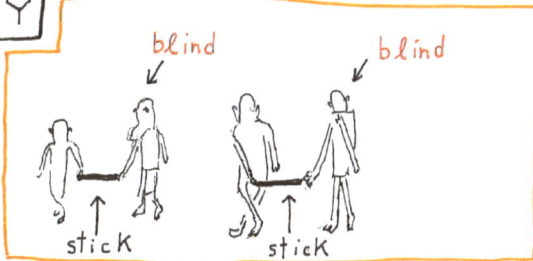

← black flies   ← villagers

river

chomp

blind   blind

stick   stick

Blind being led in rural Africa
(adapted from Wikipedia - Onchocerciasis)

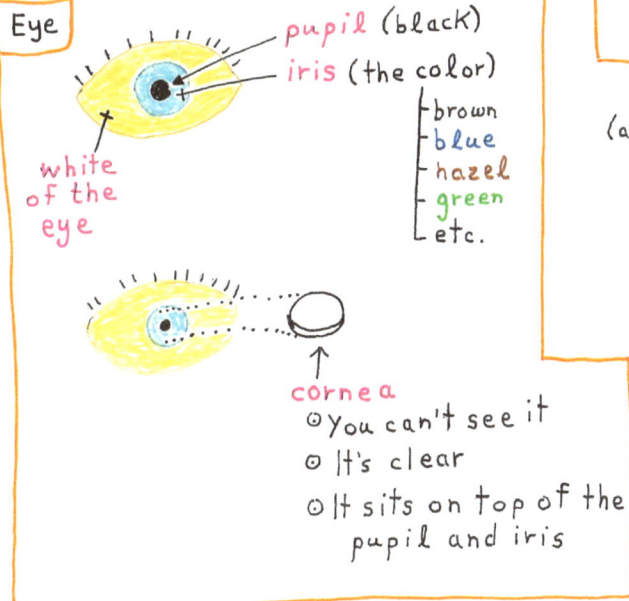

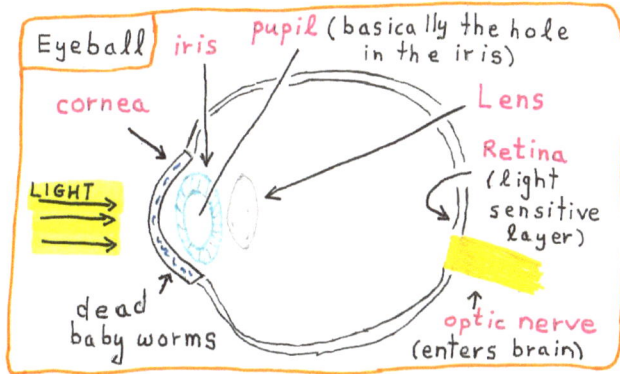

Eye

pupil (black)
iris (the color)

brown
blue
hazel
green
etc.

white of the eye

cornea
○ You can't see it
○ It's clear
○ It sits on top of the pupil and iris

Eyeball

iris   pupil (basically the hole in the iris)

cornea   Lens

LIGHT   Retina (light sensitive layer)

dead baby worms   optic nerve (enters brain)

- 80% of incoming light is bent by the cornea. The lens does fine-tuning.
- If there are dead worms in your cornea, you can't see.

- The lens is cloudy in Cataracts (totally different problem).

Plot Spoiler

Conjunctiva
○ Sits on top of the white of the eye
○ Clear ...
   unless you have blood-shot eyes
○ Coronavirus can enter through the conjunctiva. Maybe. See page 148.

That was a long night. Too many shots of JD

White of the eye
○ It's actually very tough.
○ Effort required to puncture.

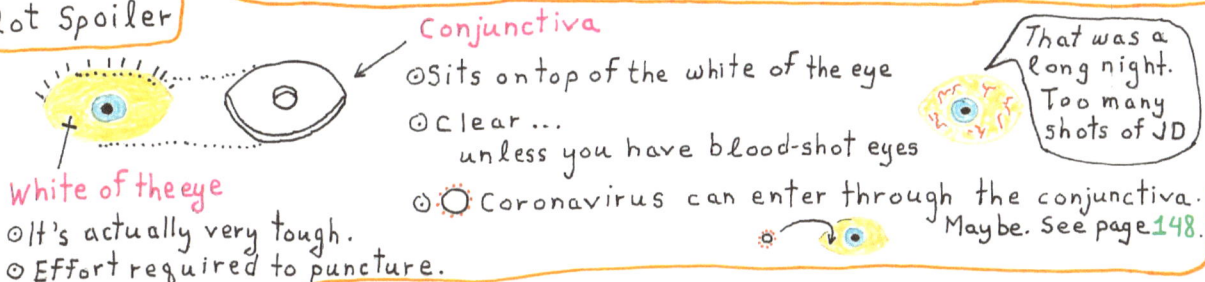

Generous Pharmaceutical Company

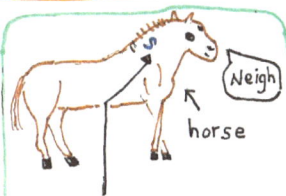

Neigh

horse

Onchocerca cervicalis
○ Close cousin of River blindness worm
○ Dermatitis in horses
○ Treated with a drug called ivermectin

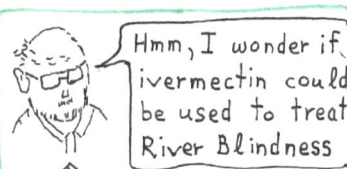

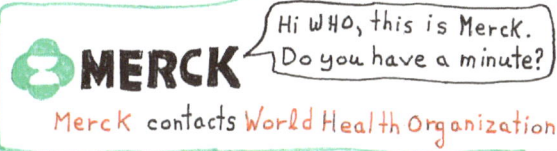

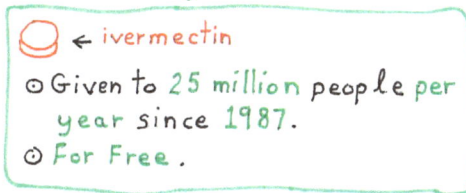

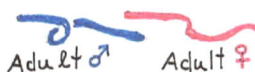

Hmm, I wonder if ivermectin could be used to treat River Blindness

Dr. William Campbell
○ Scientist in animal research division of pharmaceutical giant Merck
○ Nobel Prize

MERCK

Hi WHO, this is Merck. Do you have a minute?

Merck contacts World Health Organization

← ivermectin
○ Given to 25 million people per year since 1987.
○ For Free.

Adult ♂   Adult ♀

○ ivermectin has no effect.
○ Keep on making babies.

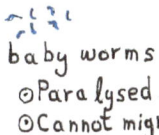

baby worms
○ Paralysed.
○ Cannot migrate to eye → ∅ blindness

- ivermectin is given until the adult worms die of old age. Wow.

♀ - Generous pharmaceutical company - is that an oxymoron?

♀ - Hmm, not this time

TAPEWORMS

☺ - Tapeworms live in our small intestine, anchored to its inner lining.

tapeworm head

tapeworm body

small intestine

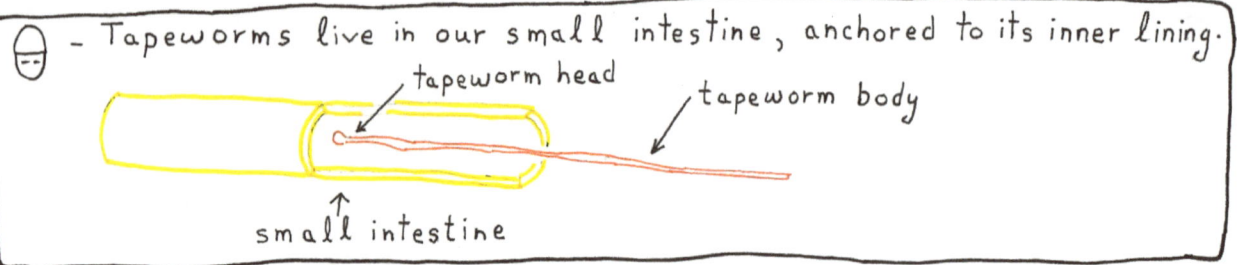

☺ - Here are the options for staying attached:

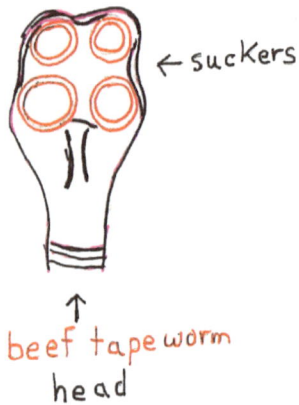

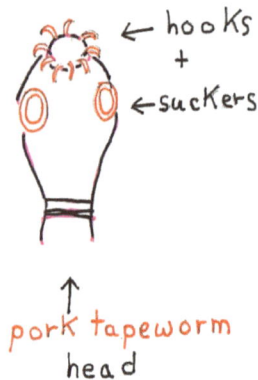

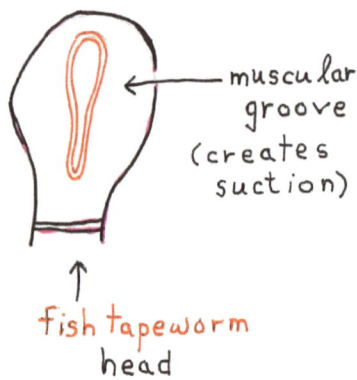

← suckers

← hooks
+
← suckers

muscular groove
(creates suction)

beef tapeworm head

pork tapeworm head

fish tapeworm head

♀ - Those look like scary sci-fi monsters

☿ - Eeek

☺ - The tapeworm head plus hold-fast structures is called the SCOLEX (worth 15 points in Scrabble, apparently).

Fish tapeworm - a model of efficiency

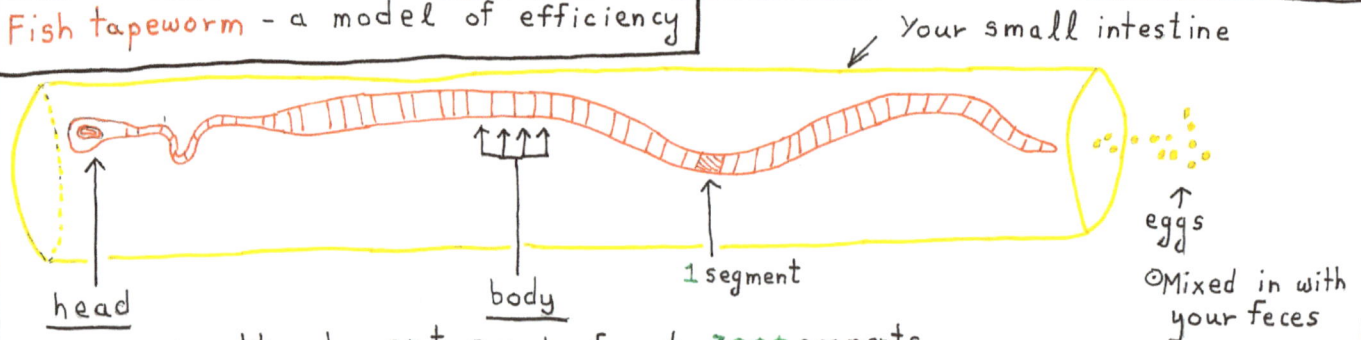

Your small intestine

head

body

1 segment

eggs
⊙ Mixed in with your feces

head
⊙ Purpose is attachment
⊙ No mouth
⊙ No eyes
  (it's dark inside the small intestine)

body
⊙ Made of up to 3000 segments.
  ⊙ 9 to 30 feet long !
    (~3 to 10 meters)
  ⊙ Each segment contains ⟨ ♀ sex organs ⟩ Self-
                            ♂ sex organs ⟩ fertilizes
                                            a.k.a.
  ⊙ Absorbs nutrients across its skin   herm-aphrodite
    (read, steals your food)

☺ - The fish tapeworm <u>out-competes</u> the human gut for Vitamin B-12.
   Vitamin B-12 is required to make our Red Blood Cells (RBCs). ∞

↳ **Vitamin B-12 Deficiency** a.k.a. **Pernicious Anemia**

→ feel tired   ☺ - "Pernicious" means nasty.

☺ - Tapeworms evolved 270 million years ago. They've had time to get efficient.

⊖ - The fish tapeworm, typical of many parasitic worms, has an elaborate life cycle.

Small Intestine (S.I.)
adult fish tapeworm
⑩ raw fish
⑪ sea gull ① ← eggs

⊖ - The Greek letter delta △ is the scientific symbol for change.

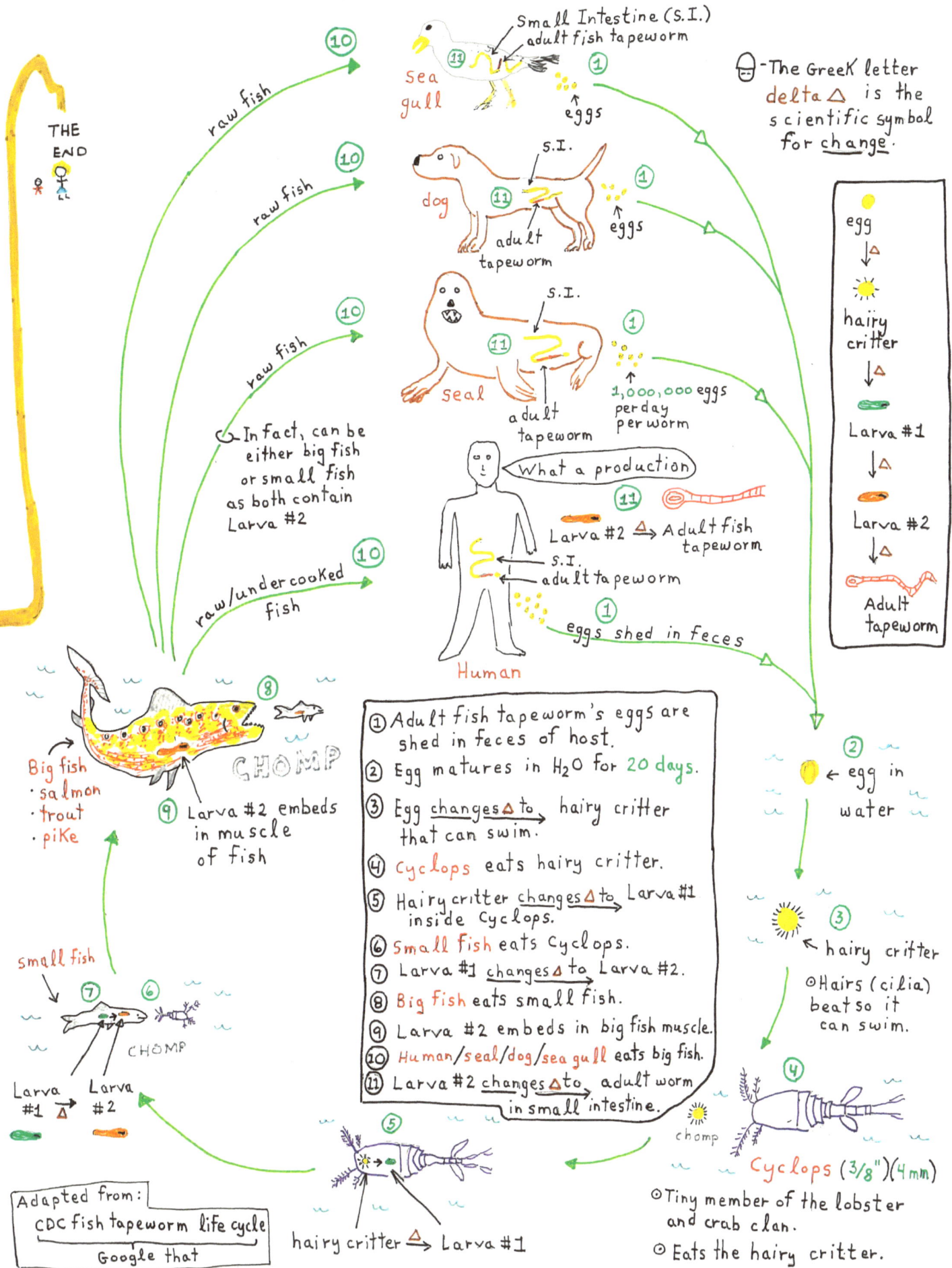

⑩ raw fish
S.I.
dog ⑪ ①
adult tapeworm ← eggs

egg
↓△
hairy critter
↓△
Larva #1
↓△
Larva #2
↓△
Adult tapeworm

THE END

⑩ raw fish
S.I.
⑪ seal ①
adult tapeworm
1,000,000 eggs per day per worm

↪ In fact, can be either big fish or small fish as both contain Larva #2

What a production
⑪
Larva #2 △→ Adult fish tapeworm
S.I.
adult tapeworm
Human
① eggs shed in feces

⑩ raw/undercooked fish

Big fish
• salmon
• trout
• pike

CHOMP
⑨ Larva #2 embeds in muscle of fish

② ← egg in water

① Adult fish tapeworm's eggs are shed in feces of host.
② Egg matures in H₂O for 20 days.
③ Egg changes △ to → hairy critter that can swim.
④ Cyclops eats hairy critter.
⑤ Hairy critter changes △ to → Larva #1 inside Cyclops.
⑥ Small fish eats Cyclops.
⑦ Larva #1 changes △ to Larva #2.
⑧ Big fish eats small fish.
⑨ Larva #2 embeds in big fish muscle.
⑩ Human/seal/dog/sea gull eats big fish.
⑪ Larva #2 changes △ to → adult worm in small intestine.

③ ← hairy critter
⊙ Hairs (cilia) beat so it can swim.

④
chomp
Cyclops (3/8")(4mm)
⊙ Tiny member of the lobster and crab clan.
⊙ Eats the hairy critter.

small fish
⑦ ⑥
CHOMP
Larva #1 △→ Larva #2

⑤
hairy critter △→ Larva #1

Adapted from:
CDC fish tapeworm life cycle
Google that

Post-Zoo Debrief

😐 – Let's recap the zoo tour by looking at how the germs got into your precious body.

Into your mouth and swallowed a.k.a. ingested

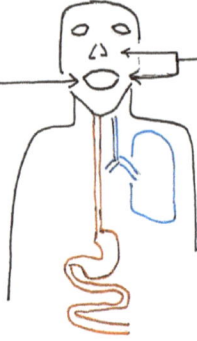

Salmonella
- Typhoid Mary who won't wash her hands causes Typhoid Fever. Because it went from her feces to your mouth, this is called Fecal-Oral Transmission.
- Infected eggs cause Food Poisoning at family picnic.

Cholera
- Infected pump water in Soho. Thank you, Dr Snow.

Botulism Nasty Cousin #2
- Toxin accumulates in poorly-canned food.

Entamoeba
- Alexander the Great drinks infected water and his Large Intestine is mangled.

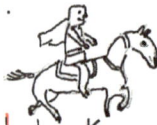

Toxoplasma
- Pregnant woman touches infected cat poop in cat litter box.

- Fish tapeworm larva in uncooked/raw fish changes into adult form (the long worm) in your Small Intestine.

Coronavirus
- Yes, this happens. (details later)

Inhaled into your lungs (via your mouth and nose)

Plague — Wolfgang / Otto
- Specifically, Pneumonic Plague.
- Yersinia pestis spreads person-to-person in airborne droplets.

Anthrax — goat hide
- Specifically, Pulmonary Anthrax.
- Those bacterial spores dormant in the soil come to life in your lungs.

TB (Tuberculosis) — droplet
- By the way, the author Robert Louis Stevenson who wrote 'Treasure Island' may have died of TB. That's disputed.

Aspergillus
- 2 micron fungal spores are airborne and settle all over the place.

Influenza virus
- It is absolutely tiny.
- Found inside the droplets the person beside you sneezed into the air.

Smallpox virus
- The victim has sores in the mouth and throat. When they cough or sneeze, infective droplets are produced: to be inhaled by the next Aztec.

Coronavirus
- Yes, this definitely happens.

♀ – Is the foodpipe beside the windpipe?
☿ – No. Behind it.

– More ways to enter.

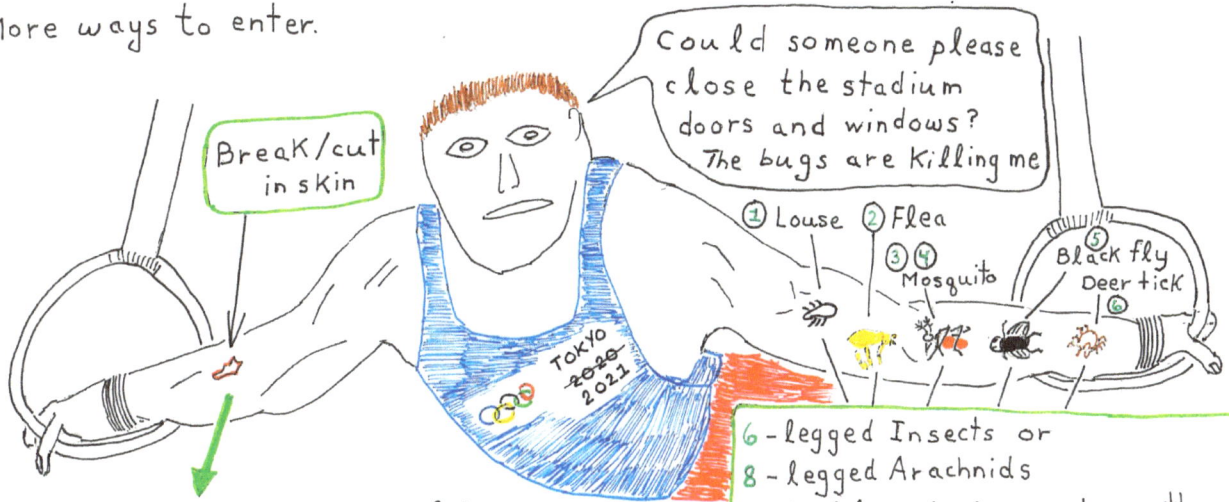

Break/cut in skin

Could someone please close the stadium doors and windows? The bugs are killing me

① Louse ② Flea
③ ④ Mosquito
⑤ Black fly Deer tick ⑥

6-legged Insects or 8-legged Arachnids drill a hole or chomp through the skin. They are Vectors.

Gangrene – Nasty Cousin #1
◦ Lives in soil and gets into wounds.

Tetanus – Nasty Cousin #3
Lockjaw
◦ Also gets into wounds.

ScuBA diver skin infection
◦ Vibrio vulnificus gets into wound
◦ Cousin of Cholera

Group A Strep (GAS)
Fascia
◦ Flesh-Eating Disease
◦ The wound is often trivial
... but consequences severe

Rose Handler's/Grower's Disease
◦ The fungus gets into the wound

Cat Scratch Disease
◦ The cat claws create the wound
◦ Bartonella

Cat bite ▽ ▽
◦ The cat teeth create the wound
◦ Pasteurella

① **Typhus = Louse bite ⟨430 B.C.⟩**
◦ The bacteria is in the louse crap and you scratch it into the break in the skin

② **Plague = Oriental rat flea bite**
◦ The bacteria is in the flea barf and you scratch it into the bite

③ **Yellow Fever = mosquito 'bite'**
◦ Virus transmitted in the mosquito saliva.
Panama canal

④ **Malaria = mosquito 'bite'**
◦ Amoeba love child is in the mosquito saliva

⑤ **River Blindness = blackfly bite**
◦ Worm is transmitted via the fly bite.

⑥ **Lyme Disease = deer tick bite**
◦ Ticks, like spiders, have 8 legs

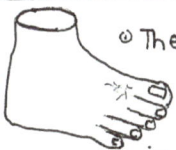

Athlete's foot
◦ The skin is intact but the moisture between the toes is a nice environment for the fungus.
But later, the skin breaks down.

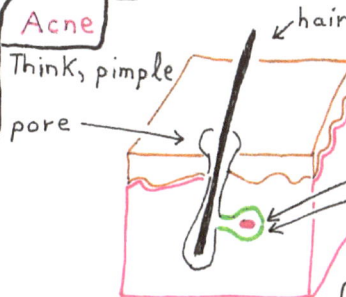

Acne
Think, pimple
pore
hair
sebaceous gland
◦ Secretes oil to protect skin
bacteria grows in the gland
The skin is intact.
SOMPOO SAYS – "seb bay shuss"

😐 - A pregnant woman can transmit a select group of bacteria, viruses and 1 amoeba to the developing fetus.
This is called Vertical Transmission.
⊙ It's not literally vertical. It's more a figure of speech.

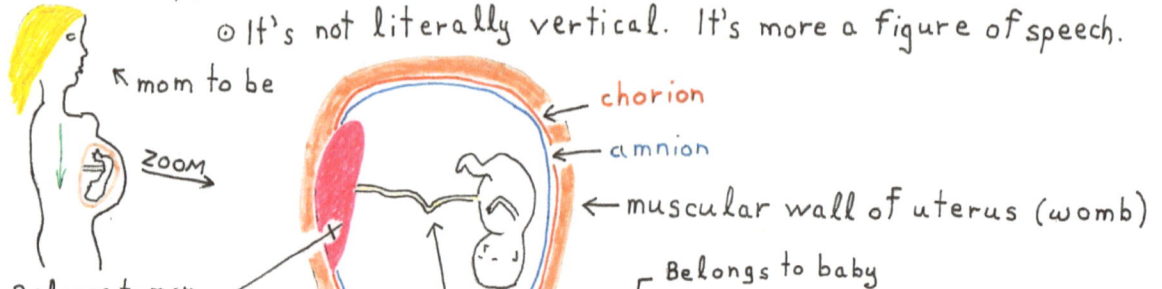

↖ mom to be

ZOOM

chorion
← amnion
← muscular wall of uterus (womb)

Belongs to baby
umbilical cord

Belongs to mom
placenta

cross-section

⊙ The placenta is the interface between mom and baby.
⊙ It allows delivery of goodies to the baby: oxygen, sugar, fat, protein.
⊙ And waste in return from the baby: carbon dioxide.
⊙ Mom's Red Blood Cells (RBCs) stay on her side.
⊙ Baby's RBCs stay on its side (in the cord and baby itself).
⊙ Do you remember Hemoglobin from the Malaria section? Well, fetal Hemoglobin has a higher affinity for oxygen than maternal Hemoglobin.
That's how O_2 gets to baby. Truly amazing.

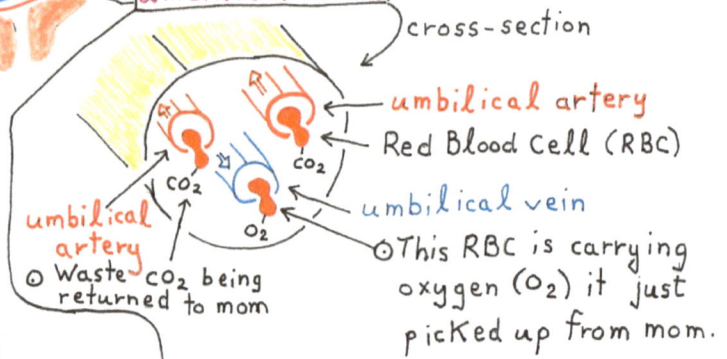

umbilical artery
Red Blood Cell (RBC)

umbilical artery
⊙ Waste CO_2 being returned to mom

umbilical vein
⊙ This RBC is carrying oxygen (O_2) it just picked up from mom.

😐 - Yes, the umbilical cord has 2 arteries and 1 vein, which can be remembered as a baby named AVA.
⊙ The 2 Arteries carry blood Away from the fetus ♡.
⊙ The 1 Vein carries blood Towards the fetus ♡.
⊙ Memory trick: AA TV

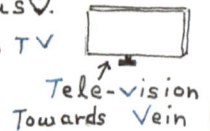

Tele-vision
Towards Vein

😐 - okay, with that as the backdrop of normal operations, some organisms get through the placenta and screw up the baby's life.
The memory trick to remember the names of the organisms is TORCH.

T = Toxoplasma : the amoeba (well, proto-zoan) in cat poop in cat litter box.

O = Other = A number of others

⚙ Zika virus
〰 Syphilis - it's a corkscrew bacteria
⚙ Coronavirus
- This occurs 3% of the time with the SARS-CoronaVirus-2 (COVID-19).
- This does not appear to occur for SARS-CoronaVirus-1 (SARS) or for MERS-CoronaVirus (MERS).

R = Rubella virus

C = Cyto-megalo virus

H = HIV virus, Hepatitis C virus, Herpex simple virus

Will those TORCH organisms pass through the placenta and travel in the umbilical vein towards the fetus? Yes.

- so that's it for the 5 Kingdoms.
` And the official names are:

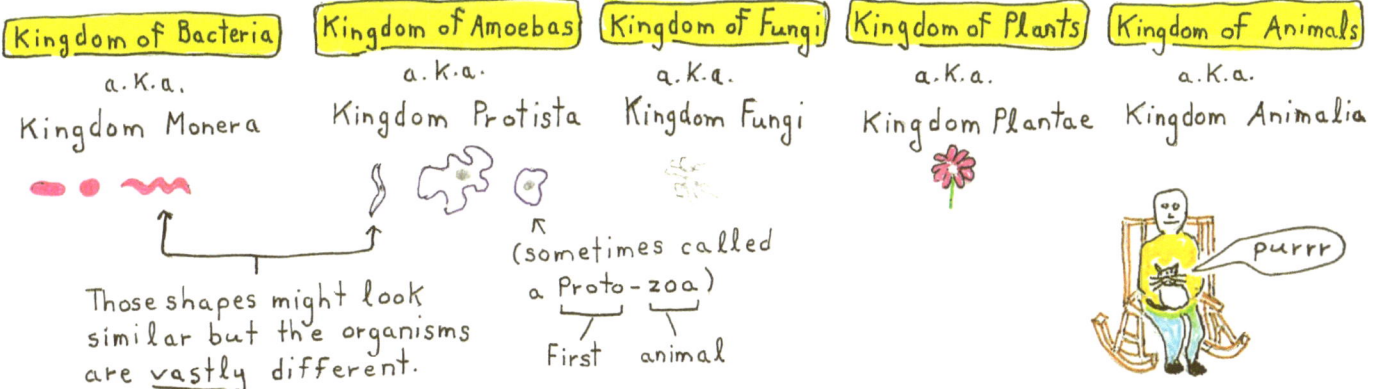

Kingdom of Bacteria	Kingdom of Amoebas	Kingdom of Fungi	Kingdom of Plants	Kingdom of Animals
a.k.a.	a.k.a.	a.k.a.	a.k.a.	a.k.a.
Kingdom Monera	Kingdom Protista	Kingdom Fungi	Kingdom Plantae	Kingdom Animalia

Those shapes might look similar but the organisms are vastly different.

(sometimes called a Proto-zoa)

First   animal

purrr

Relationships

Herman, you are a parasite

I prefer to think of myself as a micro-predator

predator: benefits
prey: Killed

- An 'apex predator' is never prey

mosquito

leech

micro-predator: benefits

Host: harmed but not Killed.
• Can be harmed many times.

bee: free sugar
plant: free pollination
Mutualism = both parties benefit

remora: benefits (food morsels)
shark: no harm no benefit
Commensalism

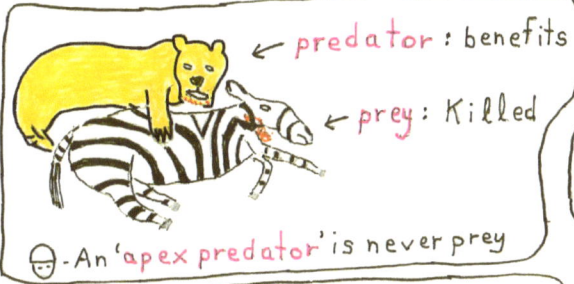

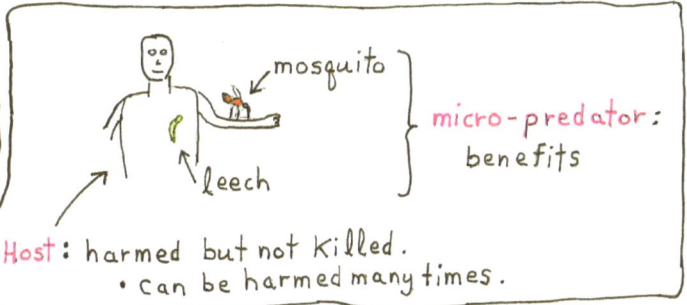

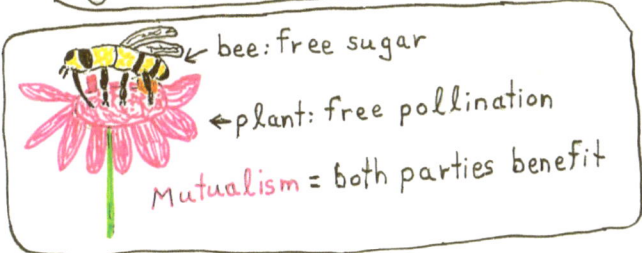

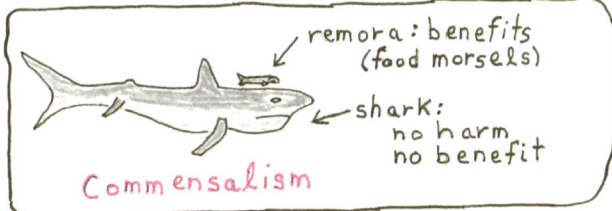

- 'Relationships' in biology/zoology/medicine have hair-splitty definitions.
(sometimes conflicting)
` So please accept the following conventions in Medicine:

Parasitology = the study of parasites
Amoebas
Worms
Ticks + lice

Virology = the study of viruses

Mycology = the study of fungi

← virologist
I ♥

Bacteriology = the study of bacteria

Infectious Disease (ID) = the medical specialty concerned with all of the above

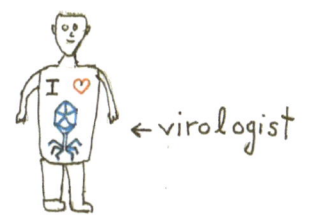

Pages 86-87 are dedicated to people who group their socks according to color, fold towels so only the round parts show, ensure the salad fork is outside the dinner fork, organize their spices alphabetically (THYME) (TURMERIC), buy index tabs, gasp in horror if the 1st and 2nd violins trade places, and slap you hard across the face if you mix up DC versus Marvel heroes. They are generally obsessed with how things are named ("Krav Maga is not Wing Chun")...

... which makes them instant fans of TAXONOMY which is the set of dresser drawers to organize the creatures within a Kingdom.

\ A Kingdom is organized like a computer path.

Animal Kingdom >	Phylum >	Class >	Order >	Family >	Genus >	species
My Computer >	Folders >	Music >	Pop >	Rihanna >	Unapologetic >	stay

\ A Phylum is a huge division within a Kingdom.
\ Let's look at the Animal Kingdom. († means extinct)

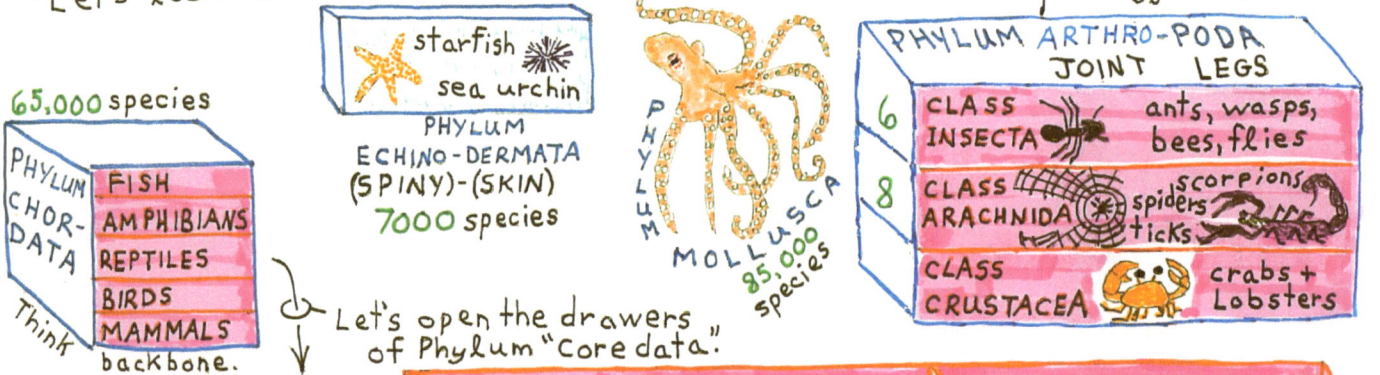

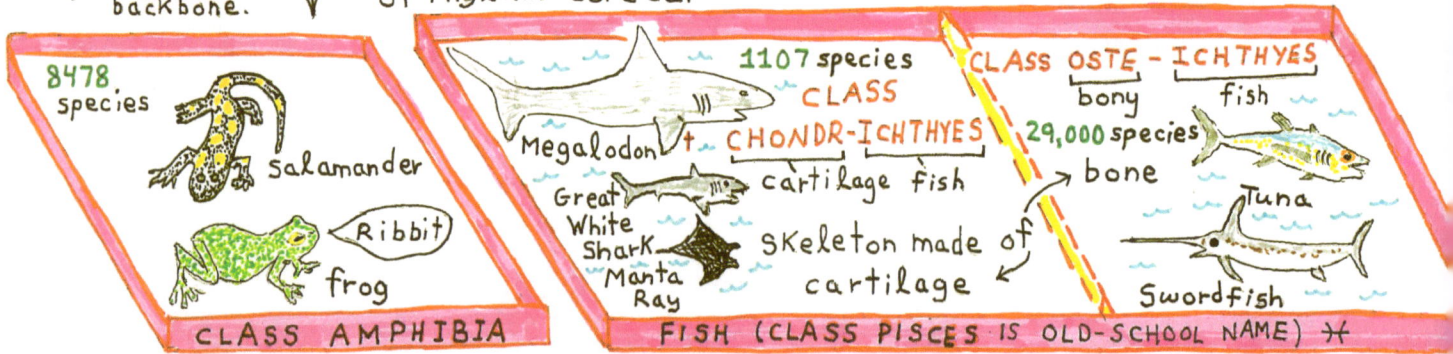

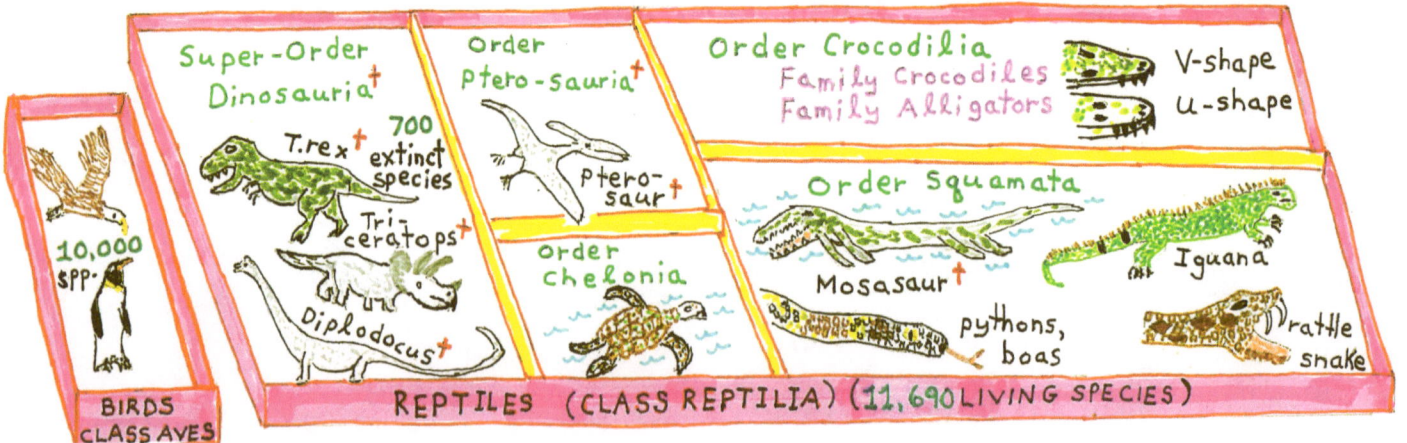

65,000 species
PHYLUM CHOR-DATA
FISH
AMPHIBIANS
REPTILES
BIRDS
MAMMALS
Think backbone.

starfish
sea urchin
PHYLUM ECHINO-DERMATA
(SPINY)-(SKIN)
7000 species

PHYLUM MOLLUSCA
85,000 species

7,000,000 species (biggest Phylum)
PHYLUM ARTHRO-PODA
JOINT LEGS
6 CLASS INSECTA — ants, wasps, bees, flies
8 CLASS ARACHNIDA — spiders, ticks, scorpions
CLASS CRUSTACEA — crabs + Lobsters

Let's open the drawers of Phylum "Core data."

8478 species
Salamander
Ribbit
frog
CLASS AMPHIBIA

1107 species
CLASS CHONDR-ICHTHYES
cartilage fish
Megalodon †
Great White Shark
Manta Ray
Skeleton made of cartilage
FISH (CLASS PISCES IS OLD-SCHOOL NAME) ♓

CLASS OSTE-ICHTHYES
bony fish
29,000 species
bone
Tuna
Swordfish

10,000 spp.
BIRDS CLASS AVES

Super-Order Dinosauria †
T. rex †
700 extinct species
Tri-ceratops †
Diplodocus †

Order Ptero-sauria †
Ptero-saur †
order Chelonia

Order Crocodilia
Family Crocodiles
Family Alligators
V-shape
U-shape

Order Squamata
Mosasaur †
pythons, boas
Iguana
rattle snake

REPTILES (CLASS REPTILIA) (11,690 LIVING SPECIES)

Meat Eaters (Order Carnivora)   bears   Wolverines, badgers, weasels

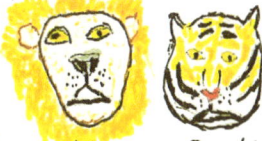 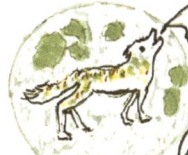 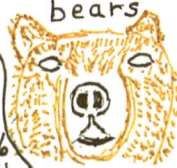

I am standing on the Apollo 16 landing site

Panthera leo   Panthera tigris   Canis lupus   Ursus arctos   Gulo gulo

Ursa major Bear great a.k.a.

Big Dipper

Kinda sorta Carnivores

Walrus + seals (Pinnipeds)   Whales (Order Cetacea)   dolphin

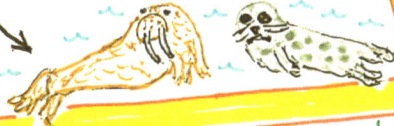 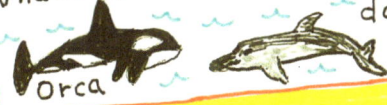

Orca

Bats (Order Chiro-ptera) (Hand-wing)   Rodents (Order Rodentia)   Lemmings

squirrels rats, mice

1400 species

Even-toed Herbivores (Order Artio-dactyla)   giraffe   Odd-toed Herbivores (Order Perisso-dactyla)

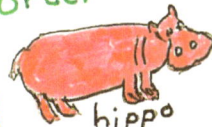 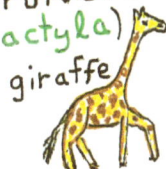 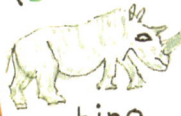 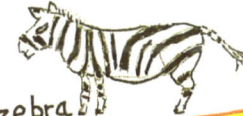

hippo   rhino   zebra

Elephants   trunk a.k.a. proboscis (Order Proboscidea)   Marsupials   Mono-tremes   egg!

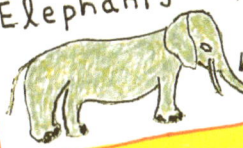 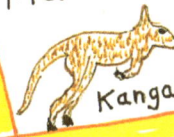 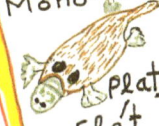

Kangaroos   Platy-pus Flat foot

☠-Only 4 of the 35 Phyla of the Animal Kingdom are shown. (Phylum is singular. Phyla is plural)

✳ Family Hominidae ("hom-in-id-day")

⚥ Which 2 classes of Animals does Coronavirus like to infect?

⚥ Birds and Mammals. See pages 112 and 129-132 for details.

Primates (Order Primates)   baboon (think, Africa)

→ Old World monkeys
→ New World monkeys → capuchin monkey (think, Central & South America)
→ Lesser Apes → gibbon (long, slender arms)
→ Great Apes ✳

• Gorillas
• Orangutangs
• Chimpanzees
• Australo-pithecus afarensis a.k.a. "Lucy" → walked upright
• Homo habilis † } → walked upright a.k.a. bi-pedal
• Homo erectus †
• Homo sapiens neanderthalensis †   My bones were discovered in the Neander Valley in Germany.
• Homo sapiens sapiens →
I have no idea how these work   ← Bluetooth headphones ⌗

MAMMALS (CLASS MAMMALIA)(warm blood, milk, placenta)
→ 6400 species (including the 1400 bat species)

☺ -'Zoonosis' means a disease can spread from animal to human or in the opposite direction, from human to animal.

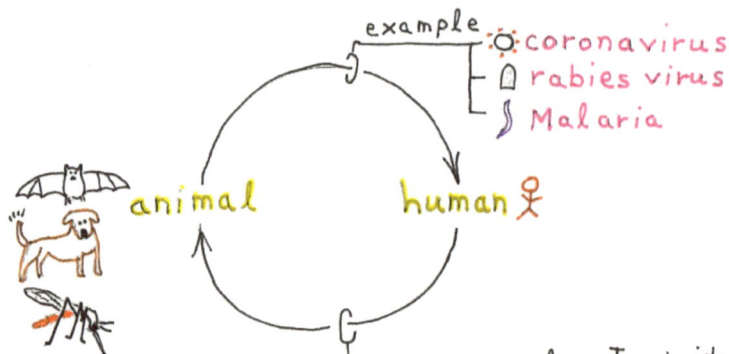

example
⊙ coronavirus
⌂ rabies virus
§ Malaria

animal   human ♀

[For example, I visited Rwanda in 2005 and saw the famous mountain gorillas in the Virunga Mountains. Amazing! If you have to sneeze, you turn away. Why? You don't want to infect the gorillas with a human virus.]

＼ Zoonosis is kind of a confusing word, maybe because of the weird spelling.
  ⊙ zoonosis - singular
  ⊙ zoonoses - plural
  ⊙ zoonotic diseases - adjective

♀ - Explain it to me in 1 sentence.
♂ - Coronavirus COVID-19 is a zoonotic disease transmitted from bats to humans, and the pangolin is probably the intermediate host. (page 140)

＼ Technically, humans are animals - a member of the Animal Kingdom - but for the purposes of this definition, humans and animals are considered separate.

＼ An easier way to think of it is 'species jumping.'

☺ - Okay, congratulations. You've learned a ton of information. And if you've already forgotten ¾ of it, that's normal. Read it again!
＼ Relax for a while and watch the koi fish.
＼ Then we can explore viruses and coronavirus.

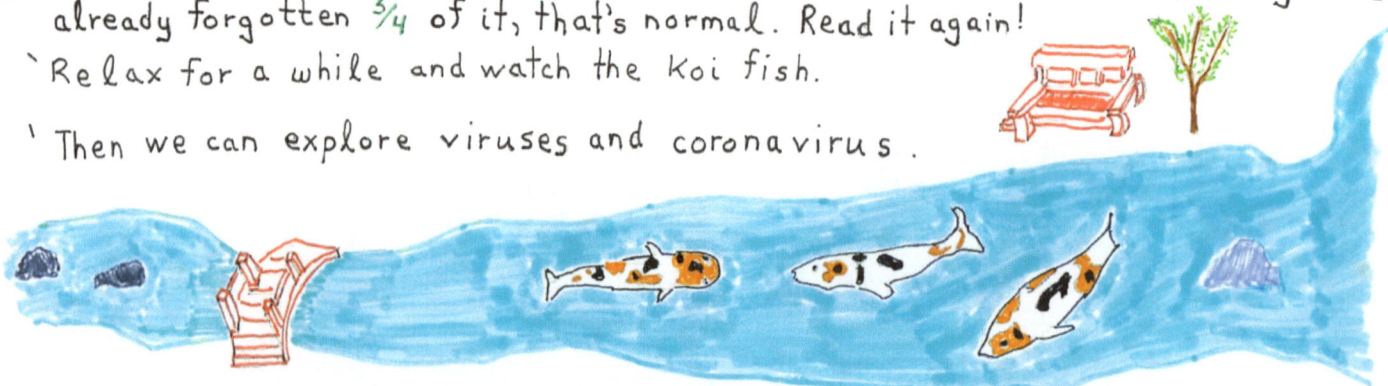

Chapter 3
Meet the Viruses

Across — Down

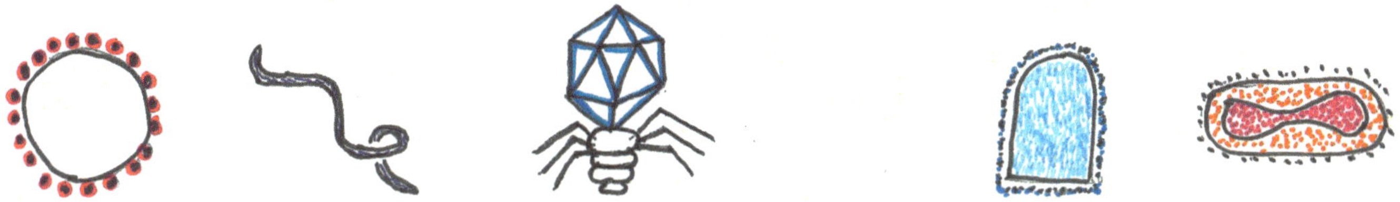

Across: 1 2 3

Down: 1 2

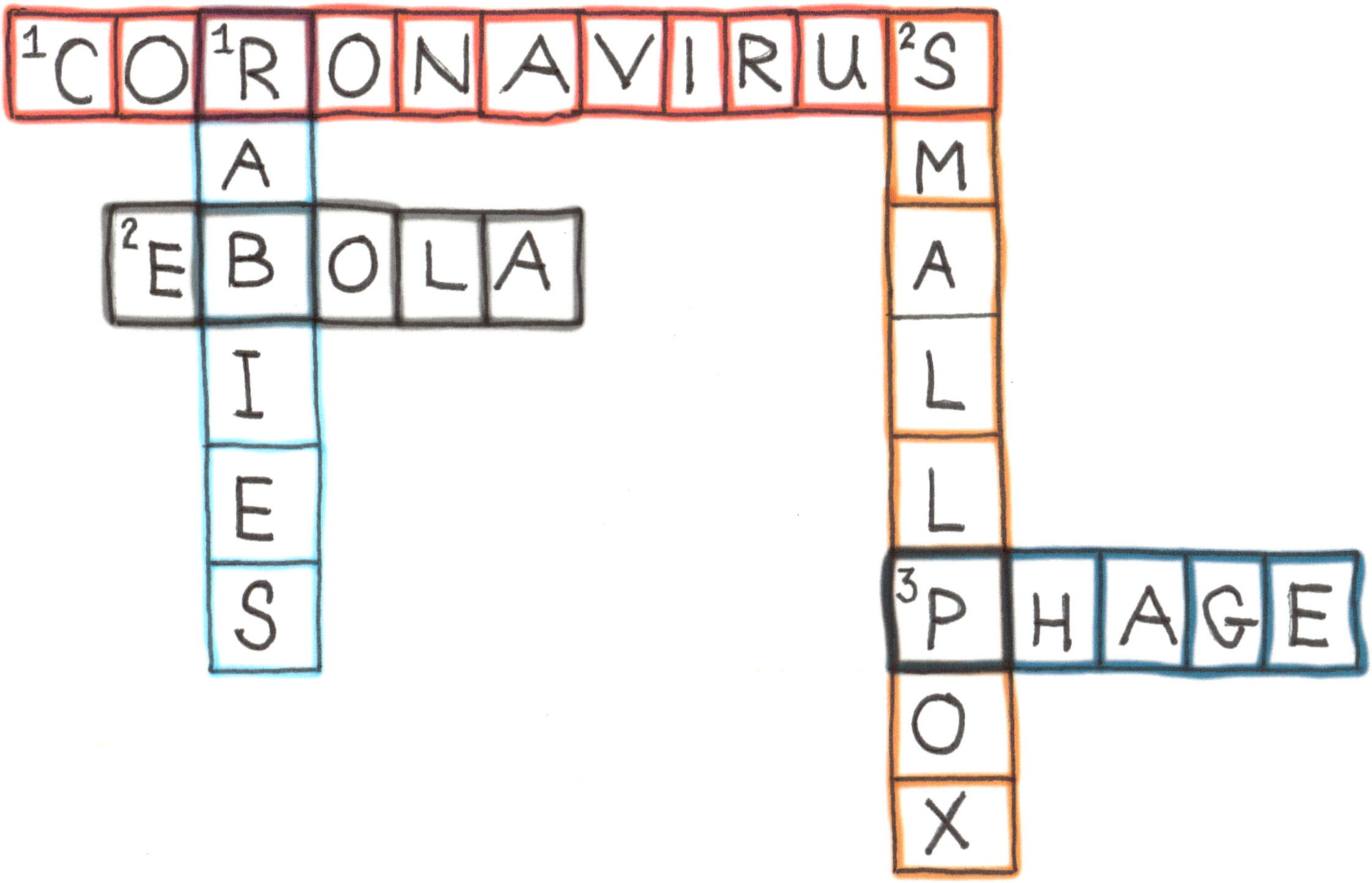
1 CORONAVIRUS
1 RABIES
2 EBOLA
2 SMALLPOX
3 PHAGE

PAUSE FOR STATION IDENTIFICATION

- There are 5 **Kingdoms** of Life (but other classification systems exist).
    - All these creatures are made of cells.

\ A virus is not a cell. It's just a scrap of genetic code minus everything else.

\ Viruses occupy the hinterland between Life and non-Life.

\ Viruses are tiny because they don't have to haul around the machinery to reproduce. They simply hijack it. They travel light, like Johnny Appleseed.

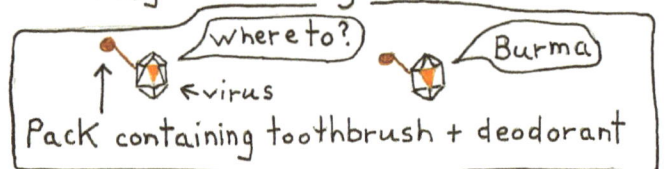

where to? Burma
← virus
Pack containing toothbrush + deodorant

\ Viruses infect the cells of all 5 **Kingdoms**. The task of the virus is to get from <u>outside</u> a cell to <u>inside</u> it.

\ A virus is not interested in you personally. It is interested in your cells.

\ Humans belong to the **Animal Kingdom**

\ ☼ Corona-virus is 1 of 219 viruses that infect Humans.

\ ☼ Corona-virus does not restrict itself to Humans.

VIRUS versus CELL

🙂 - A cell is a little city specialized for a job. Muscle cells contract, stomach cells make acid, eye cells capture light, bone cells make bone, etc., etc. All of this is accomplished by proteins. Regardless of cell type, they all have the same basic layout.

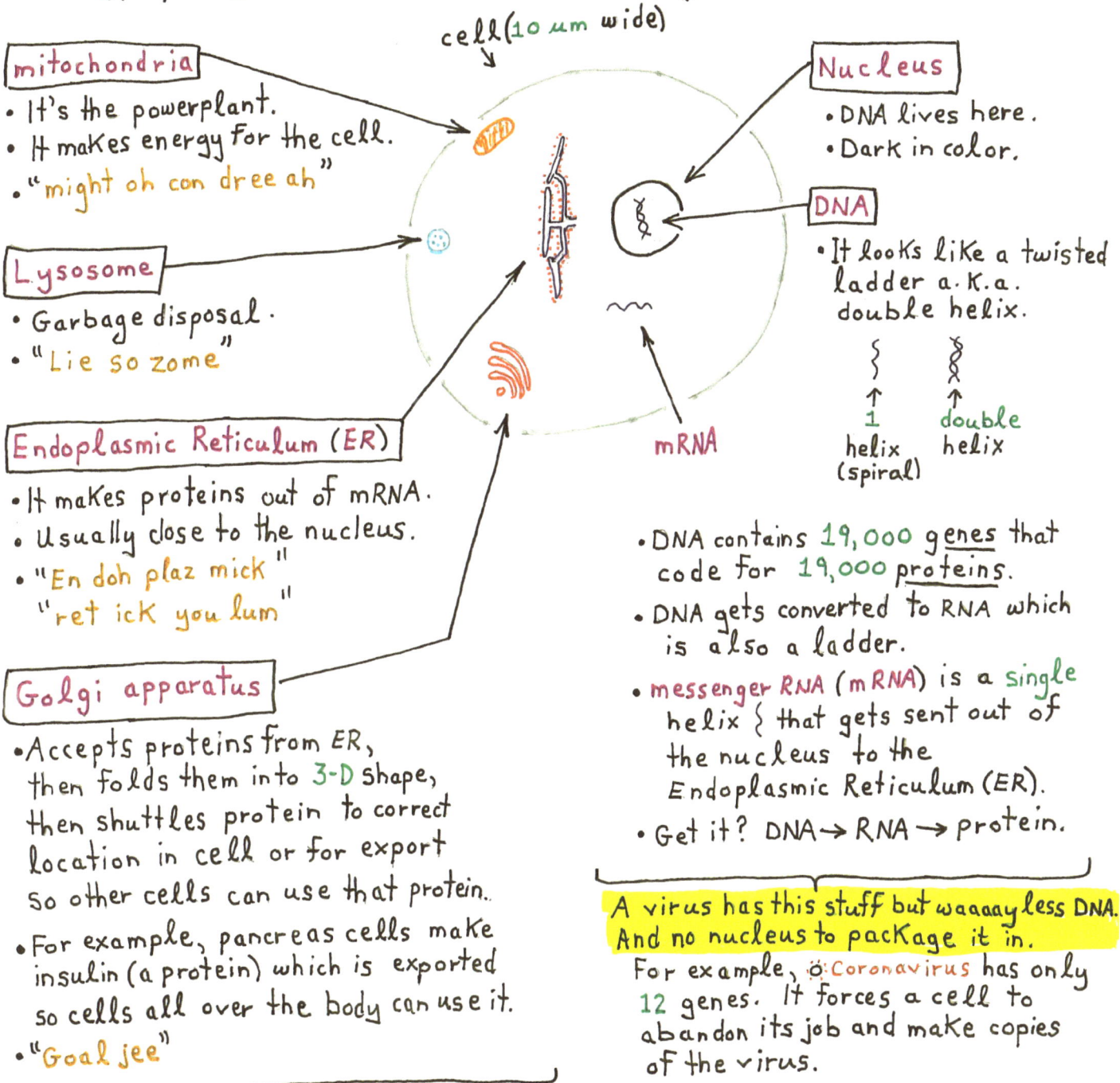

cell (10 μm wide)

mitochondria
- It's the powerplant.
- It makes energy for the cell.
- "might oh con dree ah"

Lysosome
- Garbage disposal.
- "Lie so zome"

Endoplasmic Reticulum (ER)
- It makes proteins out of mRNA.
- Usually close to the nucleus.
- "En doh plaz mick"
  "ret ick you lum"

Golgi apparatus
- Accepts proteins from ER, then folds them into 3-D shape, then shuttles protein to correct location in cell or for export so other cells can use that protein.
- For example, pancreas cells make insulin (a protein) which is exported so cells all over the body can use it.
- "Goal jee"

==A virus has none of this stuff==

Nucleus
- DNA lives here.
- Dark in color.

DNA
- It looks like a twisted ladder a.k.a. double helix.

1 helix (spiral)   double helix

- DNA contains 19,000 genes that code for 19,000 proteins.
- DNA gets converted to RNA which is also a ladder.
- messenger RNA (mRNA) is a single helix that gets sent out of the nucleus to the Endoplasmic Reticulum (ER).
- Get it? DNA → RNA → protein.

mRNA

==A virus has this stuff but waaaay less DNA. And no nucleus to package it in.==
For example, Coronavirus has only 12 genes. It forces a cell to abandon its job and make copies of the virus.

Coronavirus
0.1 μm

🙂 - The moral of the story is: A hijacker does not have to know how to fly the plane.

♀ - What is a virus made of?
♂ - Time for some geometry!

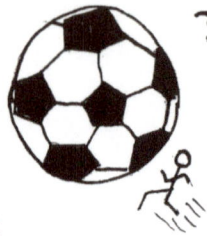

♂ - A soccer ball (European football) is made of hexagons surrounding pentagons. There are a total of 32 faces.

♀ - A typical virus is made of 20 triangles. The geometry shape is called an icosa-hedron.

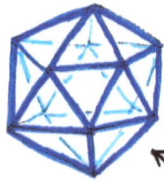

♂ - Okey dokey.

♂ - But let's consider it in 3 dimensions. It is a hollow structure made of protein. It protects the genetic code of the virus. It is called a capsid.

← capsid

♀ - What is the genetic code?
♂ - In you and me it's DNA but in viruses it can be DNA or RNA. Here are the options:

← 1 strand of DNA a.k.a. single stranded DNA (ss DNA)
← 2 strands of DNA a.k.a. double stranded DNA (ds DNA)
← 1 strand of RNA a.k.a single stranded RNA (ss RNA)
← 2 strands of RNA a.k.a. double stranded RNA (ds RNA)

This is called the 'Baltimore classification' but it's more involved than this.

♂ - Sometimes there is also an envelope (made of fat) for further protection.

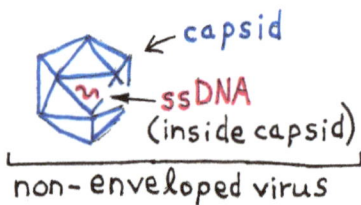

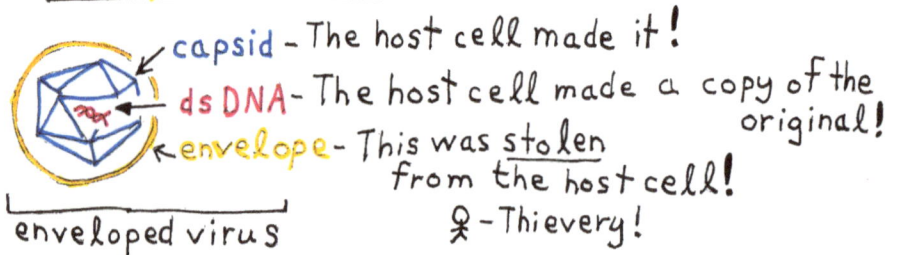

← capsid
← ss DNA (inside capsid)

non-enveloped virus

capsid - The host cell made it!
ds DNA - The host cell made a copy of the original!
← envelope - This was stolen from the host cell!
♂ - Thievery!

enveloped virus

♀ - Get it? A virus is a protein capsid + genetic code +/- fatty envelope.   ♂ - Got it.

♀ - Sometimes the capsid is a twisty, tubular shape called a helical capsid.

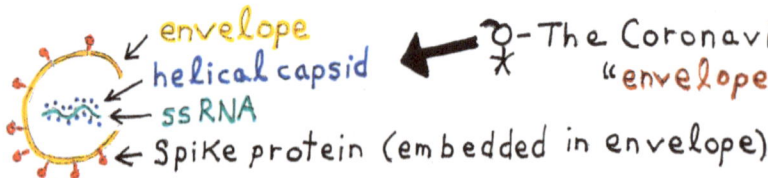

envelope
helical capsid
ss RNA
Spike protein (embedded in envelope)

♂ - The Coronavirus is an "enveloped single stranded RNA virus."

yes! Too slow sucka!

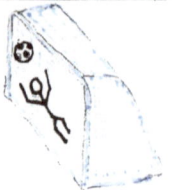

VIRUS ATTACK

⊖ Viruses infect all 5 Kingdoms of Life

Viruses infect
Bacteria

A day that started like any other...

La, la, la. What a great day to divide

↑ rod bacteria

Hi, thought I'd stop by and kill you

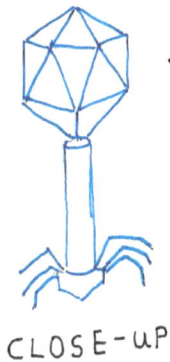

Nooooooo!

Please stop flinching. I'm trying to inject my DNA into you.

Gaaaagh!

← bacterio-phage

bacteria | eat

⊙ It's a virus that infects bacteria.
⊙ Has a unique appearance.
⊙ No harm to human cells.

CLOSE-UP

Later that day

←new viruses

↑ dead bacteria

♀ - Does it actually eat bacteria?

♂ - No. But it kills them

♀ - Are those legs?

♂ - No. Viruses don't walk. They are called tail fibers to bind to the bacteria.

⊖ "back tee ree oh fage"
SOMPOO SAYS
⌐ rhymes with page

♀ - And viruses infect and kill even something as small as a bacteria?

♂ - Yup

⊖ - This is more accurate in terms of relative size

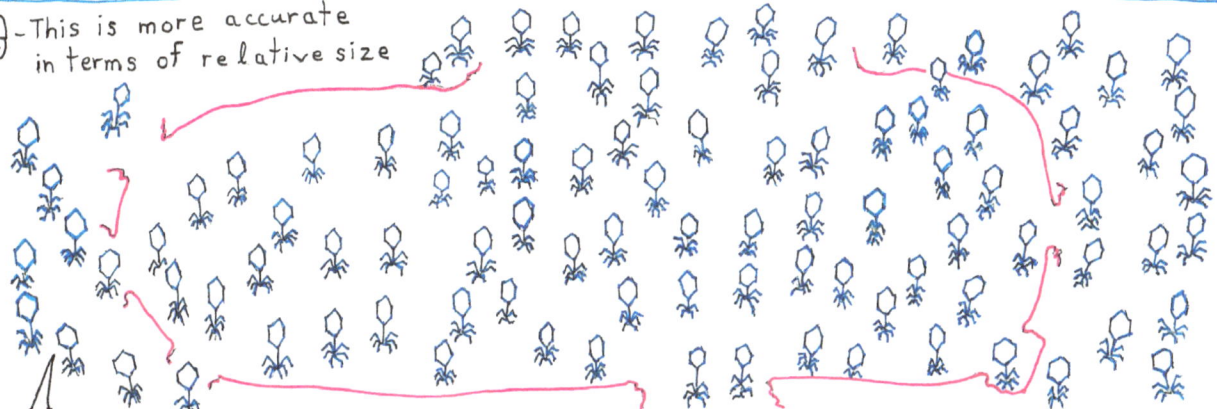

We bacteriophages outnumber everything on Earth

↑ bacteria splits apart, releasing 100 to 150 new viruses

dead

⊖ - Do you remember E.coli the bacteria in our intestines? That's 1 E.coli.

Matryoshka virus

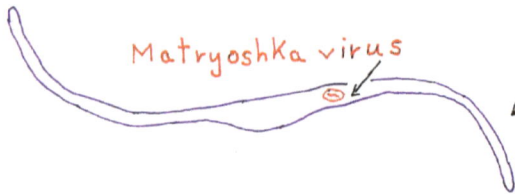

Plasmodium
- The amoeba causing Malaria.
- It's a <u>single</u> cell.

- This virus has been described as "a virus infecting a parasite infecting an animal" and therefore likened to a Russian matryoshka doll.

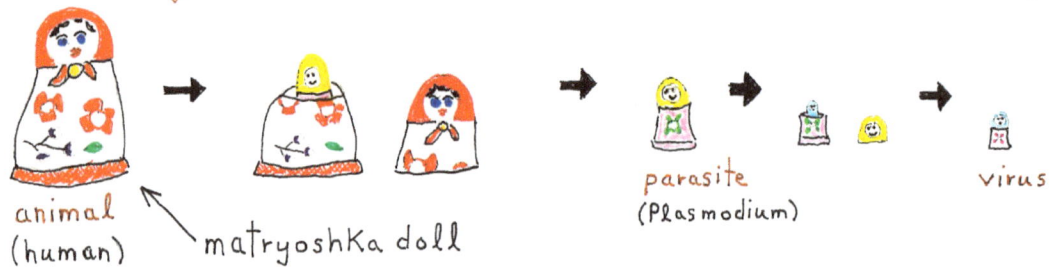

animal
(human)

matryoshka doll

parasite
(Plasmodium)

virus

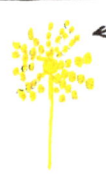

←Aspergillus
- Remember the fungus ball growing in a cavity in the lung? (Aspergilloma)

←Aspergillus fumigatus poly-myco-virus-1
- It's a virus of the fungus
- Not drawn to scale (it's way smaller)

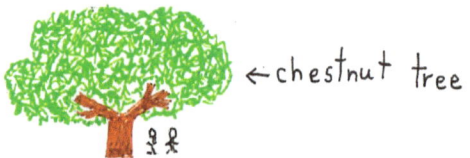

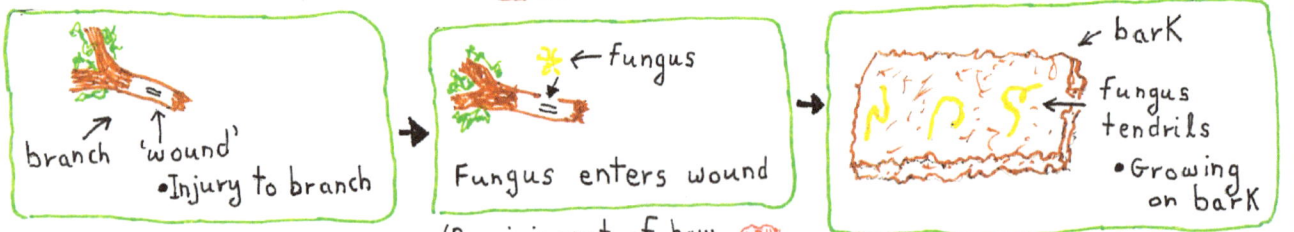

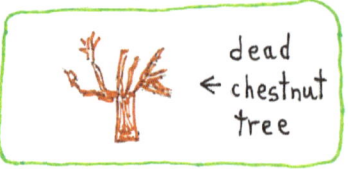

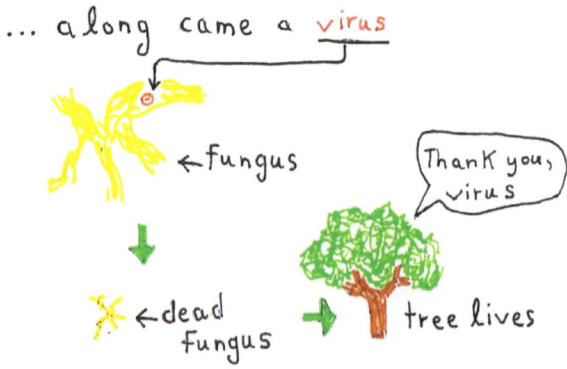

←chestnut tree

branch 'wound'
- Injury to branch

←fungus
Fungus enters wound

(Reminiscent of how fungus enters wound of rose handler)

←bark
fungus tendrils
- Growing on bark

(Adapted from Global Invasive Species Database) (GISD)

dead ←chestnut tree

... along came a <u>virus</u>

←fungus

Thank you, virus

←dead Fungus

tree lives

- Fancy schmancy names:

Crypho-nectria parasitica (fungus)
Crypho-nectria Hypo-Virus-1 (CHV-1)

Viruses infect ... you guessed it ... Plants

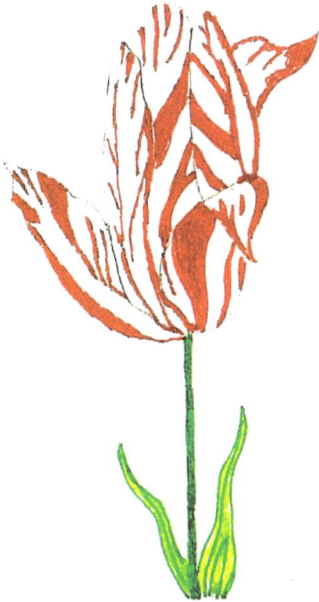

Tulip-Breaking virus

Rembrandt Tulip-Breaking virus

(yes, that's the real name)

'Semper Augustus' tulip

o This tulip was painted in 1640 during the Tulip Mania that seized the Netherlands (Holland) in the 1600s.

o The price for a single flower was 3000 Guilders, whereas the annual salary of a skilled craftsman was 300 Guilders.

⊙ The painting (unknown artist) is in the Norton Simon Museum in Pasadena, California.

☻ - These single-color tulips have an unbroken color.

The Tulip-Breaking Virus 'breaks' the color scheme, resulting in streaks and stripes.

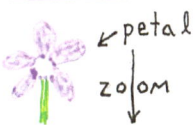

← petal
zoom

! A petal is a modified leaf !

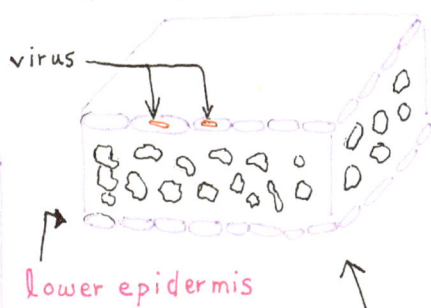

← upper epidermis

virus

• The virus gets in these cells and screws up the distribution of a pigment called antho-cyanin.

lower epidermis

petal cross-section

• There is no dermis like in human skin.

Rembrandt

Dutch painter

1606 - 1669

He painted these streaked tulips

♀ - So if I buy tulips with streaks are they infected with the virus?

♂ - No. Streaks can be produced by selective breeding.

Worms

Orsay virus
(not to scale)
(way smaller)

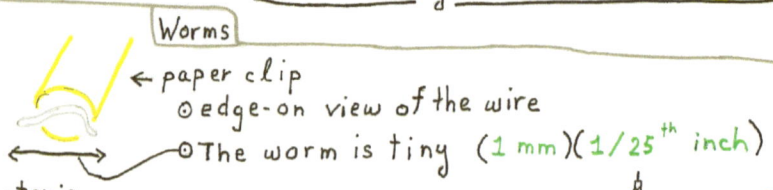

← paper clip
⊙ edge-on view of the wire
⊙ The worm is tiny (1 mm) (1/25th inch)

↑
C. elegans
⊙ This worm feeds on bacteria.
⊙ It is the lab rat of worms - massively studied.
⊙ The Orsay virus infects it (which was surprising).

☻ - The virus was found
in a c. elegans worm
in a rotting apple in the city of Orsay.

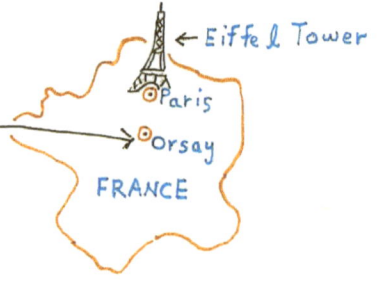

← Eiffel Tower
⊙ Paris
→ ⊙ Orsay
FRANCE

♀ - Okay, seriously, who
is looking that hard
for a virus?
♀ - Someone who lives
with Passion, like
Anthony Robbins says
you should be

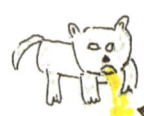

Cats

← Kitten
← vomiting
Feline Distemper virus
(Feline Pan-leukemia virus)
⊙ Death due to severe dehydration

← water dish
kitten won't
drink H₂O

Dogs

← dog

↑
Rabies virus

Cows

← dairy
cow
(♀)

⊙
↑
Cowpox virus

udder

Pustules (blisters
filled with pus)
+ raw skin on
udder and teats.

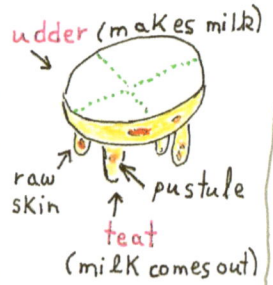

udder (makes milk)
raw
skin
pustule
teat
(milk comes out)

☻ - An udder has
4 ¼ s and 4 teats.

` 400 liters of
blood pass
through the
udder to make
1 liter of milk.
(400:1 ratio)

Bees

← honey bee

← lavender

JOHNNY
BEE
April 2020
-
June 2020

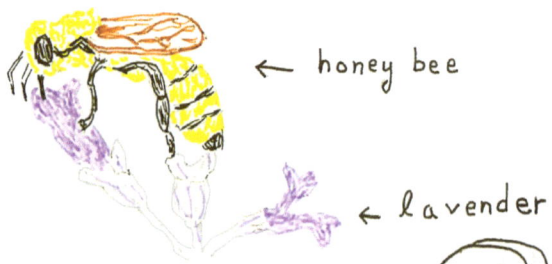

↑
Chronic Bee Paralysis Virus
⊙ Irregular shape

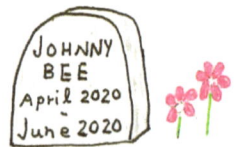

Infected worker bee →

loses hair →
cannot fly →

← trembles + crawls on ground

← abdomen bulges with honey

1,000,000,000,000 viruses per bee
(that's 1 trillion) (1 Tera-virus)

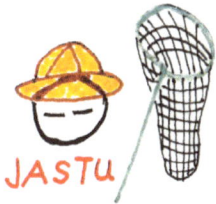

SPECIAL GUEST APPEARANCE

JASTU - Udders, milk... how unspeakably boring. What the world needs is more dragonflies! Dragonflies are it!!

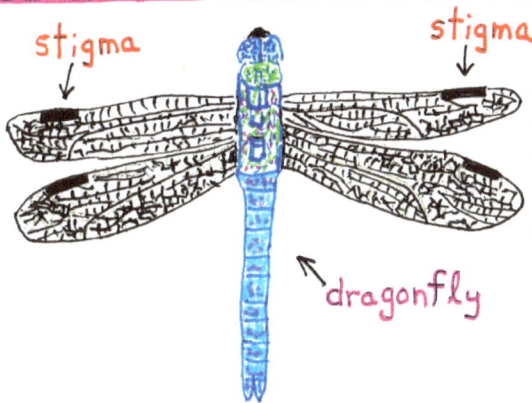

stigma

stigma

← dragonfly

↕ Narrow front wings
↕ Broad rear wings
} That's why dragonflies are called **An-iso-ptera.** **Not-same-wing**

SOMPOO SAYS - If I may interrupt, that's pronounced, "An-eyes-op-terra."

- The stigma adds weight to the outer wing.
- Its purpose is to ↓vibrations called flutter that would prevent the dragonfly from gliding.
- Also called the ptero-stigma. The plural is stigmata.
  wing mark

- Dragonflies are infected by amoebas, mites, worms, and viruses. How dreadful that this lovely flier must endure nasty organisms.

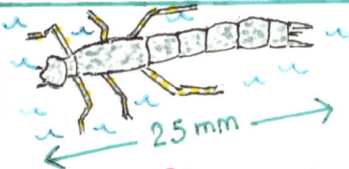

← 25 mm →

Dragonfly nymph
- Lives in water.
- Gills in rectum!
- 6 legs (Class Insecta).
- Turns into adult.

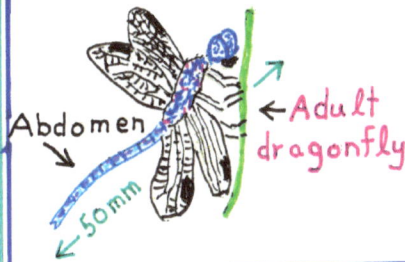

↑ 1 mm ↓ ← water mite

- Infects dragonfly nymph.
- 8 legs (Class Arachnida) page 86

Abdomen ←Adult dragonfly
←50mm→

- 6 legs (same as nymph).
- Breathes air. Pumps its abdomen faster if there is low oxygen (Hypoxia).
- Abdomen has 10 segments.

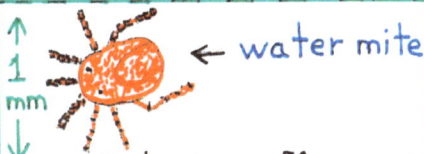

← Gregarina
- Single cell.
- Think, amoeba.
- Lives in dragonfly abdomen.
- Causes decrease in power of flight muscles.

← Dragonfly Cyclo-virus (DrCyV)
- Lives in dragonfly abdomen.
- Effect unclear.

← Bullfrog lung fluke
- It's a type of worm that lives in the frog lung.
- Immature worms infect both Dragonfly nymph + adult.

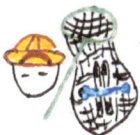

- Unlike my sibling SOMPOO, my data comes packaged in tidy rectangles with 90° corners.
- That will be $40 USD. e-transfer or bitcoin is accepted.

- What the?

Viruses infect Humans (who belong to the Animal Kingdom)

Rhino-virus ○
- Causes the **Common Cold** (runny nose, stuffed up, itchy eyes, sore throat)
- 'Rhino' means nose

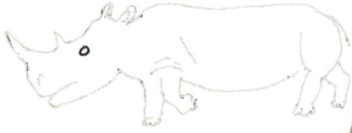

human

Corona virus

Influenza A virus

- Remember that 'pox' or 'poc' means skin lesion?

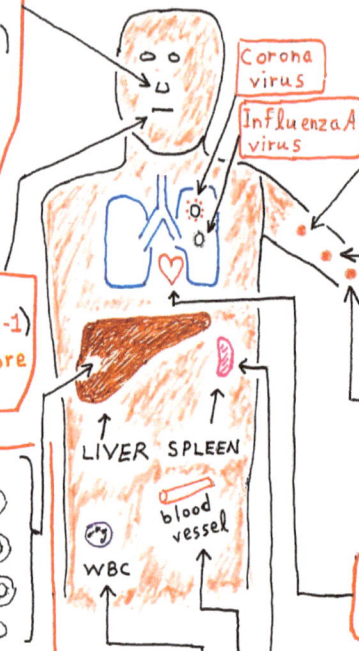

Chickenpox virus ☼
- Has nothing to do with chickens.
- Official name is:
  Varicella Zoster Virus (VZV)
- Can reactivate as **Shingles** (usually in people **50 years** or older).

Herpes Simplex Virus-1 (HSV-1) ☼
- **Oral Herpes** a.k.a. **cold sore** a.k.a. **fever blister**

Cowpox virus ○
- Milkmaids used to get this by milking cows with Cowpox.

Smallpox virus ○
- Related to cowpox virus but much nastier.

Hepatitis
- A virus (HAV) ○
- B virus (HBV) ○
- C virus (HCV) ○
- D virus (HDV) ○
- E virus (HEV) ○

LIVER   SPLEEN

blood vessel

WBC

Coxsackie virus ○
- It can infect heart muscle ♡, sometimes.

Epstein-Barr virus (EBV) ☼
- It causes 'Mono' a.k.a. **Mono-nucleosis** a.k.a. **Kissing Disease.** 👄
- Contact sports must be avoided for **8 weeks** because spleen can rupture.

- Hepatitis B and Hepatitis C are the nasty ones. Can progress to **Liver Cancer.**
  - If you inject drugs and share needles, you stand a **90%** chance of acquiring Hep C in **1 year.**

  `Hepatitis A causes **Traveller's Hepatitis.**
  It rarely kills (CFR **0.3%**) (**3** deaths per **1000** cases) but will ruin your vacation.

Ebola virus ∿
- Die of wacky blood complications

HIV/AIDS virus ✳
- Destroys immune system
- Die of 'opportunistic infections' because germs (like Tuberculosis - TB bacteria ▬) have an <u>opportunity</u>.

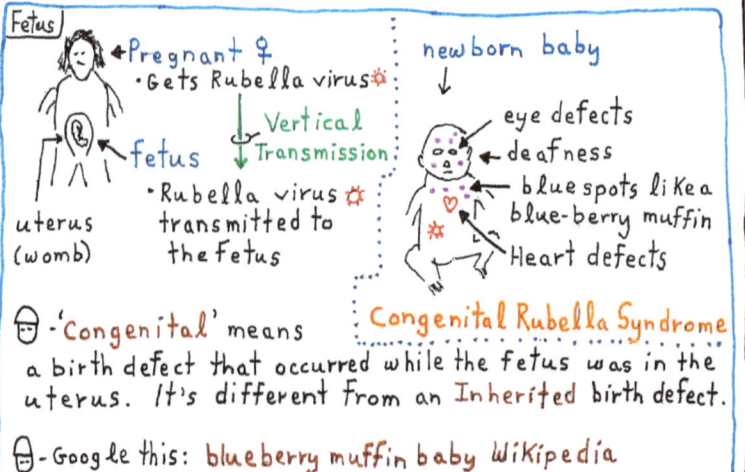

Yellow Fever virus ☀ infects the liver (think, mosquitoes when building the **Panama Canal**)

- 'Jaune' is the French word for <mark>yellow</mark> → 'Jaundice' means you turn yellow in Liver Failure (but there are many other causes of Jaundice).

Fetus

Pregnant ♀
- Gets Rubella virus ☼

newborn baby
↓
- eye defects
- deafness
- blue spots like a blue-berry muffin
- Heart defects

↓ **Vertical Transmission**

Fetus
- Rubella virus ☼ transmitted to the Fetus

uterus (womb)

Congenital Rubella Syndrome

Children
- **Measles virus** ☼
- **Mumps virus** ☼
- **Rubella virus** ☼
  - a.k.a. **German measles**
  - Get a skin rash for **3 days** then it's all good

But this is bad

- 'Congenital' means a birth defect that occurred while the fetus was in the uterus. It's different from an Inherited birth defect.

- Google this: **blueberry muffin baby Wikipedia**

Polio virus ☼

This man has Polio

cough, cough

droplets
· contain virus

into her mouth →

He touches his feces ... then prepares salad

feces
· contain virus

into her mouth

↑ tossed salad

swallows virus →

70% → nothing happens (asymptomatic) (but can shed virus in feces)

$\frac{1 \text{ in}}{200}$ (0.5%) → **Paralysis**
↳ Virus moves to spinal cord!!

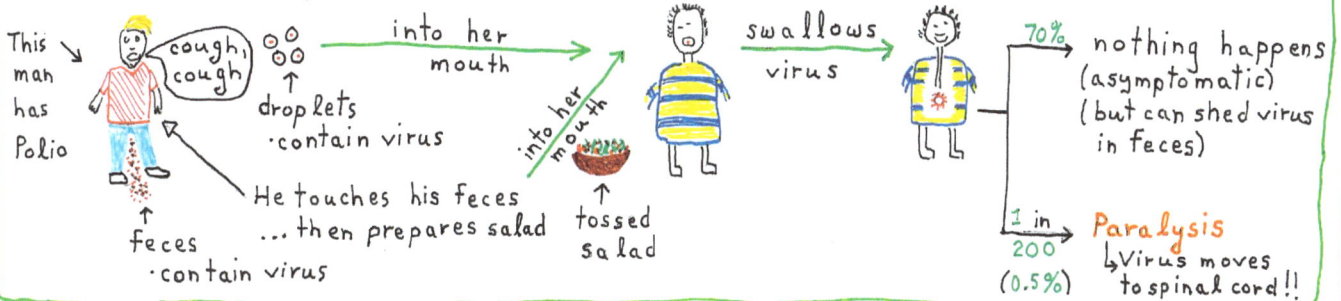

☻ - Let's check out that paralysis.

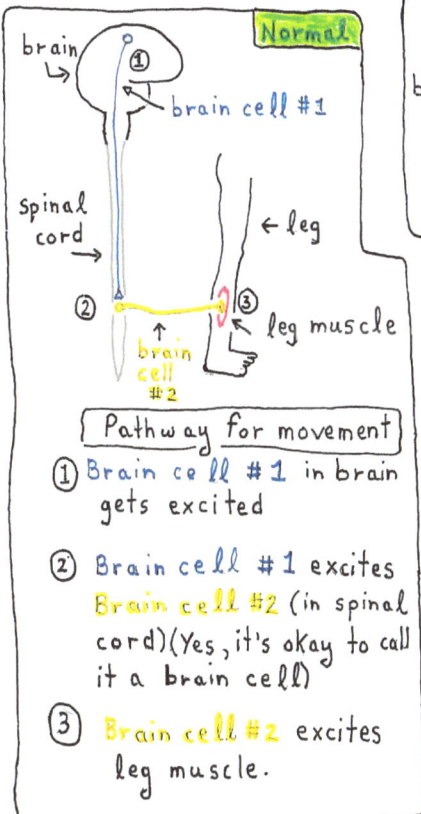

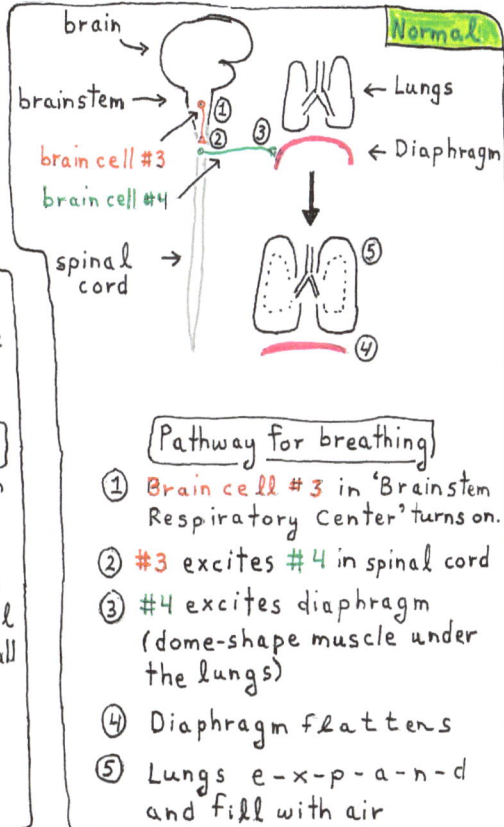

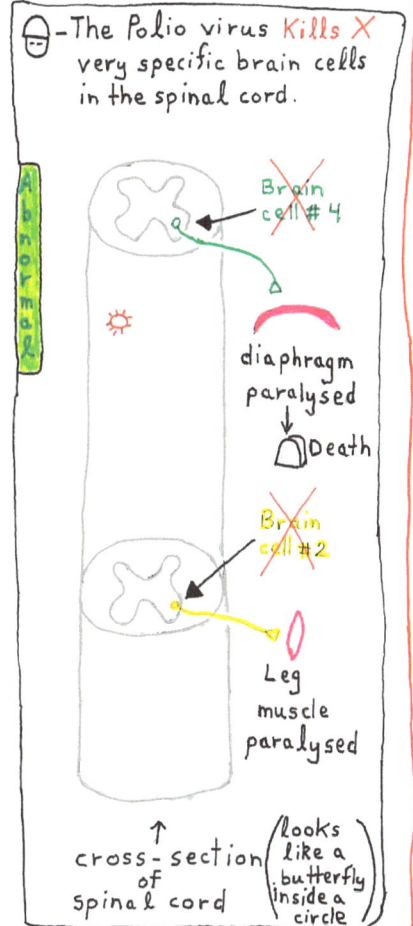

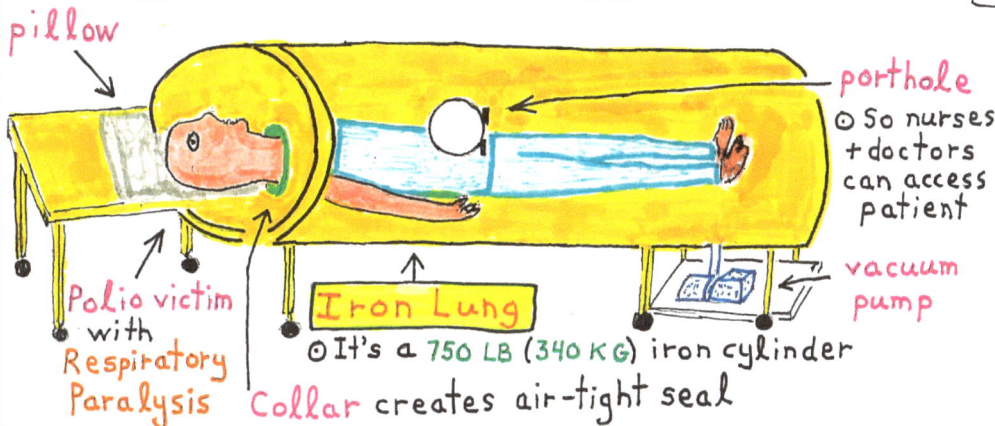

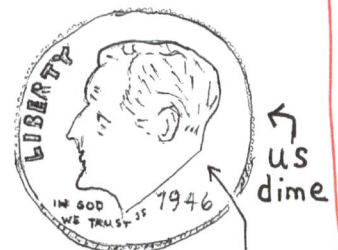

Normal

brain → ① brain cell #1

spinal cord →

② brain cell #2

← leg

③ ← leg muscle

Pathway for movement

① Brain cell #1 in brain gets excited

② Brain cell #1 excites Brain cell #2 (in spinal cord) (Yes, it's okay to call it a brain cell)

③ Brain cell #2 excites leg muscle.

Normal

brain →

brainstem → ①
② ③

brain cell #3
brain cell #4

spinal cord →

← Lungs
← Diaphragm

⑤
④

Pathway for breathing

① Brain cell #3 in 'Brainstem Respiratory Center' turns on.

② #3 excites #4 in spinal cord

③ #4 excites diaphragm (dome-shape muscle under the lungs)

④ Diaphragm flattens

⑤ Lungs e-x-p-a-n-d and fill with air

☻ - The Polio virus **Kills ✗** very specific brain cells in the spinal cord.

Abnormal

Brain cell #4 ✗

☼

diaphragm paralysed
↓
Death ✗

Brain cell #2 ✗

Leg muscle paralysed

↑ cross-section of spinal cord

(looks like a butterfly inside a circle)

---

pillow →

porthole →

◉ So nurses + doctors can access patient

Iron Lung

← Polio victim with **Respiratory Paralysis**

Collar creates air-tight seal

vacuum pump →

◉ It's a 750 LB (340 KG) iron cylinder

☿ - How does an iron lung work?

☿ - A vacuum is created inside the cylinder ➤ so Pressure↓ ➤ so lungs expand (Volume↑) ➤ so atmospheric air (in the room) at higher P flows into mouth/nose ➤ into lungs ➤ pump reverses ➤ exhale ➤ cycle starts again.

LIBERTY
IN GOD WE TRUST 1946
← US dime

Franklin Delano Roosevelt (FDR)
◉ President of the United States 1933-1945

◉ FDR had Polio.
◉ FDR wore **leg braces.**

Rabies virus →

brain → ③ Rabies virus enters brain → 99.99% Fatal
② Rabies virus travels in nerve upwards towards brain
① Rabid dog bites your arm

Rabies virus   nerve   ← rabid dog

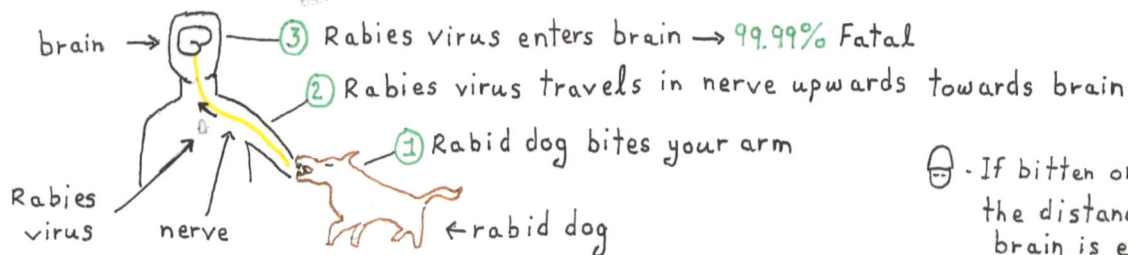

☺ - If bitten on the face, the distance to the brain is even shorter.

Multiple Choice Question

If you are bitten by a rabid dog you should:
a. Refuse to round up 99.99% to 100% and insist you'll be the exception.
b. Photograph the dog and post to Instagram #isthisyourrabiddog
c. Seek medical attention for Rabies vaccine and Rabies Immune Globulin.

ans - c.

Rabies

↑ Rabies virus

Worldwide
• 59,000 Human Rabies deaths per year.
• 99% due to dog bites (the rabies virus is in the dog saliva).

Bats are a 'natural reservoir' for rabies. It has to bite you to transmit the virus.

Plot Spoiler: Travis →

Somebody in this story gets rabies.

Old Yeller →

OLD YELLER by FRED GIPSON
Harper Publishing 1956

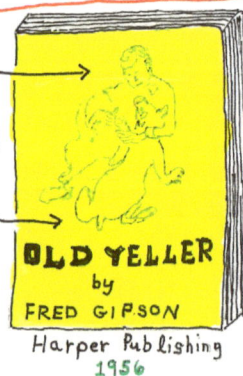

Human Rabies deaths per year in USA.

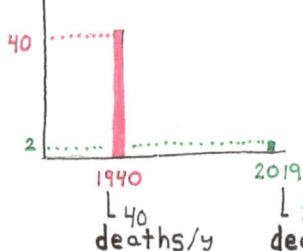

40
2
1940   2019
└ 40   └ 2
deaths/y   deaths/y (in a country of 328 million people)

☺ - Why the dramatic decline?
1. Vaccination of dogs!!
   rabies vaccine →   dog
2. Rabies anti-bodies Y
   • You get this if you're bitten by a rabid animal.

← Rabies virus
⊙ Bullet shape
⊙ The earliest written record of rabies was 2300 B.C. in Babylon.

Size comparison

100 nm (nano-meter) scale bar ↳ p.53

180 nm

60 nm
Rabies virus

100 nm (on average)
Coronavirus

☽ - Do you think any of the animals on Noah's ark had rabies?

☿ - Hmm, they seemed to march up the ramp politely, so I vote No.

BATS ON TRIAL

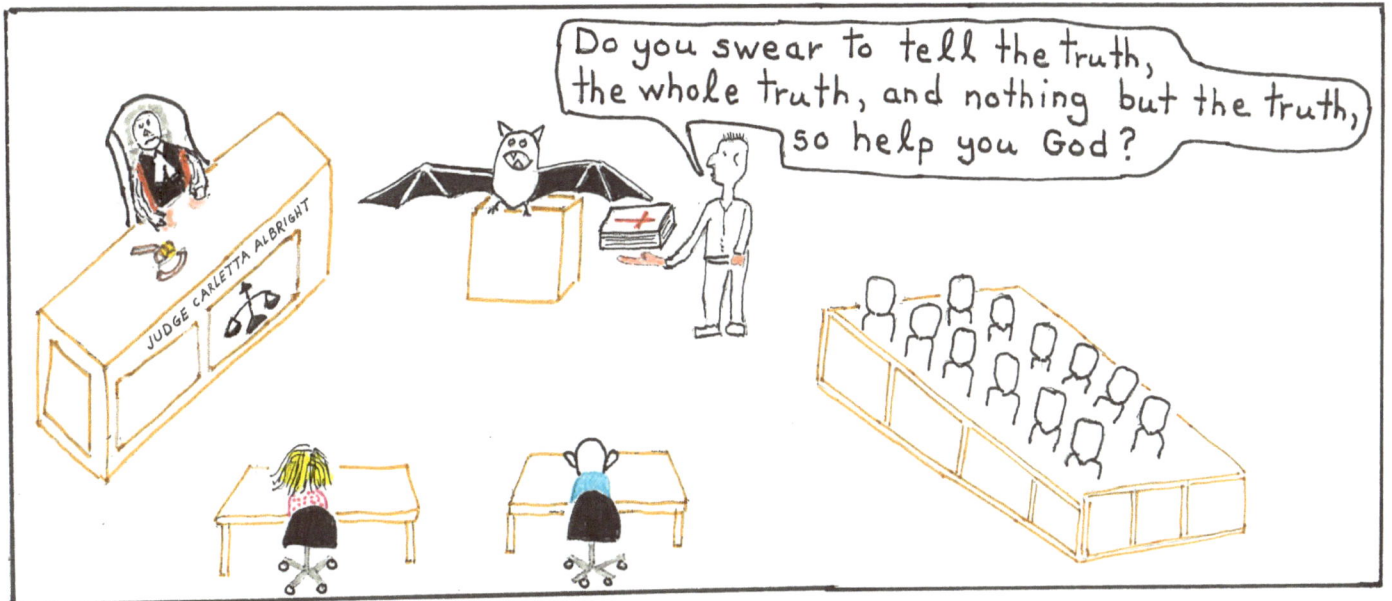

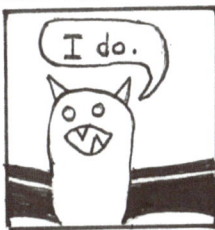 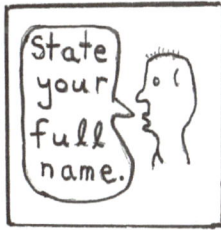 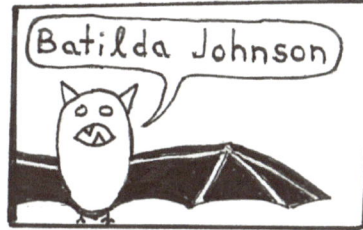

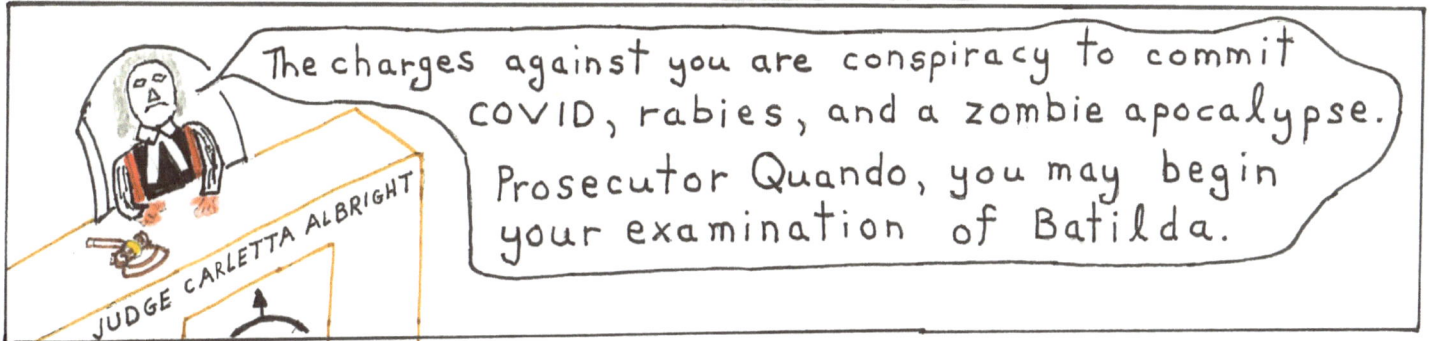

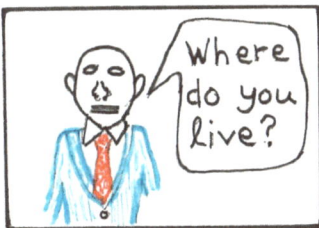 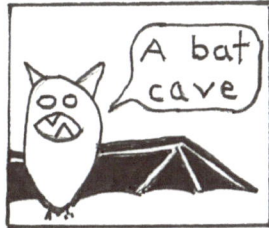 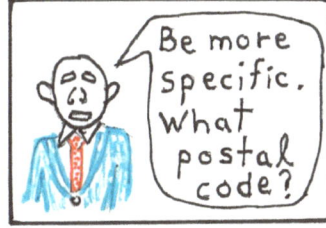 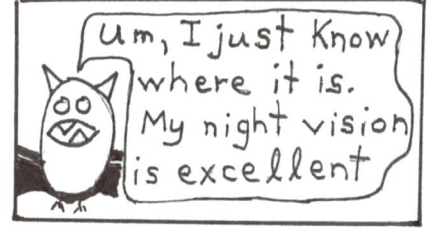

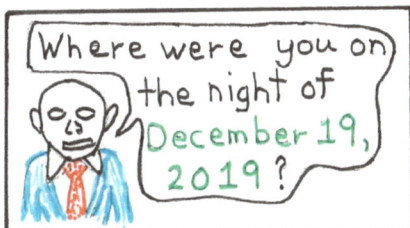 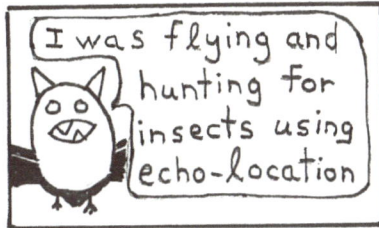 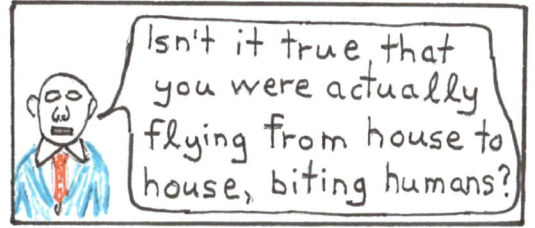

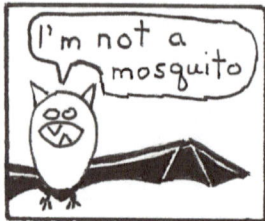

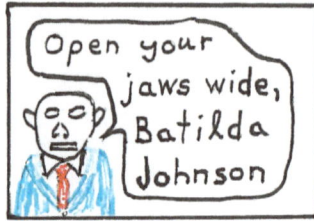

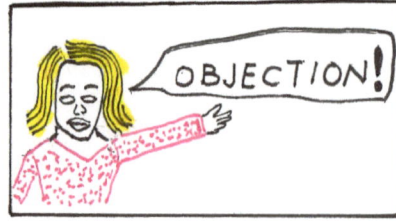

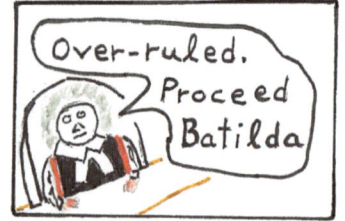

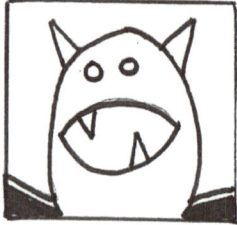

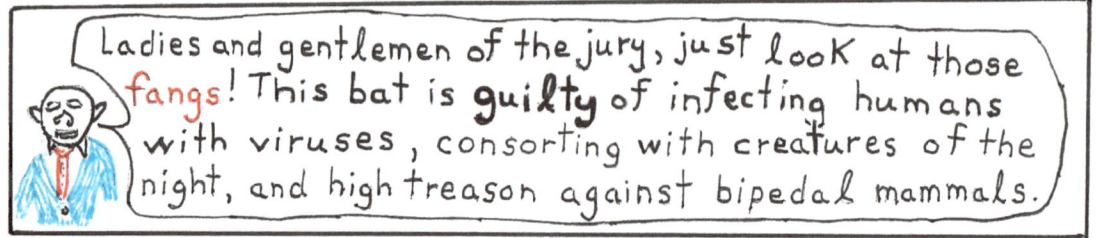

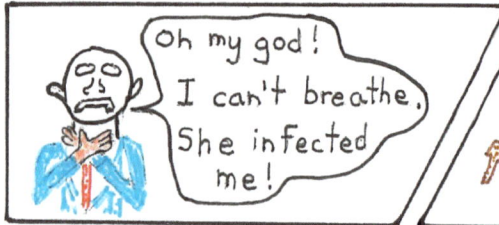

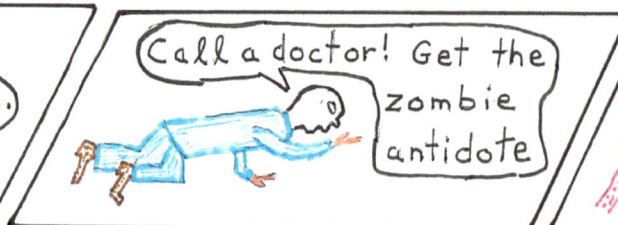

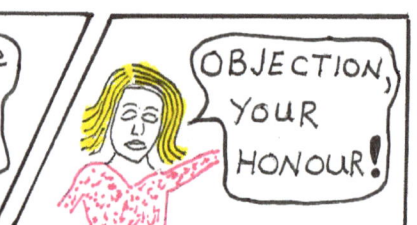

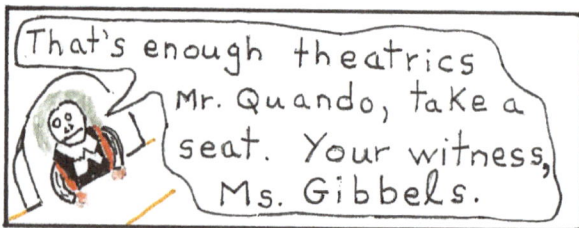

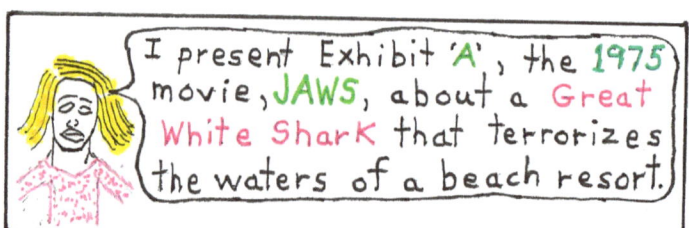

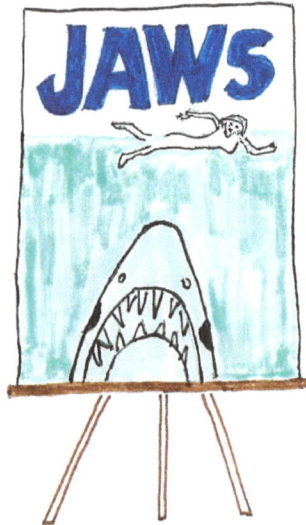

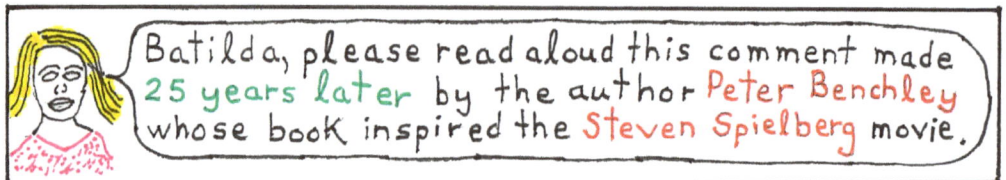

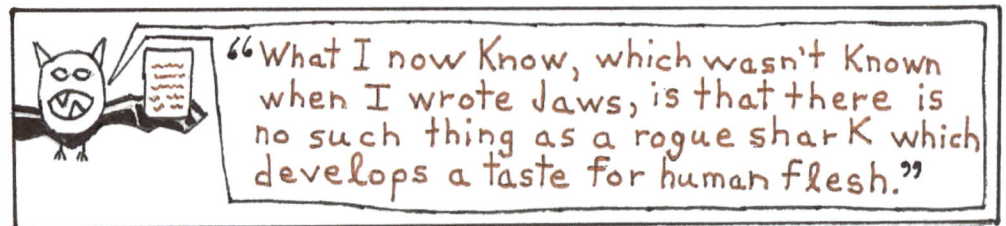

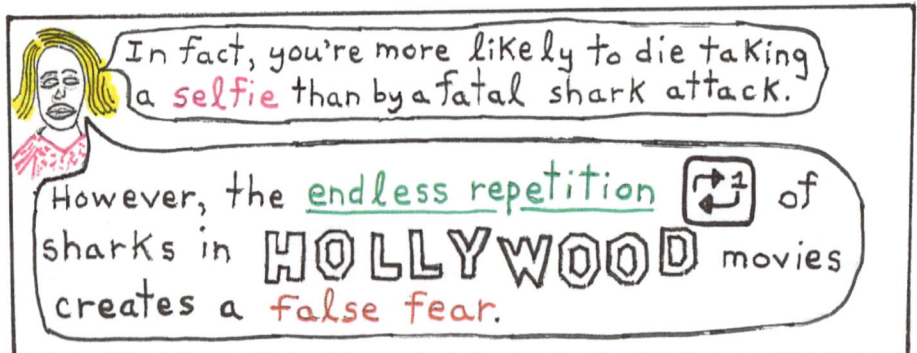

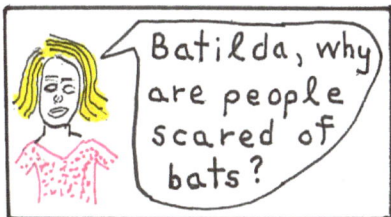

Batilda, why are people scared of bats?

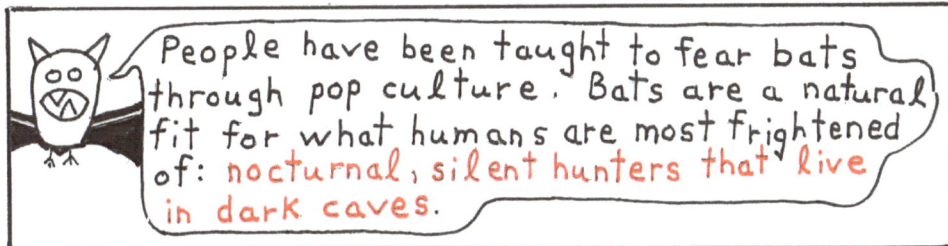

People have been taught to fear bats through pop culture. Bats are a natural fit for what humans are most frightened of: nocturnal, silent hunters that live in dark caves.

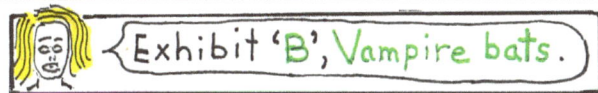

Exhibit 'B', Vampire bats.

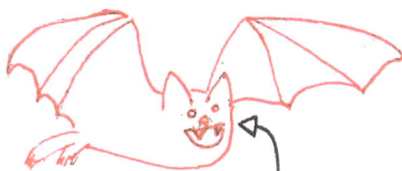

Common vampire bat

Thermo-receptors in face detect (sleeping) mammal!

pig

cow

horse

Human (rare)

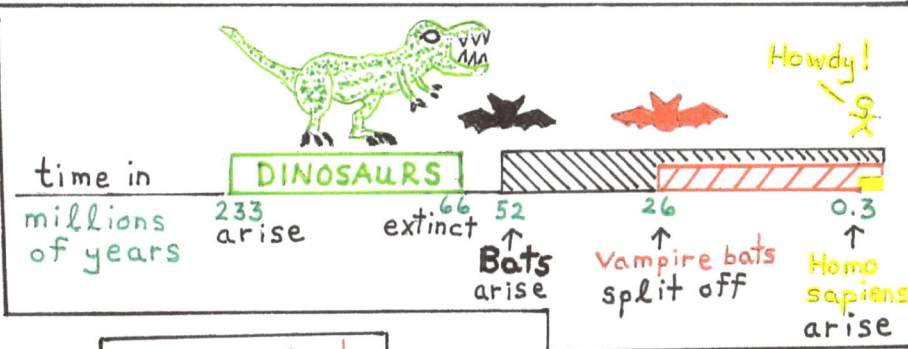

time in millions of years

DINOSAURS

233 arise

66 extinct

52 Bats arise

26 Vampire bats split off

0.3 Homo sapiens arise

Howdy!

Vampire bats

◆ They are mammals (warm blooded, live birth).
◆ They are the only mammals that feed exclusively on blood.
◆ There are 3 species of vampire bat.

Common vampire bat | Hairy-legged vampire bat | White-winged vampire bat

Feeds on blood of mammals

Feed on the blood of birds

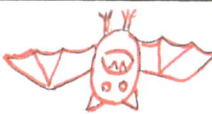

sleeping chicken

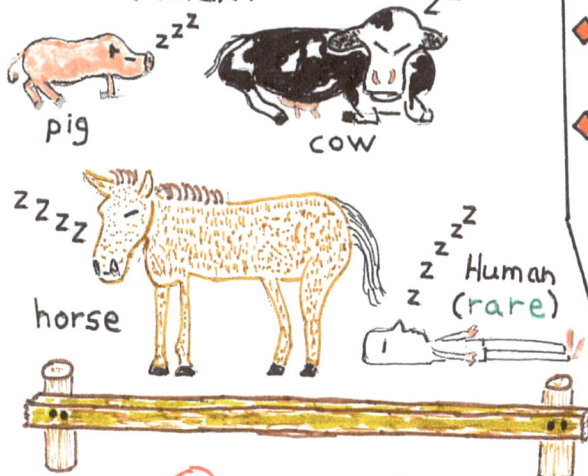

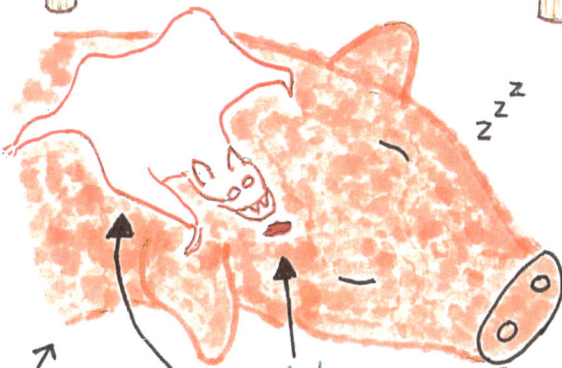

sleeping pig

Bat sitting on pig

ear

1 teaspoon of pig blood (5 ml)

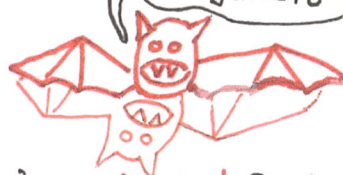

Isabella, I'm dying

I'll regurgitate some blood, Alejandro

Dies if no blood for 2 days

2 days

'Donor' vampire bat feeds blood to starving bat!

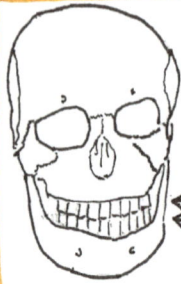

Exhibit 'C', Fangs

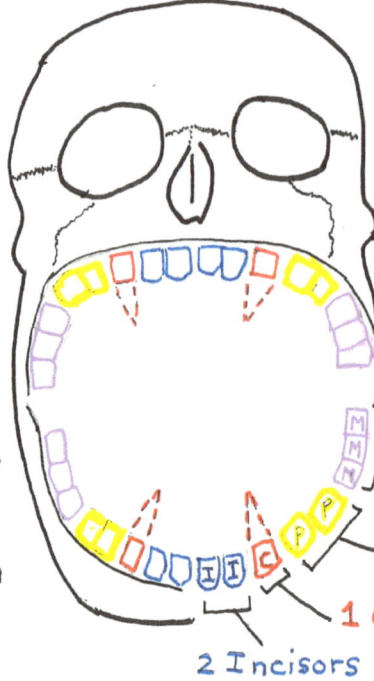

← Human skull

← 16 teeth upper jaw
← 16 teeth lower jaw
_____
32 teeth

Dentists (and zoologists) divide the 32 teeth into 4 'quadrants' of 8 teeth each.

The 'Dental Formula' describes the type of teeth in a quadrant.

The Dental Formula of humans is: 2, 1, 2, 3.

The 3rd (last) molar is the 'wisdom tooth.'

3 Molars

2 Pre-molars

1 Canine

2 Incisors

8 teeth
×
4 quadrants
= 32 teeth

The Dental Formula of apes, chimpanzees, orangutans, (and Dracula) is also 2, 1, 2, 3 but their canine is elongated into a 'Fang.' ⋀

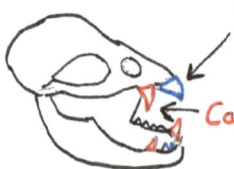

Exhibit 'D', bat fangs

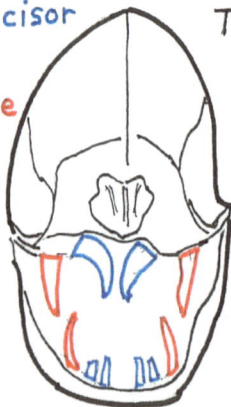

Incisor

Canine

20 teeth

☆ It is the razor-sharp upper Incisors that cut the skin. Not the canines (fangs). So every Dracula movie you've ever seen is inaccurate. ☆

The Dental Formula of the Common vampire bat is a touch complicated: $\frac{1, 1, 1, 1}{2, 1, 2, 1}$ upper jaw
lower jaw

Not shown

1 Incisor, 1 Canine, 1 Pre-molar, 1 Molar

2 Incisors, 1 Canine, 2 Pre-molars, 1 Molar

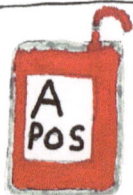

A POS

When you donate blood (450 ml), you lose 90 times more blood than by a vampire bat bite (5 ml).

← blood bag

Ladies and gentlemen of the jury, bats, like sharks, have been vilified through a century of books and film.

Things started to go badly for bats in 1897, with the publication of Bram Stoker's *Dracula* - Exhibit 'E'.

Vilified?

To be portrayed as vile. It is derived from the Latin, vilis, meaning worthless.

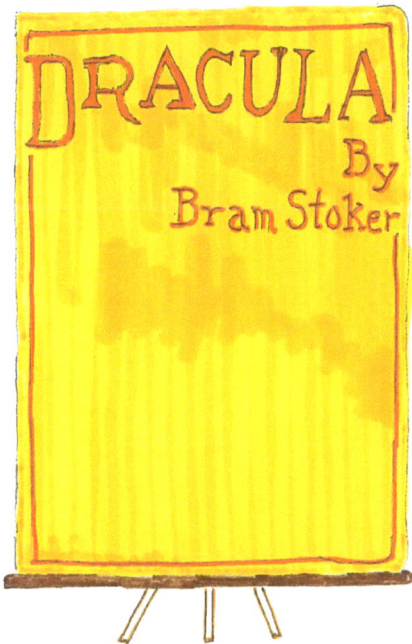

DRACULA
By
Bram Stoker

"One of those big bats that they call vampires had got at her in the night, and what with his gorge and the vein left open, there wasn't enough blood in her to let her stand up, and I had to put a bullet through her as she lay."

That comment was made by the character Quincey Morris, telling of a horse bled dry in the Pampas of Argentina. I present Exhibit 'F', Horse Blood Volume.

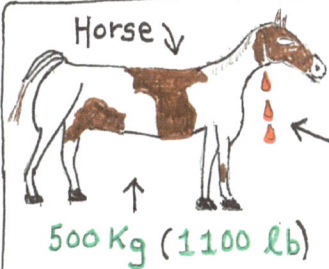

Horse ↓

← Horse blood volume = 8% of body weight (Kg)
8% x 500 Kg = 40 liters = 10 gallons

500 Kg (1100 lb)

Hemorrhagic Shock in a Horse
Grade I = 15% blood loss
Grade II = 15-30%
Grade III = 30-40%
Grade IV = Greater than 40% = High risk of death

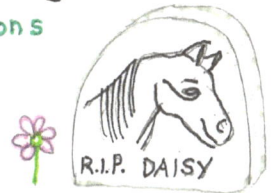

R.I.P. DAISY

So, if the horse lost 40% of its blood, that's 40% of 40 liters, which is 16 liters = 4 gallons = 3200 teaspoons.

Yet a vampire bat drinks only 1 teaspoon of blood. So that means 3199 teaspoons kept on bleeding? Nonsense!

Bram Stoker was a theatre manager, not a veterinarian.

Batilda, where do vampire bats live, geographically speaking?

From Mexico to Brazil, basically

Not in Transylvania? No

And do vampire bats carry rabies? Yes

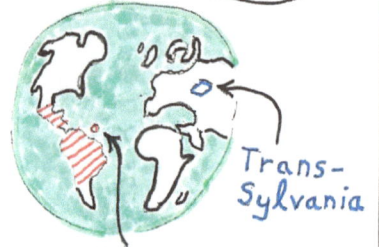

Trans-Sylvania

Trinidad

In the 1930s, there was a rabies outbreak in livestock in Trinidad. This was due to vampire bats. In response, 8000 bat caves were dynamited or poisoned. And bananas were poisoned, killing fruit bats that had nothing to do with it. In fact, only 1 in 1000 bats is a vampire bat. The other 999 eat fruit or insects, and are critical for seed dispersal in the Amazon.

And I remind the jury that 99% of Human Rabies is caused by dog bites. I present Exhibit 'G', 99:1.

Rabies virus	Stan	Sinbad	Butler	Jane	Sumo / Rapunzel
	Violet	Comfy	Gus	Pi / Razzle	Pongo / Tilly
Mandy	Niko	Pita	Ripley	Zoom	Tom / Rio
Toaster	Flo	Lee loo	Jack	Fozzie	Bolt / Vespa / Missy
Smoothie	Seoul	Pretzel	Rookie	Bluetooth	Ghost / Caffeine / Trouble

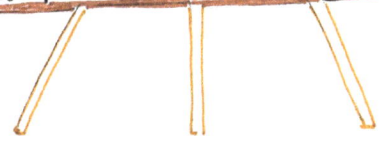

Bats ← Dies in 1-3 days!

· Of the 1400 species of bats, only 0.5% are infected by rabies.

· Tip-off ⟨ Flies in daytime / Sitting on ground → Do not touch. Call wildlife authority.

Virus changes the behaviour of the bat.

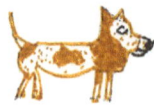

Cats Meow

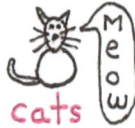
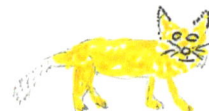

Dogs ⟨ Furious Rabies → Attacks / Paralytic Rabies

· Number 1 reservoir globally → cause 99% of Human Rabies

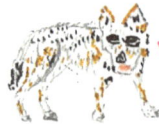

Wolf
· Northern Europe

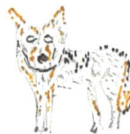
Coyote

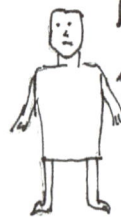
Fox

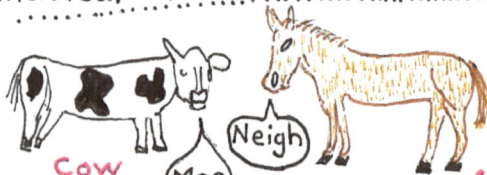

Cow

Moo / Neigh

Horse / mule

→ Very dangerous if Furious Rabies.

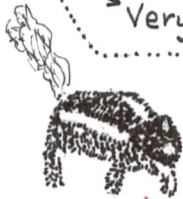
Skunk

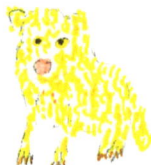
Mongoose

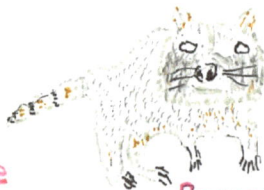
Raccoon

The Rabies virus lives in the **salivary glands** of infected animals.

99%

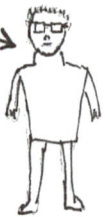

Theoretically possible but never documented

Human ⟶ **Human**

→ 80% 'Furious' Rabies, but not actually furious.
→ 20% Paralytic Rabies.
Both types die in a coma.

GUNS, GERMS, AND STEEL

— The FATES of HUMAN SOCIETIES

JARED DIAMOND

W.H. NORTON 1997

Exhibit 'J' - HOLLYWOOD

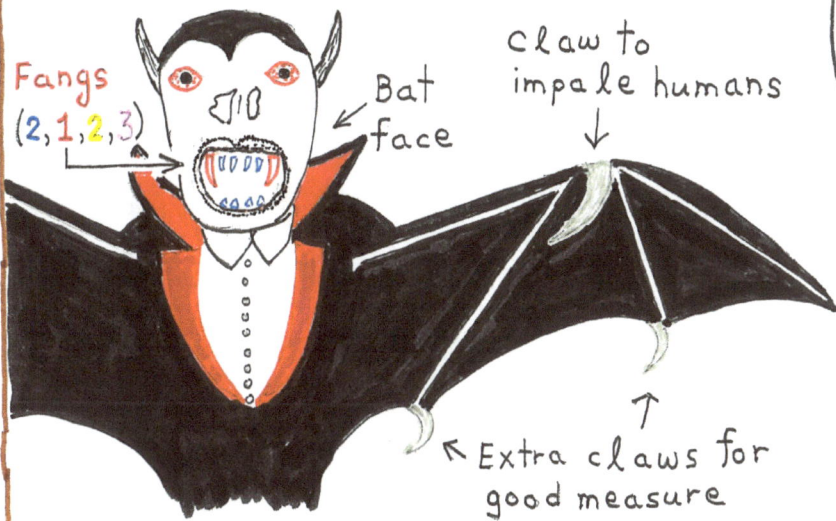

Fangs (2, 1, 2, 3)

Bat face

Claw to impale humans

← Extra claws for good measure

Dracula

♪ popcorn

movie screen →

↑ Human **wants** to be scared, and will pay $ for it.

Suspenseful music is **essential**. If it was

Row, row, row your boat
Gently down the stream
the suspense would be ruined.

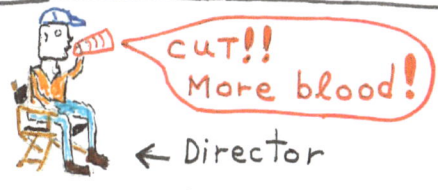

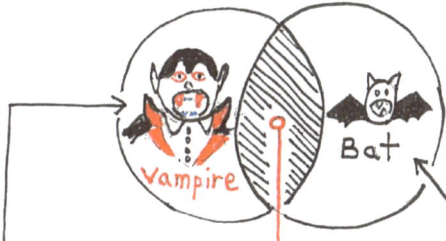

CUT!! More blood!

← Director

Vampire

Bat

Does not exist. No more real than Chewbacca.

Fear
Suspicion
Blood
Horror
Evil
Undead

Ø Dead

The fear created by the movie is **transferred** to what is real ... the bat.

HOLLYWOOD

+ IGNORANCE

= Misguided

Bats are dangerous. I need to kill bats.

← Your only source of information on bats is a HOLLYWOOD screenwriter who would get 20% on a MCQ exam (due to chance alone) and 1% on a fill-in-the-blank exam on bat biology.

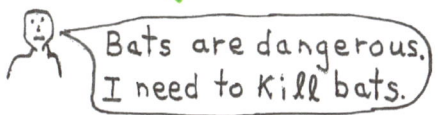

43 Ⓐ Ⓑ Ⓒ Ⓓ Ⓔ

Bats belong to Order _____.

Finally, Exhibits 'K', 'L', 'M', and 'N' - Reductio ad absurdum.

If you want to kill ==all bats== (which actually doesn't make sense as they only cause 590 of 59,000 Human Rabies deaths annually) ... then it would make more sense to kill ==all dogs== (that cause 58,410 Human Rabies deaths) ... and it would make even more sense to kill ==all birds== (which still doesn't make sense, but whatever) to prevent a repeat of the 1918 Influenza Pandemic (that killed 50,000,000 people).

Even if humans successfully killed ==all animals==, we'd still be left with the Kingdom Bacteria.

* It is the human proximity to bat caves, wet markets, and the illegal wildlife trade that promotes corona-virus transmission to humans. The problem is humans. Not bats.

Anti-biotic Resistant bacteria kill 5,000,000 humans every year.
1) Staph aureus — 1,100,000
2) E. coli — 950,000
3) Strep pneumoniae — 829,000
4) Klebsiella pneumoniae — 790,000
5) Pseudomonas aeruginosa — 559,000
And 28 other bacteria.
Are bats on this list? No.
THE LANCET 19 Jan 2021

Even if we killed ==all bacteria==, we'd still be left with smoking, which kills 2,500,000 people yearly due to COPD (Chronic Obstructive Pulmonary Disease). That's not even including Lung Cancer.
If you really want to save humans, put your efforts here, not bats.
2.5m

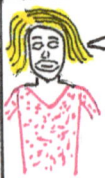

Batilda, did you ever offer cigarettes to humans? And do you sit on the Board of Directors of any tobacco company?

No and No.

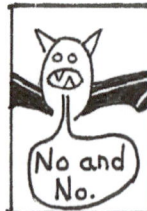

Very well. In conclusion, Prosecutor Quando's argument is falsely predicated on fangs and cheezy movies.

OBJECTION! Ms. Gibbels loved *The Notebook*

Don't read into it, Quando. You kiss like a dying fish.

That was catty but I'll allow it. Objection over-ruled. I declare this a mis-trial.

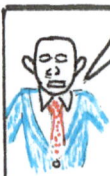

Pound Pound

Batilda Johnson, you are a free bat.

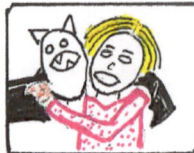

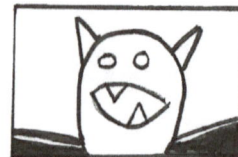

Chapter 4

Coronavirus –
it has more personality
than you thought

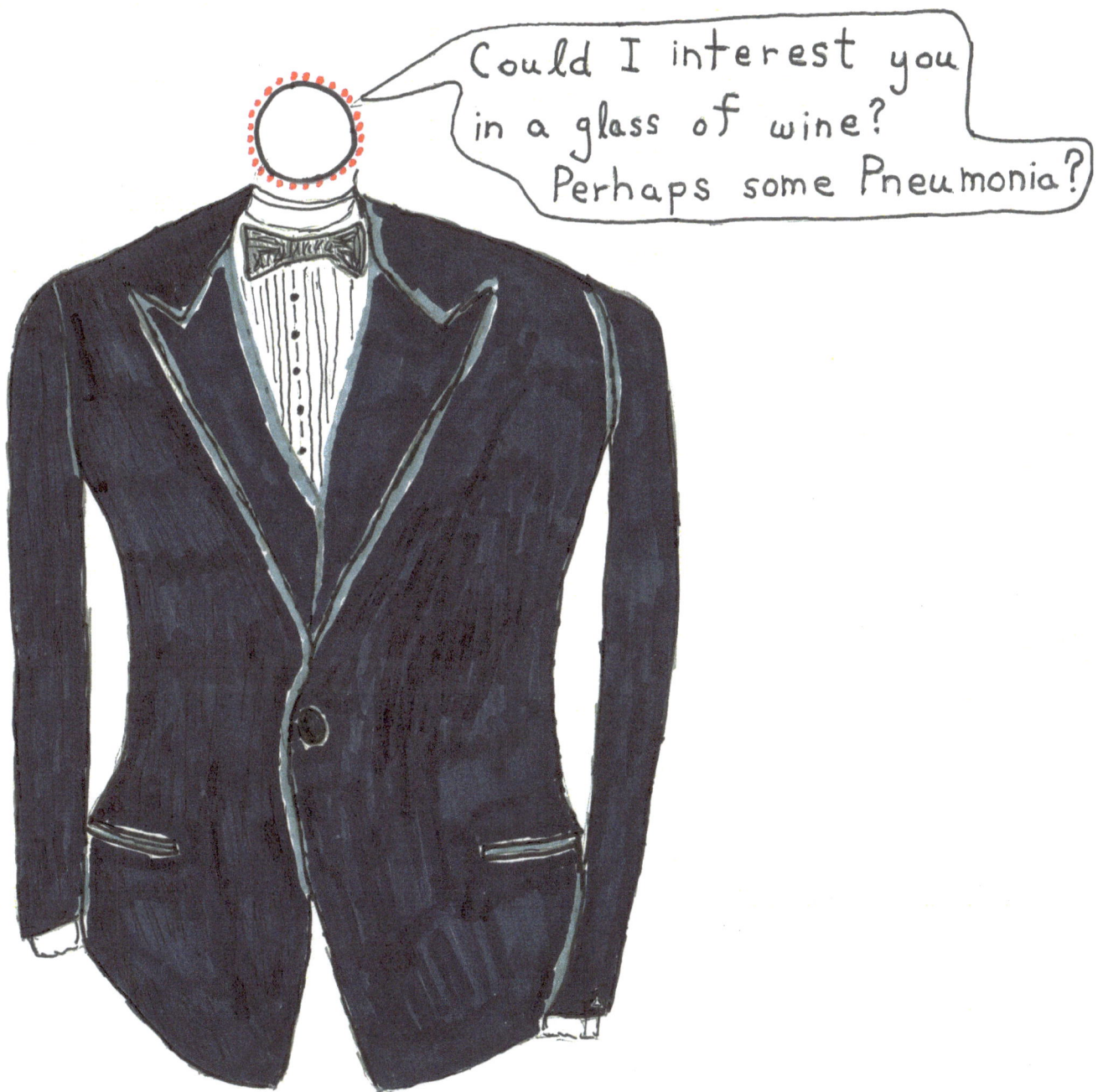

Could I interest you in a glass of wine? Perhaps some Pneumonia?

WHO DOES CORONAVIRUS INFECT?

⊖ – Lots of different animals

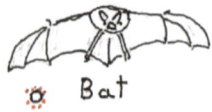

Bat
Miniopterus bat coronavirus
Pipistrellus bat coronavirus
Rhinolophus bat coronavirus
Rousettus bat coronavirus
Tylonycteris bat coronavirus

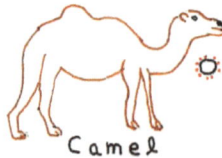

Bulbul
Bulbul coronavirus
• A bulbul is a bird

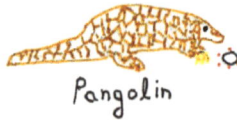

Chicken
Avian coronavirus
• A chicken is a bird

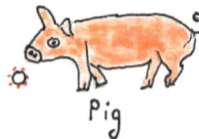

Cat
Feline coronavirus

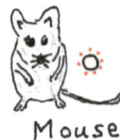

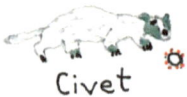

Cheetah
Feline coronavirus

Civet
Civet coronavirus
• This jumped from civet to human in 2003, causing the SARS Coronavirus Pandemic

Dog
Canine coronavirus

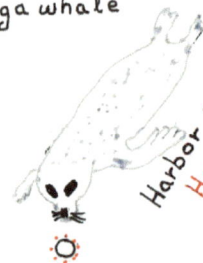

Hedgehog
Hedgehog coronavirus

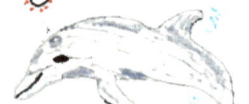

Camel
Camel coronavirus
• This jumped from camel to human in 2012, causing the MERS Coronavirus Pandemic

Pangolin
Pangolin coronavirus
• This jumped from pangolin to human in 2019. Maybe.

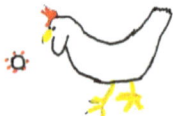

Pig
Porcine coronavirus
Porcine epidemic diarrhea virus
• It's a coronavirus
Transmissable gastro-enteritis coronavirus

Mouse
Murine coronavirus

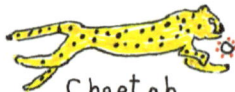

Beluga whale
Beluga whale coronavirus

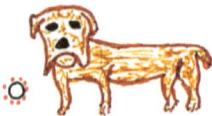

Harbor seal
Harbor seal coronavirus

Bottlenose dolphin
Bottlenose dolphin coronavirus

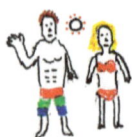

Human

Full name	Short name	Transmission	Disease
Human CoronaVirus 229E	HCoV-229E		
Human CoronaVirus NL63	HCoV-NL63		
Human CoronaVirus HKU1	HCoV-HKU1		
Human CoronaVirus OC43	HCoV-OC43		
Severe Acute Respiratory Syndrome CoronaVirus	SARS-CoV-1 ⊗	bat → civet → human	SARS
Middle East Respiratory Syndrome CoronaVirus	MERS-CoV	bat → camel → human	MERS
Severe Acute Respiratory Syndrome CoronaVirus-2	SARS-CoV-2	bat → pangolin? → human	COVID-19

CoronaVirus Disease 2019

⊖ – ⊗ To ↓ risk of confusion, let's refer to it as SARS-CoV-1.

☺ - This is <u>exactly</u> the same information as the previous page ... but reorganized into 4 groups based on genetic similarities of ☼ Coronavirus strains.

Group 1 : alpha (α) : Genus Alpha-coronavirus

bat — Miniopterus bat coronavirus
       Rhinolophus bat coronavirus
cat (Meow) — Feline coronavirus
cheetah — Feline coronavirus
dog — Canine coronavirus
harbor seal — Harbor seal coronavirus
human — Human CoronaVirus 229E (HCoV-229E)
        Human CoronaVirus NL63 (HCoV-NL63)
pig (oink, oink) — Porcine epidemic diarrhea virus
       Transmissable gastro-enteritis coronavirus

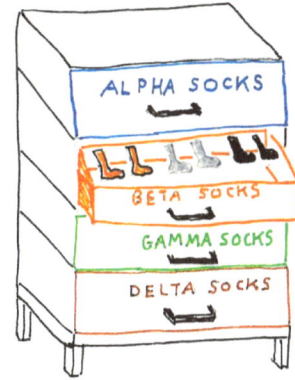

Group 2 : beta (β) : Genus Beta-coronavirus

bat — Pipistrellus bat coronavirus
       Rousettus bat coronavirus
       Tylonycterus bat coronavirus
camel — Camel coronavirus
civet — Civet coronavirus
hedgehog — Hedgehog coronavirus
human — Human CoronaVirus HKU1 (HCoV-HKU1)
        Human CoronaVirus OC43 (HCoV-OC43)
        SARS CoronaVirus (SARS-CoV-1)
        MERS CoronaVirus (MERS-CoV)
        COVID-19 CoronaVirus (SARS-CoV-2)
mouse — Murine coronavirus
pangolin — Pangolin coronavirus

Group 3 : gamma (γ) : Genus Gamma-coronavirus

chicken — Avian coronavirus
beluga — Beluga whale coronavirus
dolphin — Bottlenose dolphin coronavirus

Group 4 : delta (Δ) : Genus Delta coronavirus

bulbul — Bulbul coronavirus
pig — Porcine coronavirus

☺ - The use of Δ here has nothing to do with change. It's just a letter in a list.

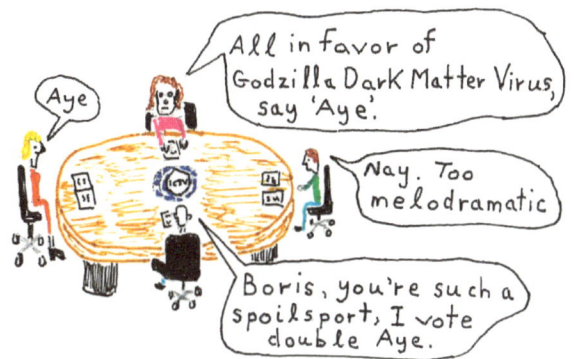

ALPHA SOCKS
BETA SOCKS
GAMMA SOCKS
DELTA SOCKS

☺ - The first four letters of the Greek alphabet are:
alpha α
beta   β
gamma γ
delta Δ

♀ - Who comes up with all these virus names?

♂ - A bunch of virologists from the International Committee on Taxonomy of Viruses (ICTV)

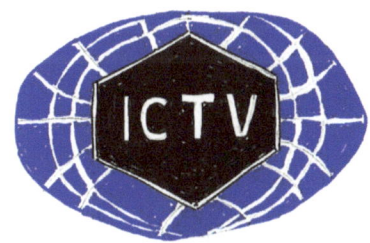

ICTV

All in favor of Godzilla Dark Matter Virus, say 'Aye'.
Aye
Nay. Too melodramatic
Boris, you're such a spoilsport, I vote double Aye.

CORONAVIRUS ZOO

Roit, ya! Folks this is a zoo. Di-ver-sity is what it's all about. That means many species of bats, many species of coronavirus, many species, period.

I like to eat moths

○ ← **Miniopterus bat coronavirus**
- This does not infect humans.
- Some strains of this virus are endemic to bats in Hong Kong. That means it is continuously found in them.

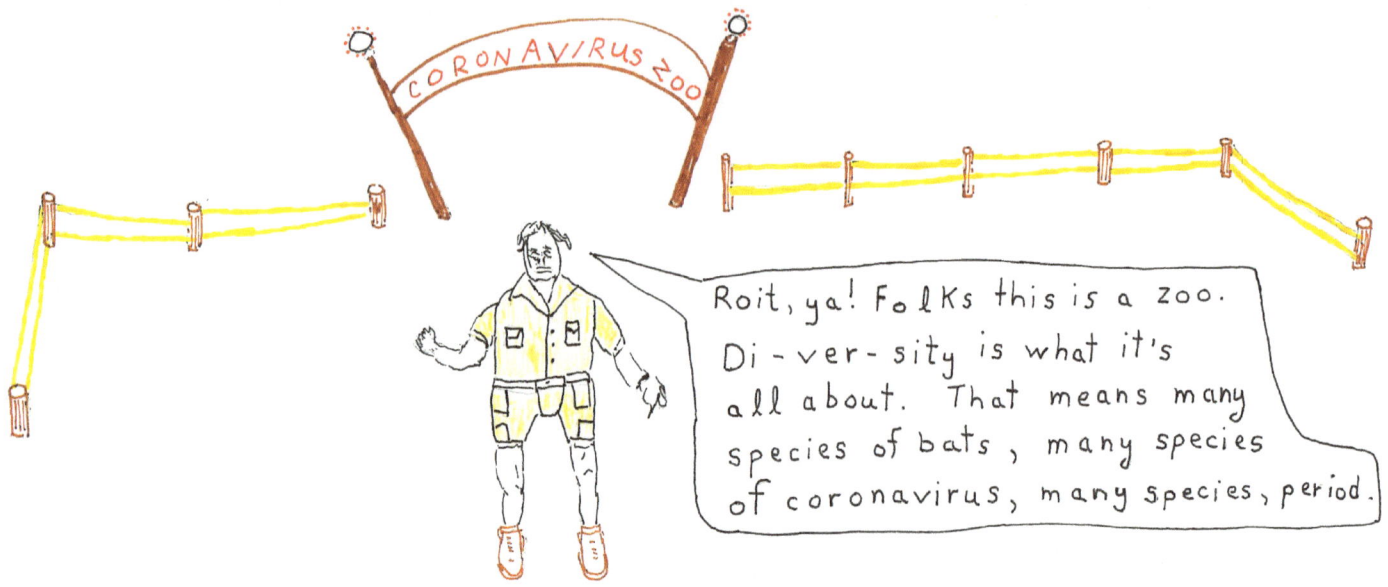

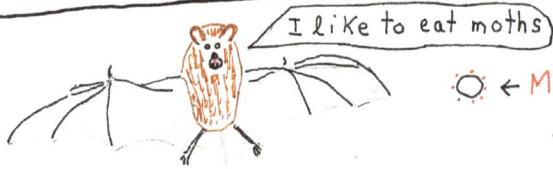

Bat lives in Asia and Middle East

Common bent-wing bat

Miniopterus   *schreibersii*
↑   ↑
Genus   species

itty bitty lungs
· 2 lungs →

Long
pinky
Ⓛ hand

← If a human hand became a bat wing

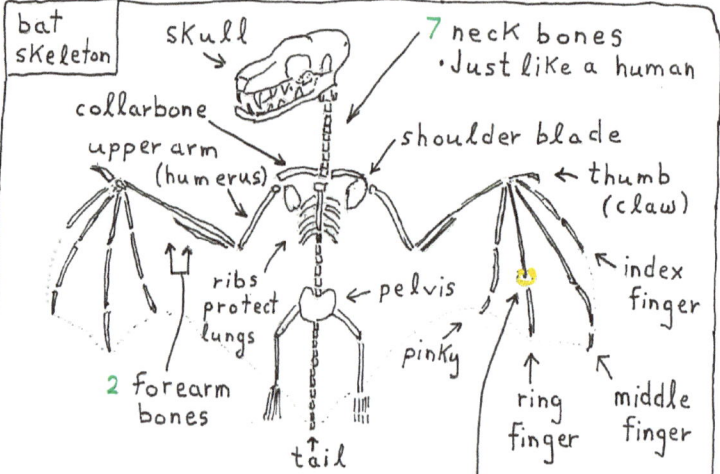

bat skeleton

skull →

7 neck bones
· Just like a human

collarbone
upper arm (humerus)
shoulder blade
thumb (claw)
ribs protect lungs
pelvis
index finger
2 forearm bones
pinky
ring finger
middle finger
tail

wedding ring (if bats got married)

☺ - Are you surprised there is a bat called the **dog-faced bat**?

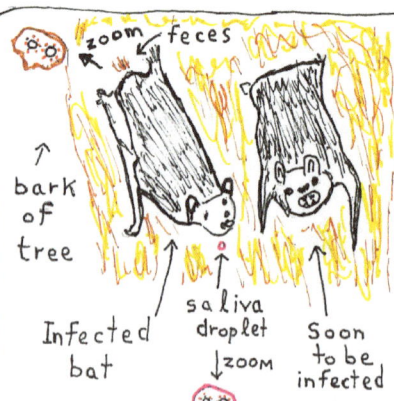

Roosting

zoom feces

bark of tree

Infected bat

saliva droplet ↓zoom

Soon to be infected

- Bats are chummy. The roost is where they chill out
- Bent-wing bat colonies can have **1,000,000** bats

saliva

Coronavirus is transmitted in bat feces

Drawing adapted from Bat Conservation Trust
www.bats.org.uk

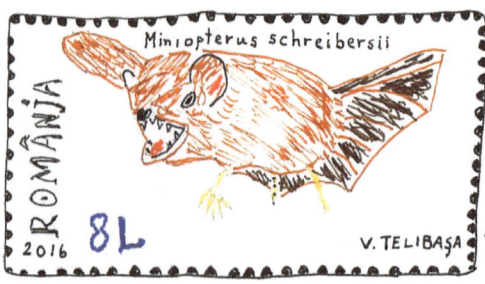

ROMÂNIA 2016 **8L**
Miniopterus schreibersii
V. TELIBAŞA

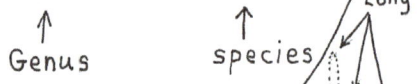

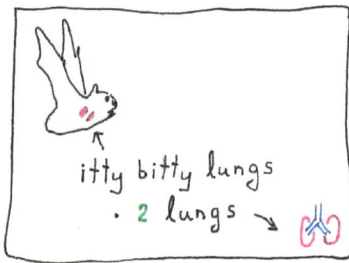

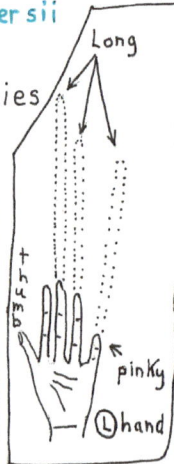

← stamp from **Romania** [I bought it]

Artist is Victor Telibaşa

☺ - The currency in **Romania** is the **Leu** (**L**).

moth ⊗

Lives in Europe

Echo-location at 55,000 pulses per second
(55 kiloHertz)(55 KHz)
• It's a burst lasting $6/1000^{th}$ of a second

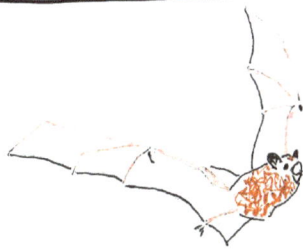

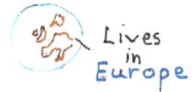

Soprano pipistrelle

Pipistrellus pygmaeus

• It hunts and eats while flying, which is called 'aerial hawking.'

⊗

Moths have 3 evasion tactics:
1. Slow turn
2. Erratic flight
3. Literally cease flying and drop to the ground

Does coronavirus infect the soprano pipistrelle? Yes.

☼ ← Bat coronavirus P. pyg.

If you want to listen, Google this:
soprano pipistrelle school of biological sciences

There is an < echolocation call } You can
social call } listen to both

? human hearing range
20,000 Hertz (high)
20 Hertz (low)

So how can I hear the sounds of the soprano pipistrelle?

Answer:
You can't.
The bat chirp recordings were slowed down 10 times.
So 55,000 Hertz became 5500 Hertz.
We can't hear that   We can hear that

(Thank you to the:
Bat Ecology and Bio-acoustics Lab at the University of Bristol)

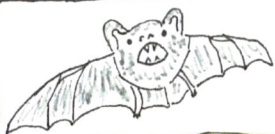

Japanese house bat

日本の家のバット
"Ni hon ie no batto"
Pipistrellus abramus

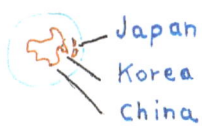

Japan
Korea
China

☼ ← Pipistrellus bat coronavirus HKU5
• This is closely related to the MERS Coronavirus that caused a pandemic in 2012.

♀ - Those bat drawings all look the same to me
♂ - Not if you're a bat

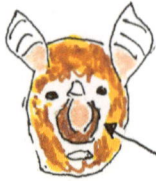

weird nose shaped like a horseshoe

Chinese rufous horseshoe bat

Rhinolophus sinicus

horseshoe

☺ - rufous means reddish

☺ ← Bat SARS-like Coronavirus WIV1

Lives in
China, Nepal, Vietnam

☺ - Guess what that means?

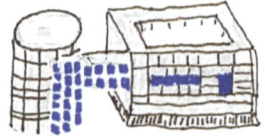

(W I V)

Wuhan Institute of Virology

☺ - This was an important discovery.
The coronavirus was isolated from a Chinese rufous horseshoe bat.
Then at the Wuhan Institute of Virology, they did some cool experiments.

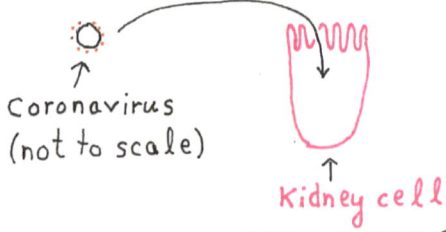

Coronavirus
(not to scale)

Kidney cell

☺ - A kidney cell was deliberately
infected with the virus.
- But this kidney cell came from
a green monkey in 1962 in Japan

green
monkey →
(its fur has a
hint of green)

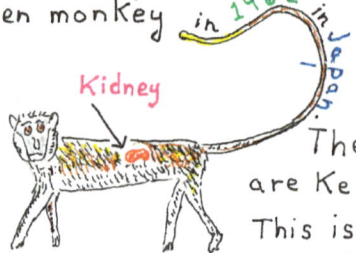

Kidney

These cells
are kept alive.
This is called
a cell line.

☺ - The point of all that
was a discovery about
the virus's spike.

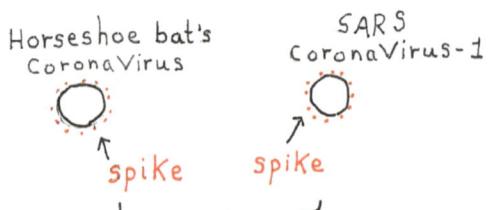

Horseshoe bat's
CoronaVirus

SARS
CoronaVirus-1

spike   spike

⊙ 99.9 % similar
⊙ Both use ACE2 to enter
cells (details later)

¹ Are the 2 viruses identical? No.
Are the 2 viruses similar? Yes
Hence the name:

Bat SARS-like CoronaVirus WIV1
a.k.a.
Bat SL-CoV-WIV1

- This particular cell line from the
Green monkey is called the
Vero cell line because
verda is the Esperanto word for
green but Esperanto is an
artificial language invented by
an eye doctor who obviously
took the Spanish word for
green which is
verde from which we get
verdure which is lush
greenery.

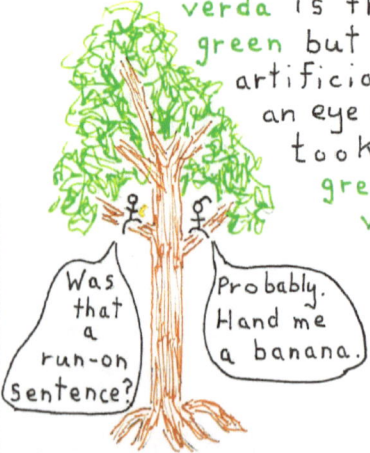

Was
that
a
run-on
sentence?

Probably.
Hand me
a banana.

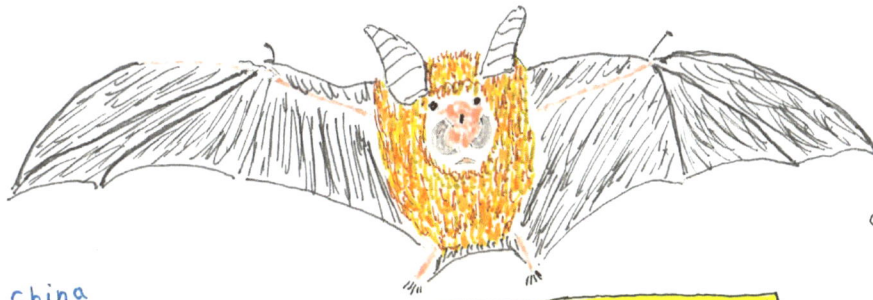

China
South-East Asia

==Intermediate horseshoe bat==

Rhinolophus affinus

○ It roosts in caves, sometimes with other species of bats.

○ Looks very similar to Chinese rufous horseshoe bat

⭐ This bat may be the 'natural reservoir' of the
☼ SARS-CoronaVirus-2 of our current coronavirus pandemic. ⭐

⊖ - Let's review some important facts.

🦇 Chinese rufous horseshoe bat
  ○ Definitely carries a SARS-like CoronaVirus
  ○ Probably associated with SARS CoronaVirus-1 (2003)

🦇 Intermediate horseshoe bat
  ○ Probably the reservoir for SARS CoronaVirus-2 (2019)

` At the very least, horseshoe bats are implicated.

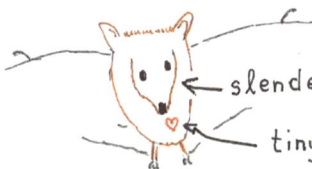

← slender face
tiny little heart beats ⟨ 248 beats per minute - at rest
                         444 beats per minute - while flying

==Egyptian fruit bat== sometimes called a ==flying fox== or ==dog-faced fruit bat==

Rousettus aegyptiacus

○ Squabbles with others in colony.
○ May steal their fruit.
○ Cleans fruit pulp off chest fur with hindfeet then licks toes.
○ Hangs upright by thumbs to ⟨ pee
                               poop
○ Uses echo-location to assist flying.

☼ ← Rousettus bat coronavirus
○ Has similarity to the MERS Coronavirus.

Middle East
Africa (including Egypt)

That's an adult!

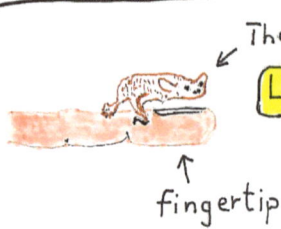

Lesser bamboo bat   *Tylonycteris pachypus*

- Does it eat bamboo? No.
- It roosts in bamboo.
- Echo-locates and eats insects in flight.
- Female usually has non-identical twins.

↑ fingertip

↑ *Sarah*   ↑ *William*

☉ ←Tylonycteris bat coronavirus HKU4
- Closely related to MERS Coronavirus

Lives in
- China
- South-East Asia
- India

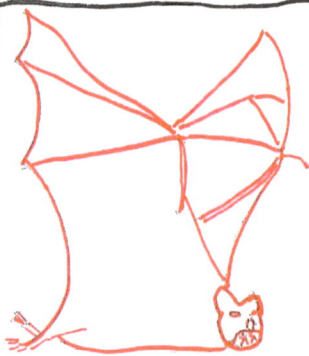

☉ ←Coronavirus
- It infects the bat.
- It was isolated from the intestines of a Common vampire bat in Brazil.

◉ - Remember the sock drawers? (p. 113)

LL ← Alpha (α) socks
↖ The ☉ Coronavirus from the Common vampire bat was in this drawer.

LL ← Beta (β) socks
↖ The ☉ SARS-Coronavirus-2 that causes COVID is in this drawer.

Common vampire bat
Desmodus rotundus

←Rabies virus
☉ It infects the Common vampire bat, also (p. 108).

◉ - There are more bats with coronavirus but I think you get the picture.

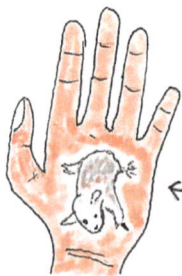

♀ - Do mother bats produce milk?

♀ - Yes. Bats are mammals, and mammals make milk.
- Making milk requires a lot of energy, so roosting (close together in a colony) saves body heat → this ↓ energy expended by 50%.

← baby bat (very cute)

(drawing adapted from Wikipedia - common pipistrelle)

◉ - Bats are infected by 130 viruses
- Not in a single bat, mind you.

eg. Coronavirus
eg. Rabies virus
eg. Plant viruses

400 strains of coronavirus have been found in bats in China.

◉ - Humans are infected by 219 viruses.

– Moving on ...

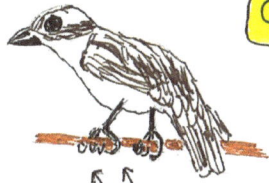

Chinese bulbul a.k.a. light-vented bulbul

Pycnonotus sinensis

– 'Sino' means Chinese
○ eg. Pycnontus sinensis
 is a Chinese bulbul
○ eg. Sino-Tibetan languages

1 toe points backwards } = Hold onto branch
3 toes point forwards } more firmly

○ Bulbul coronavirus

Chinese bulbul lives in
china
shanghai especially

wee-wee-der-wee

○ That's the song of the Chinese bulbul.

The Cornell Lab of Ornithology

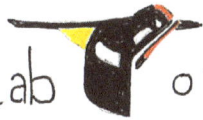

↖ The coolest logo, ever

– You can listen to a Chinese bulbul (and a ton
 of other birds) on their website.

' Google this:

Cornell laboratory of ornithology light vented bulbul

↓

Then scroll down a bit and click on 'Recordings'

– There are 10,000 species of birds
 ○ 6500 species have toes like the bulbul

– Ornith - ology is the study of birds

bird in Greek

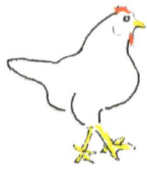

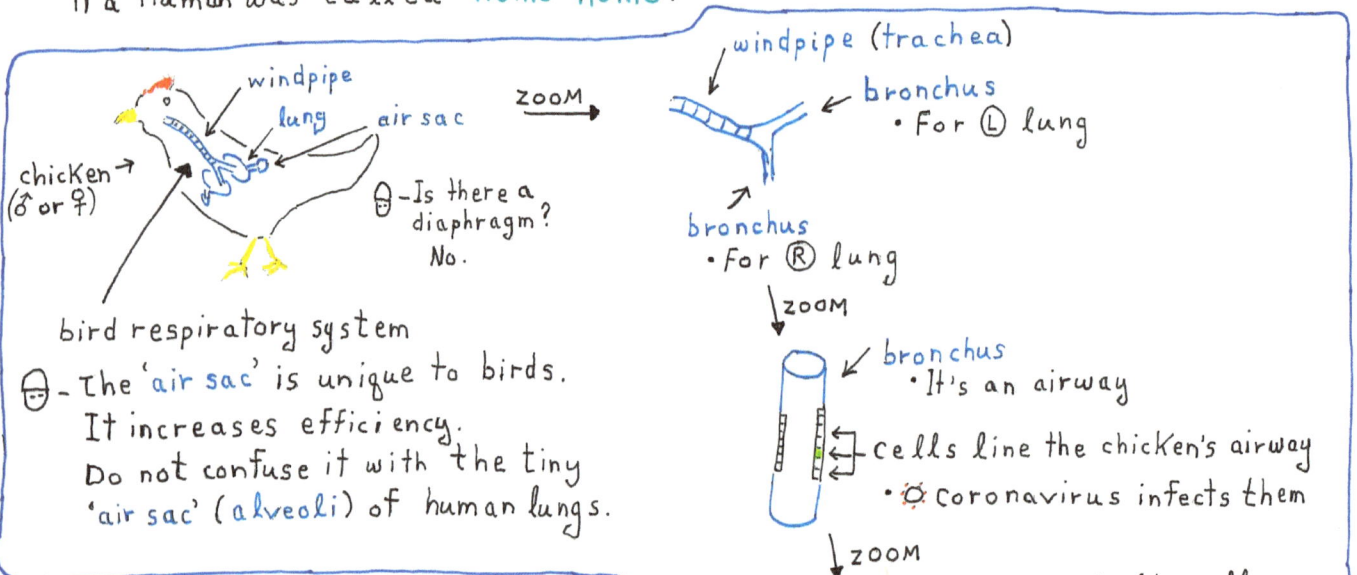

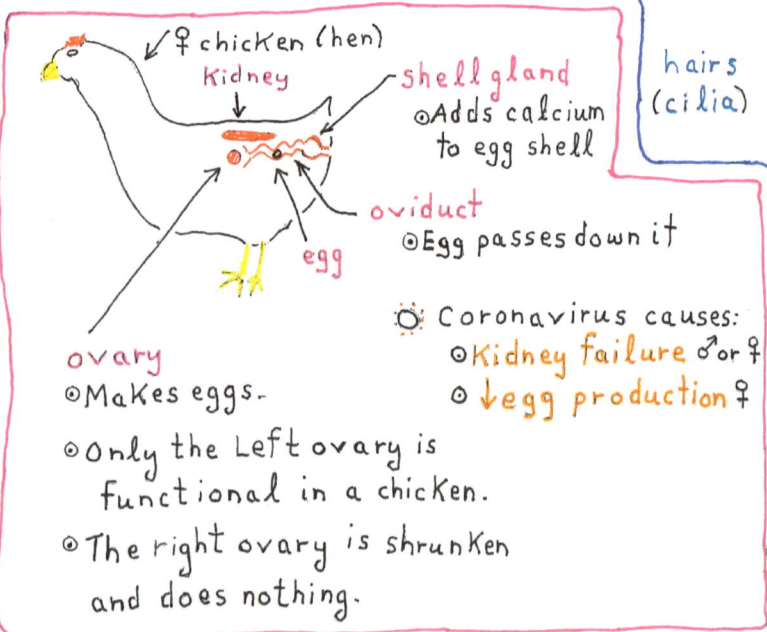

Meow

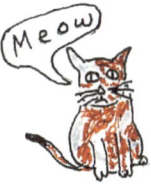

Cat Felis catus
- Basically, a house cat a.k.a domestic cat
- But if it lives in the wild it's a 'feral cat'.

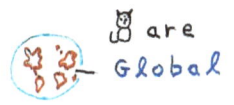

🐱 are Global

☼ Feline Coronavirus (FCoV)
- There are 2 versions of this virus - one nice, one nasty.

Nice version

☼ Feline Enteric CoronaVirus (FECV)
- It infects Kittens worldwide.

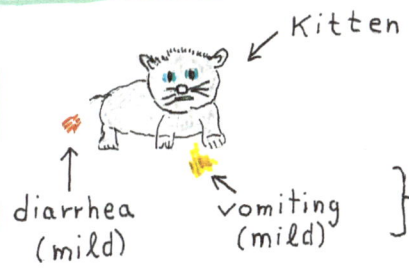

← Kitten

↑ diarrhea (mild)   ↖ vomiting (mild)

} That's Gastro-Enteritis

That means stomach   'Enteron' is the Greek word for intestines

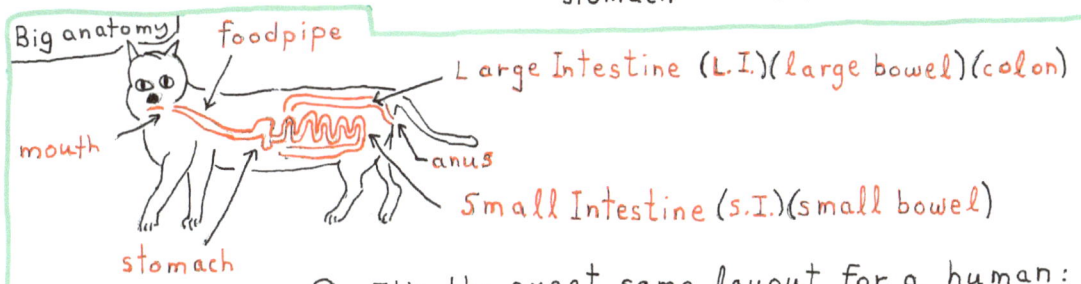

Big anatomy

foodpipe

Large Intestine (L.I.)(large bowel)(colon)

mouth   anus

stomach   Small Intestine (S.I.)(small bowel)

🧑 - It's the exact same layout for a human:
mouth → foodpipe → stomach → S.I. → L.I → anus
'Let's zoom in on the small intestine

Small anatomy

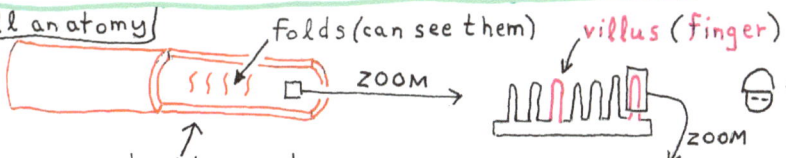

folds (can see them)   villus (finger)

ZOOM →

ZOOM

small intestine cut-away
(cat or human)

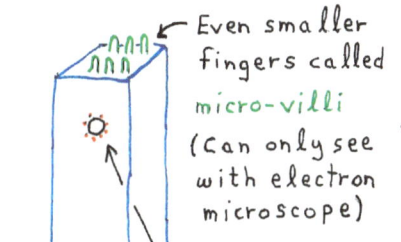

🧑 The velvet-like lining of the small intestine looks like a shag carpet.

Even smaller fingers called micro-villi
(Can only see with electron microscope)

Coronavirus (not to scale)

Food

1 mm (1/25")

blood vessel

ZOOM

BLOOD IN → ← BLOOD OUT
1 villus (1 finger)
- It is made of dozens of rectangular-shaped cells.
- Each finger has a blood supply.

← shag carpet

A villus is like an individual strand of the shag carpet (except it's a super-small strand).

- There are millions of villi in the S.I.

1 finger = villus
Many fingers = villi

entero-cyte
intestine   cell
(Can see with regular microscope)

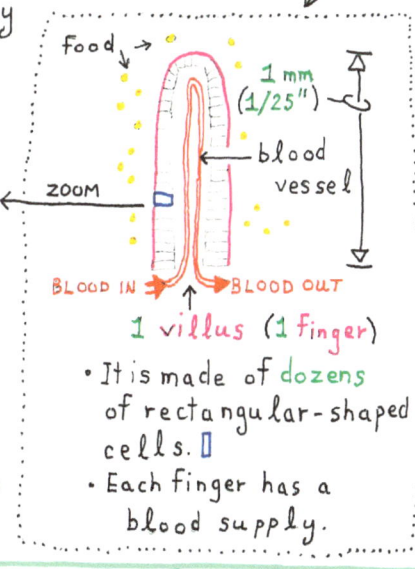

🧑 - "vill eye"
SOMPOO SAYS

Lactose
(milk sugar)

coronavirus
• It's just a shade wider than
each micro-finger

Micro-fingers
(micro-villi)
• 1000s of them

Coronavirus
• It infects and
replicates
in this cell

Entero-cyte
(small intestine cell)
(of a cat)
(could just as easily be a human)

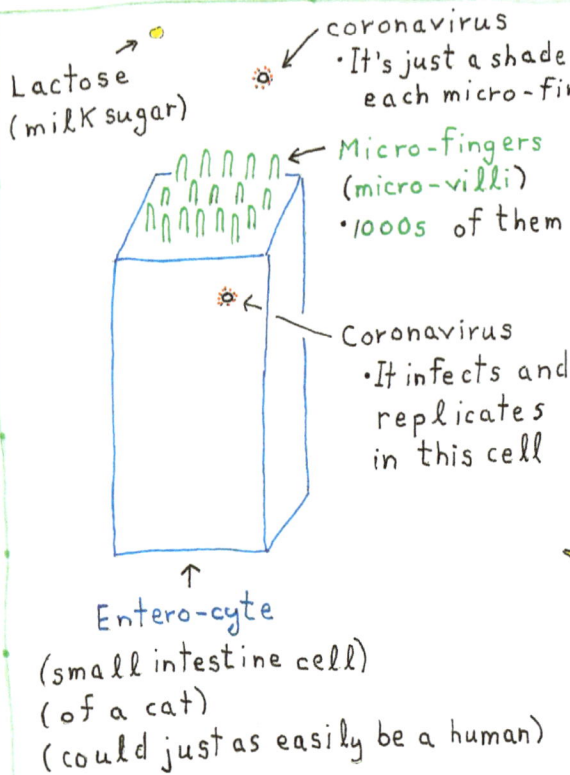

◉ - Okay, the entero-cyte is the
workhorse of the intestines.

- Those micro-villi (micro-fingers)
form the so-called 'brush-border'
where digestion occurs.

• For example, milk sugar (lactose)
gets broken down here. Or not,
resulting in discomfort.

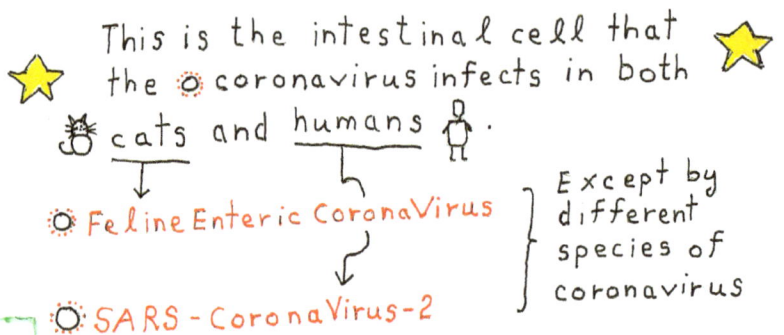

⭐ This is the intestinal cell that
the ◉ coronavirus infects in both
🐱 cats and humans 🧍. ⭐

Except by
different
species of
coronavirus

◉ Feline Enteric CoronaVirus

◉ SARS-CoronaVirus-2

⭐ Some humans only get mild diarrhea
from the coronavirus. It was their
enterocytes that were infected. ⭐

This brings us to a
Key 🔑 Point
about viruses: Tropism

- That means a virus has a preference for:
  - certain animals
  - certain cell types

◉ Coronavirus has a preference for:
  - birds 🐦
  - mammals ← bat 🦇
    cat 🐱
    human 🧍
    Everything else on page 112

Everything else on page 112

And it also likes:
  - Nasal cells ┐ nasal cavity
    cells in the airways
  - Lungs specifically ← cells in the air sacs
  - Entero-cytes in the intestine

By contrast ... the Tobacco Mosaic Virus
likes (tropism) the tobacco plant, specifically
the cells of the leaves.

◉ - "trow-pizm"
SOMPOO
SAYS   rhymes with
        crow

♂ - Do insect gut cells have
     micro-villi?
♀ - Yes. The guts of Kingdom Animalia
     are remarkably similar.

TRIVIA BOX

↙ House of lady with
100 cats
A "cattery" is a place
where cats are bred

13% of cats are carriers
of the ◉ Feline Coronavirus

The Cholera Toxin (CTX)
messes up the entero-cyte.

People with a true gluten
allergy end up losing the
villi (of the shag carpet).
That's called
villous atrophy.

Nasty version

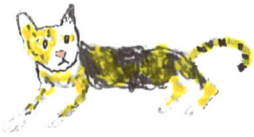

↑
1-year old cat

⊙ **Feline Infectious Peritonitis Virus** (FIPV)
- This is a ⊙ Feline Coronavirus that mutated (inside an enterocyte, it is thought) to the ⊙ Feline Infectious Peritonitis Virus.
- Basically, nice mutated to nasty.

Feline Infectious Peritonitis
- Kind of an umbrella term for lots of badness.
- Most cats are less than 1 year old, and the susceptible ones are:

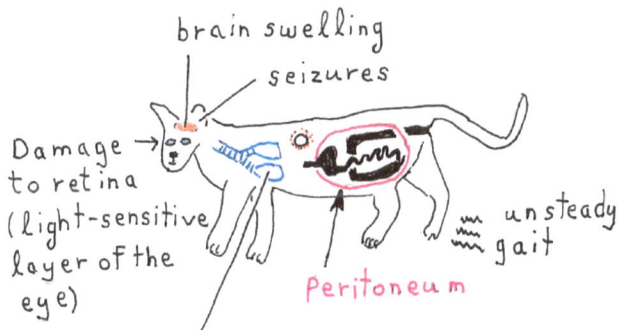

brain swelling
seizures

Damage to retina (light-sensitive layer of the eye)

Peritoneum

unsteady gait

Lungs: difficulty breathing
(= open-mouth breathing in a cat)

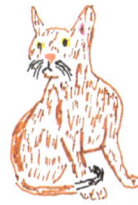

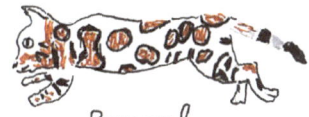

Abyssinian

Bengal

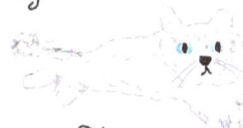

Birman

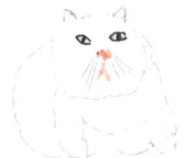

Himalayan

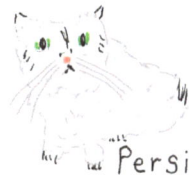

Persian

(All cat drawings from Wikipedia)
[and more or less butchered by AJ]

Peritoneum
- This is the biological Saran Wrap that wraps the abdominal organs.

Peritonitis
- This means the peritoneum is inflamed.
- If your (human) appendix acts up (Appendicitis), it can end up causing Peritonitis.
- In this cat, however, the virus is the problem.

SOMPOO SAYS ⟨ "pair it on Knee um"
"pair it on eye tiss"

Prognosis: Poor (Death in 9 days in a study of 43 cats).
Treatment: 'Supportive', meaning nothing specific. eg, Fluids to maintain hydration

- To summarize, Feline CoronaVirus (FCoV) comes in 2 flavors:

⊙ Feline Enteric CoronaVirus (FECV) → FECV-Associated Gastro-Enteritis
- mildly sick kittens

⊙ Feline Infectious Peritonitis Virus (FIPV) → Feline Infectious Peritonitis (FIP)
- seriously sick <1y old cats

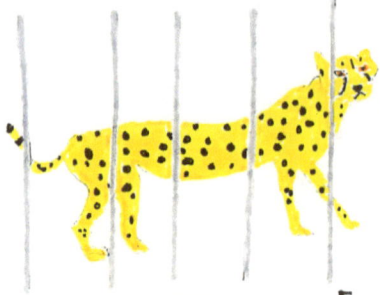

Captive cheetah
- Highly susceptible to the
  ⊙ Feline Infectious Peritonitis Virus

Listen, I'm not Ted Bundy, so set me free.
I want to kill **antelopes**

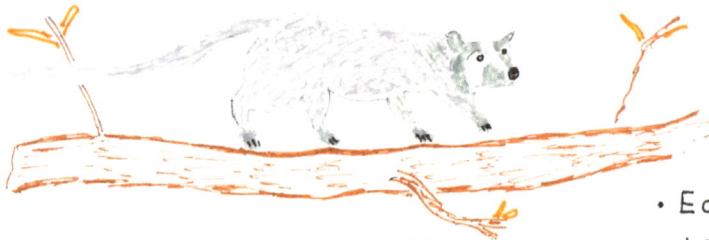

cheetah

↖ zoo bars

Acinonyx jubatus

South-East
Asia

- Eats rats and mangoes. Yum
- Lives in the forest.
- Heavily trafficked and kept
  in captivity to make 'better'
  coffee beans.

Masked palm civet

Paguma larvata

- ?
- It is fed coffee beans.
  Then the defecated
  beans are used to
  make coffee called
  Kopi luwak.

⊙ Civet coronavirus
- This is the SARS CoronaVirus (SARS-CoV-1).

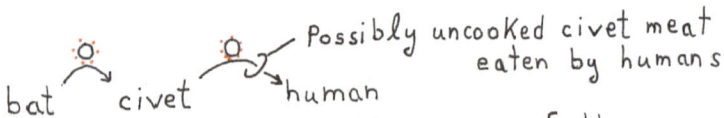

Possibly uncooked civet meat
eaten by humans

bat → civet → human

- This was the cause of the
  2003 SARS pandemic.
- SARS = Severe Acute Respiratory Syndrome

- Get it? A ⊙ coronavirus jumped from a bat to a civet, changed (mutated) in
  the civet to the ⊙ SARS CoronaVirus, then jumped to humans.

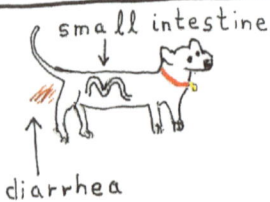

small intestine
↓

⊙ Canine coronavirus
- Infects the small intestine just like the ⊙ Feline coronavirus.
- Diarrhea

CRCoV

↑
diarrhea

dog

Canis familiaris

⊙ Canine Respiratory CoronaVirus (CRCoV)
- Cough a.k.a. Kennel Cough
- Spread by ⌐ dogs coughing and sneezing
            dog bowls
            hands of <u>human</u> handlers

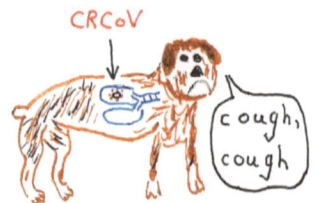

cough,
cough

- These do not
  infect humans.

intestine

European hedgehog a.k.a. Common hedgehog

— Europe

Erinaceus europaeus

- Cute? Yes
- Able to kill poisonous viper snakes?

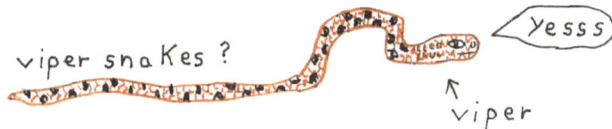

yesss

↑ viper

☼ Hedgehog coronavirus
- Found in hedgehog intestines.
- Unclear if illness results.

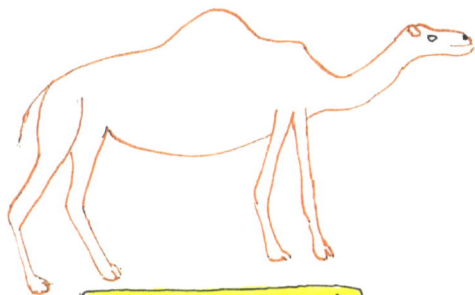

☼ Camel coronavirus
- This is the MERS CoronaVirus
(Middle East Respiratory Syndrome CoronaVirus)
- The camel is a reservoir.
- The camel does not get sick.

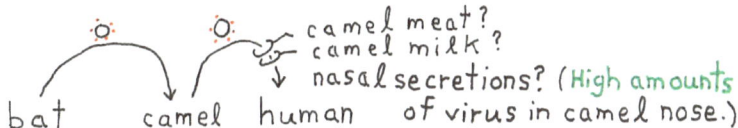

camel meat?
camel milk?
↓ nasal secretions? (High amounts
of virus in camel nose.)
bat   camel   human

- This coronavirus caused the 2012 MERS pandemic.

It spread to
27 countries

Arabian camel
a.K.a.

Dromedary

Camel bio-geography

Bactria
- This is eastern Afghanistan.
- This is about as far east as Alexander the Great
went in 350 B.C., then his men quietly revolted.

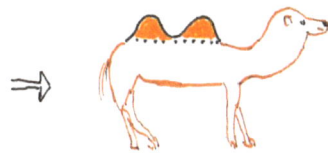

⇒

Bactrian camel
Camelus bactria

Saudi Arabia
- The ☼ MERS CoronaVirus is endemic in camels here.

↳ Meaning, continuously present, right up to today.
The only way to get rid of it would be to
kill the 1,700,000 camels ... which would
cause a huge camel revolt.

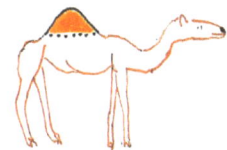

♀ - Does a pregnant 1-hump camel have a 1-hump fetus?
♀ - No. Both species have a 2-humped fetus in the
uterus. But in the Dromedary, the 2 humps fuse
into 1 hump prior to being born.

Dromedary
Camelus dromedarius
(Arabian camel)

- If you tip the B and D backwards,
you'll never forget who is who.

Pangolin

long, sticky tongue
← termite (or ant)

3 massive claws
• To tear apart ⟨ termite mound
                  ant hill

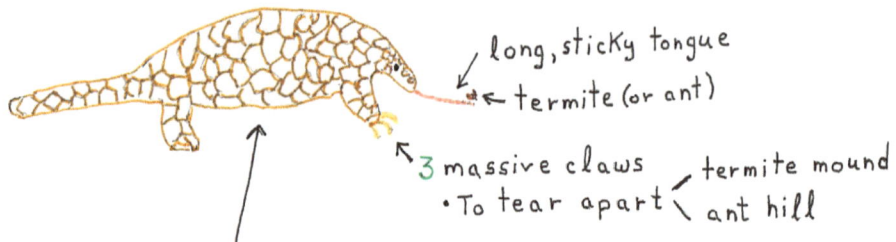

dermal plates (scales)
• 20% of body weight
• Made of the protein Keratin
  (which is the same as our
  fingernails)   ← fingernail

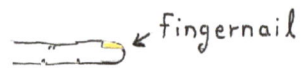

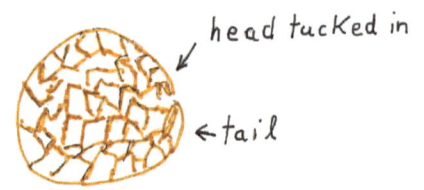

head tucked in
← tail
Pangolin rolled up in a
defensive ball

○ Pangolin coronavirus

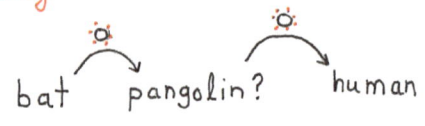

bat → pangolin? → human

• This is our current pandemic.
• But the pangolin coronavirus
  has some question marks ???

Sunda pangolin
Manis javanica
○ Coronavirus infects its lungs.

Thailand
Borneo
Sunda Islands

☺ - What exactly are virologists looking at?

☺ - You'll learn lots
about the
genetic code.

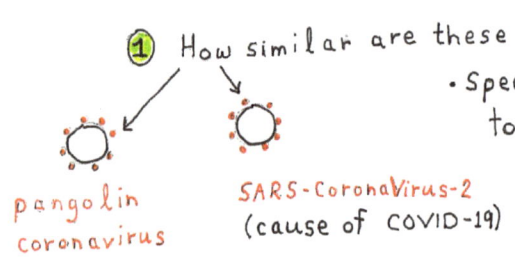

① How similar are these spike proteins?
   • Specifically, how similar is the genetic code
     to make the protein?
   99% = That's pretty close.

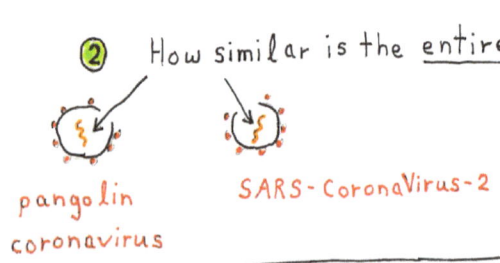

pangolin coronavirus   SARS-CoronaVirus-2
                              (cause of COVID-19)

② How similar is the entire genetic code?
   • That means all the genetic code,
     not just the code for the spike.
   92% = That's why the pangolin
         is not a "slam dunk."

pangolin coronavirus   SARS-CoronaVirus-2

Pangolin features: 38 million years old. That's old. Eats ants and termites. Fabulous
set of front claws. Scales used in herbal medicine ... which means ... drum roll please
... no better than eating your own fingernails. YET THE PANGOLIN IS THE #1 TRAFFICKED
ANIMAL IN THE WORLD.

T
R ↙ Plate tectonics causes
I   Continental Drift.
V • About 7 major plates.
I • They cause disasters.
A

December 26
2004
Earthquake
↓
Tsunami

tsunami →

INDONESIA
☺ - The Burma micro-plate
is part of the larger
Sunda plate

↳ India Plate goes under Burma Plate

[I arrived on
December 28.
It was Krazy]

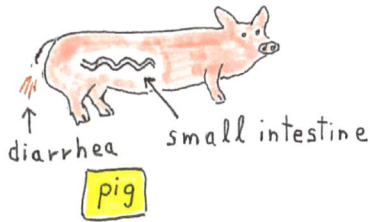

⊙ Porcine Epidemic Diarrhea Virus

nice ↗
- It's a coronavirus.
- It only infects farm pigs. Not wild pigs. And not humans.
- Diarrhea

↑ diarrhea   small intestine ↑

pig

Sus scrofa   _nasty_ ↗

⊙ Porcine Transmissable Gastro-Enteritis Coronavirus

← piglet less than 1-week old → 99% Fatal

↑ diarrhea   ↑ vomiting

(small intestine p. 121)

◉ -Guess where coronavirus lives in the pig? You guessed it - the shag carpet.
- The nasty version destroys the fingers (villi) in the carpet.   ← shag carpet
                                                                    villi (fingers)

◉ - The Latin word 'porcinus' means pig.
  ↘ If you have an infected ♡ valve or leaky ♡ valve, a ♡ surgeon can
    replace it with one from a pig. That's called a _porcine_ valve.
  ↘ If it comes from a cow, it's a _bovine_ valve.

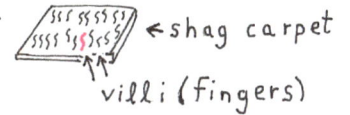

◉ SOMPOO SAYS: "poor seen"   "bow vine"

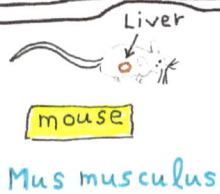

Liver

mouse

Mus musculus

◉ -The Latin word
  'murinus' means
  mouse.

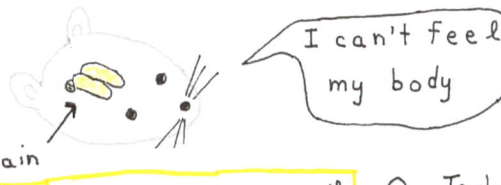

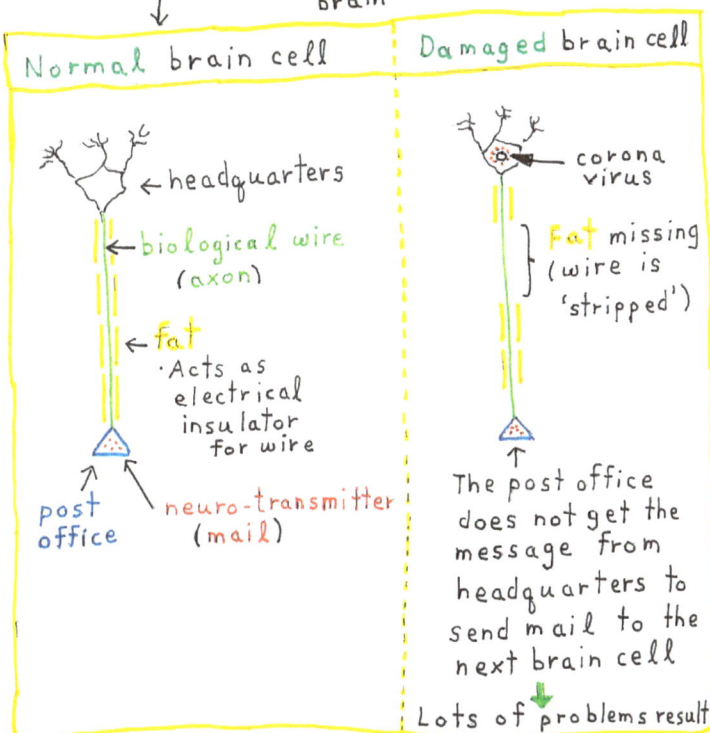

⊙ Murine coronavirus

◉ - Well, it turns out that coronavirus likes mouse liver.
  ↘ So the other name is ⊙ Murine Hepatitis Virus (MHV).
  ↘ And it also turns out that the mouse's
    brain cell wires get 'stripped.' What?

ZOOM mouse
      brain

[I can't feel my body]

Normal brain cell | **Damaged brain cell**

← headquarters

← biological wire (axon)

corona virus

← Fat · Acts as electrical insulator for wire

Fat missing (wire is 'stripped')

post office   neuro-transmitter (mail)

↑ The post office does not get the message from headquarters to send mail to the next brain cell

Lots of problems result ↓

◉ - Technically, the fat insulating the wire is called the myelin sheath (or just myelin).
- If there is damage, it's called de-myelination.
- Scientists deliberately infect the mouse with ⊙ coronavirus to act as an animal model of the human disease called Multiple Sclerosis (MS).

Multiple regions of de-myelination in the brain and spinal cord

This means there is 'hardening' (think, scar tissue) wherever the fat is damaged.

◉ - Get it? The wire is okay. It's the insulation that gets damaged.

◉ SOMPOO SAYS - "dee my Ellen nation"

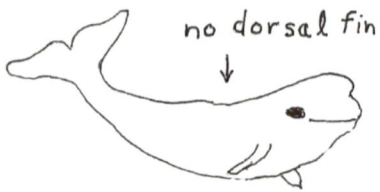

no dorsal fin
↓

☉ Beluga Whale CoronaVirus (BWCoV)

- Found in the liver of a 13-year old male beluga whale that died in captivity in 2008.
- Did the virus kill the whale? Maybe.
  It had both liver disease and lung disease.
- This is 1 reported case. Hard to draw conclusions.

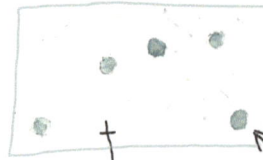

beluga whale

Delphinapterus leucas

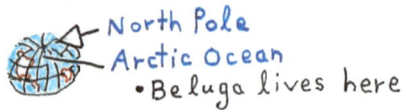

- North Pole
- Arctic Ocean
- Beluga lives here

- Likes to eat Arctic cod.

miws nac elahw aguleb A - ☉
.sdrawKcab

← fuzzy photo from electron microscope
- Magnified 129,000 x

↙ coronavirus

beluga whale liver biopsy

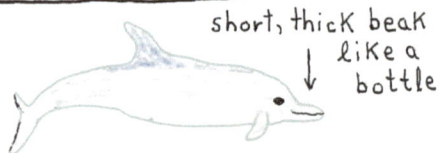

---

short, thick beak like a bottle
↓

☉ Bottlenose dolphin CoronaVirus (BdCoV)

- This was isolated from fecal samples from 3 dolphins.

'Viral load' was 1000-100,000 viruses per milli-liter (1/30th ounce) of feces.

Indo-Pacific bottlenose dolphin

Tursiops aduncus

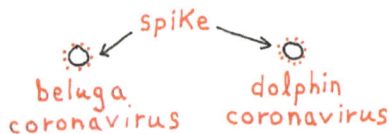

spike

beluga coronavirus → dolphin coronavirus

74% similarity of genetic code for spike protein

They both belong to Group 3, the gamma (γ) coronaviruses.
(Rember the sock drawers?)

Professor: Alright, any volunteers to collect those fecal samples?

Underling #1: Um, I can't. My mom texted me — she has a nose bleed

Underling #2: I'm having a palm reading at 3 p.m.

Underling #3: !

☉ - Whales, dolphins and seals are marine mammals.

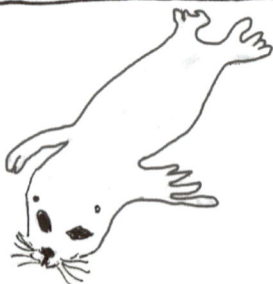

☉ Harbor Seal CoronaVirus (HSCoV)

- Isolated from 21 dead harbor seals in 2010.
- Lots of lung damage, specifically 'congestion,' meaning fluid in the lungs.
- Plus Lobar Pneumonia which is characteristic of bacteria, not viruses.
- Plus bacteria in lungs.
- Contribution of ☉ coronavirus unclear.

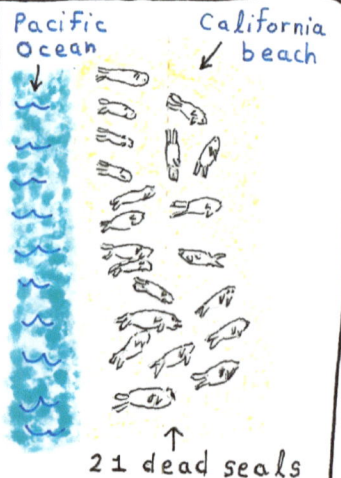

Harbor seal

Phoca vitulina

- A harbor seal pup can swim 1 hour after it is born.

Pacific Ocean

California beach

21 dead seals

- I lied.
  ` Coronavirus infects <u>lots and lots</u> of animals. Here are the rest.

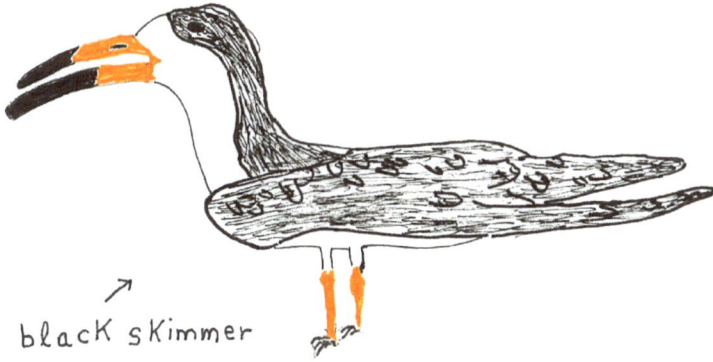

black skimmer

· Likes to lay flat on the ground.
  How strange is that?

☼ Coronavirus was found in a black skimmer
  in Brazil in 2009.

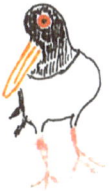

European
oystercatcher ☼

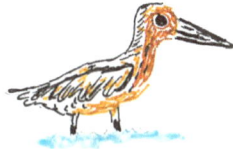

Red Knot ☼

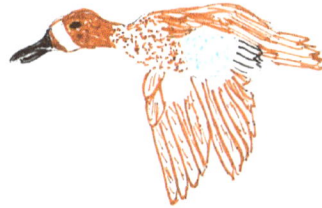

Blue-winged teal ☼

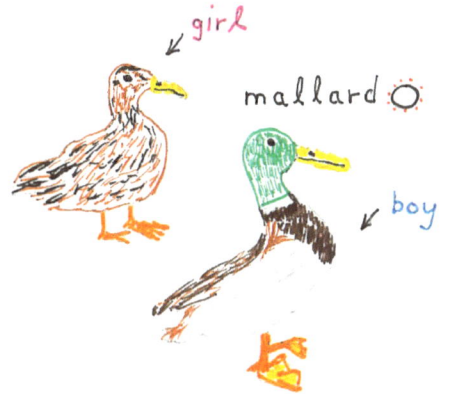

girl
mallard ☼
boy

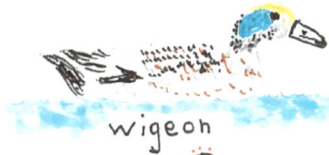

wigeon ☼

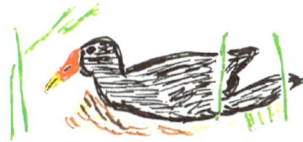

Common moorhen ☼

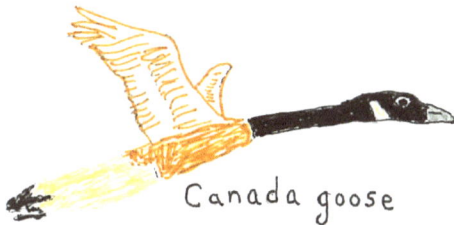

Canada goose

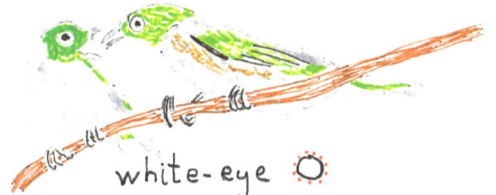

white-eye ☼
· 3 toes forward
  <u>1</u> toe backwards
  (like the Bulbul)

Victoria Island
· Canada's 2nd biggest
  island

Baffin Island
· Canada's
  biggest
  island

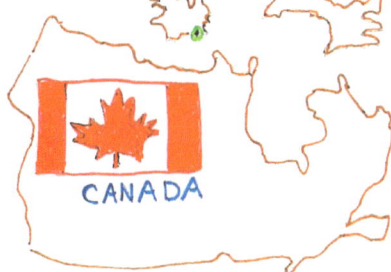

CANADA

☼ Canada goose coronavirus strain Cambridge Bay 2017

· This was isolated from a Canada goose that died
  at Cambridge Bay ● on the south coast of Victoria Island.

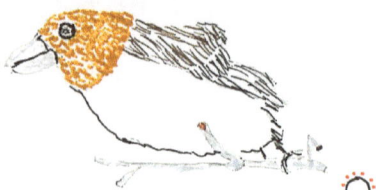

white-rumped munia
- Linguists study them because they have grammar rules when learning to sing.

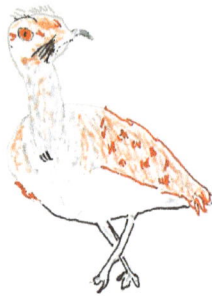

Houbara bustard

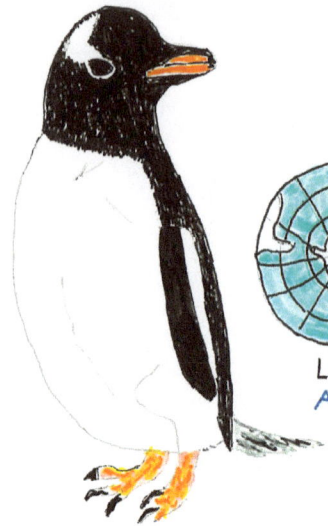

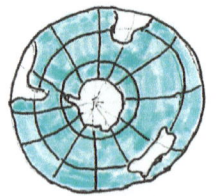

Lives in Antarctica

Gentoo penguin
Gentoo penguin virus isolate Antarctic1
- This coronavirus was discovered in Antarctica.

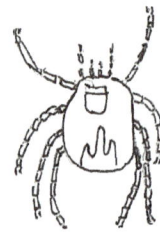

seabird tick
Ixodes uriae
- Amazingly, this sucks on gentoo penguin blood

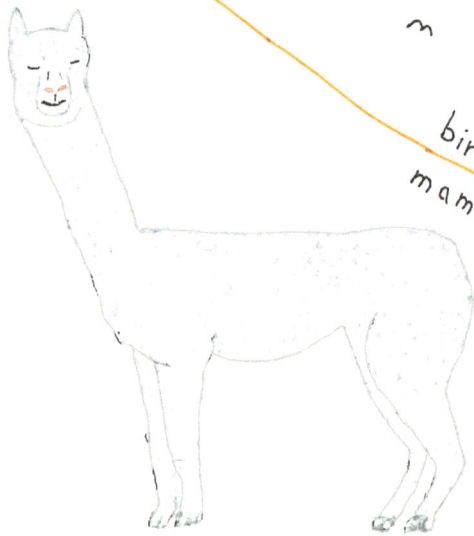

birds
mammals

alpaca
Alpaca respiratory coronavirus isolate CA08-1/2008

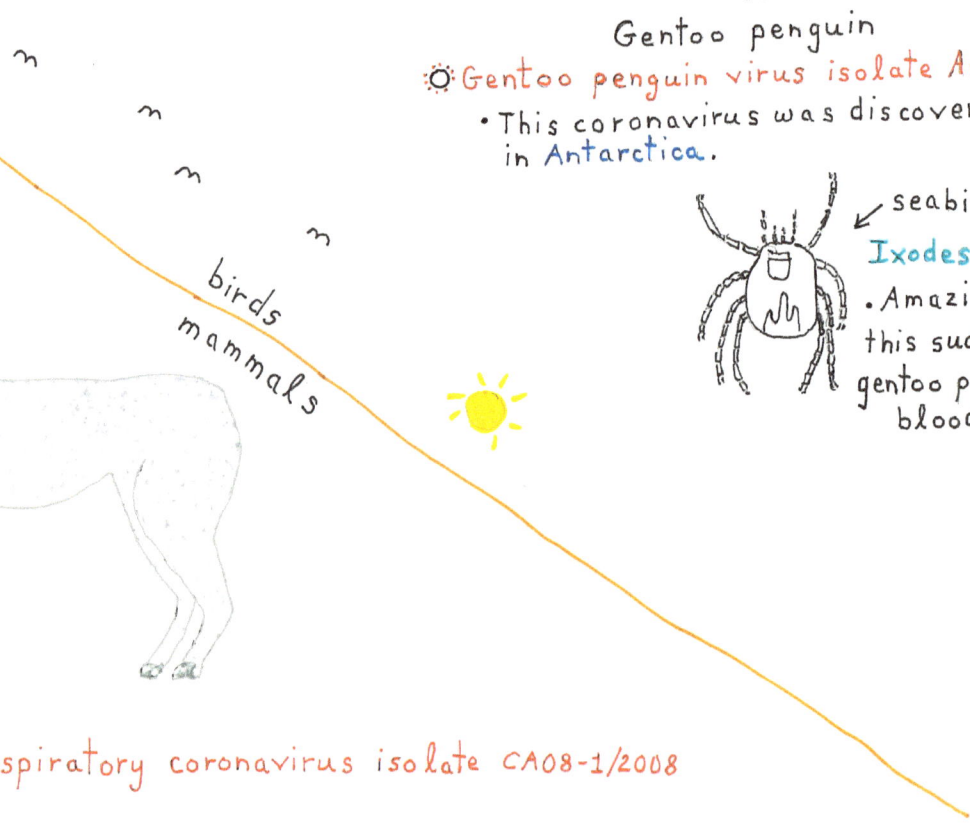

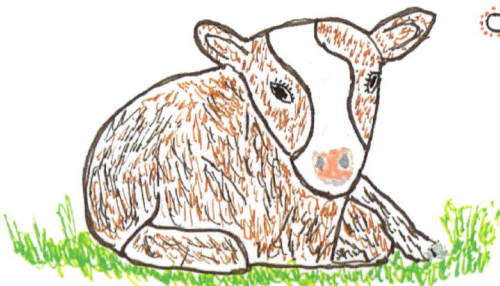

Bovine coronavirus cow/WDBR-1005/BRA/2003
species   strain
- This causes Neo-natal Diarrhea in a cow calf.
  new   born
- This one was isolated from cow feces in Brazil in 2003.

Cow calf
(cattle)
Bos taurus → If you were born April 20 to May 20, then your horoscope sign is Taurus. ♉

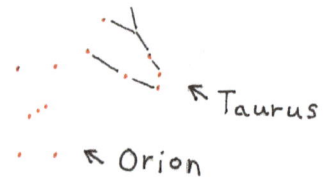

Taurus

Orion

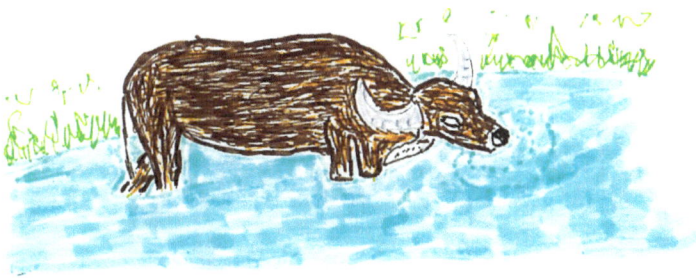

water buffalo   (Bubalus bubalis)
- There are 130 million water buffalos on planet Earth
- ☼ Bovine coronavirus Bubalus

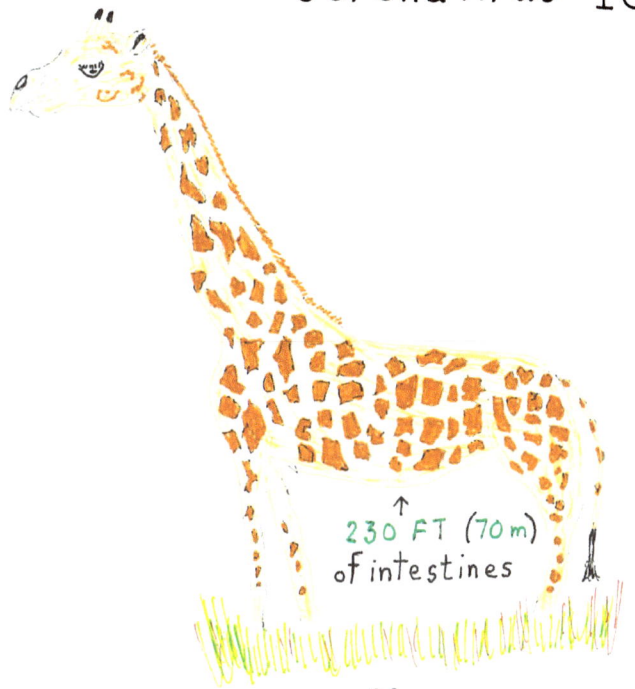

Sambar deer
- Lives in India but ☼ coronavirus was isolated from one in Ohio, USA in 1994 (presumably a game park)

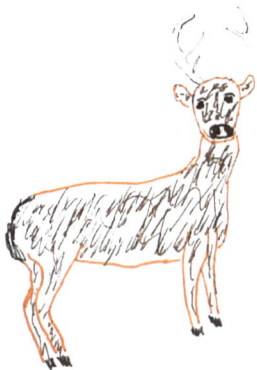

230 FT (70m) of intestines

Giraffe

☼ Giraffe CoronaVirus US/OH3/2003 (GiCoV-OH3)
- This was isolated from a giraffe in a game park in Ohio, USA in 2003.
- It causes mild to severe Diarrhea in giraffes.

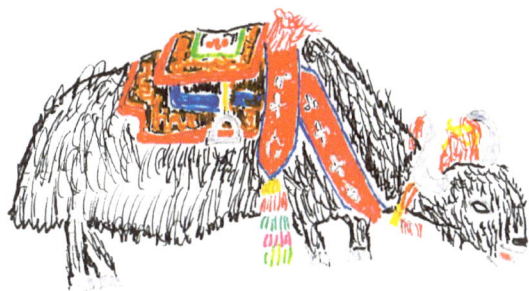

Domestic yak (this one in Tibet)

Bos grunniens
↑
Same Genus as a cow

☼ Yak coronavirus strain YAK/HY24/CH/2017
- Isolated from a yak in China in 2017.

या ω या'
↑
"yak" in Tibetan language

Grammar rules vary when it comes to the order of Subject (S), Object (O), Verb (V).

Yak eats grass = English (SVO)
Yak grass eats = Tibetan (SOV)
Grass yak eats = Yoda   (OSV)

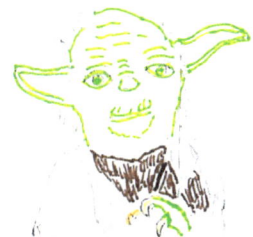

Hee, hee, hee
ha, ha, ha

⊙ Spotted hyena coronavirus
• Diarrhea

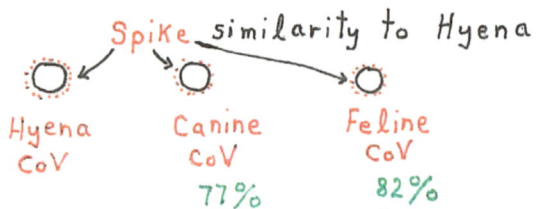

Spike similarity to Hyena

⊙ → ⊙ → ⊙

Hyena   Canine   Feline
CoV   CoV   CoV
         77%   82%

Despite the similarity, the hyena
does not suffer any illness that
resembles Feline Infectious Peritonitis
(which would be no laughing matter).

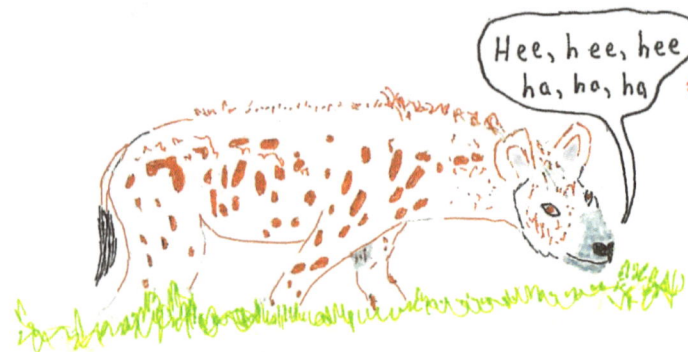

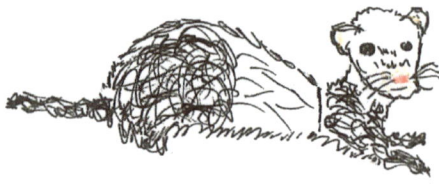

Spotted hyena a.k.a. Laughing hyena
Crocuta crocuta

Ferret

⊙ Ferret systemic coronavirus
└ That means it has spread
throughout the body.
• Can be highly fatal to ferrets.

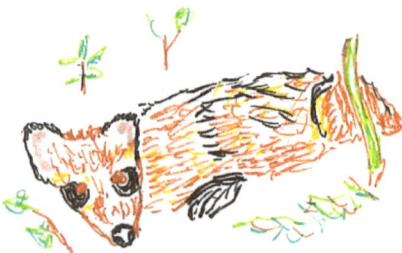

American mink
Neovison vison

⊙ Mink coronavirus 1
• Isolated from the feces of an
American mink in Denmark in 2015.
• The 'American' mink lives in:
    N America ⚥ — Europe
    S America —

raccoon dog
• Loosely implicated in
SARS pandemic of 2003

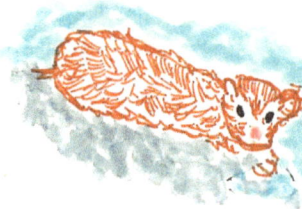

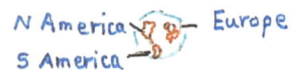

◉ - Okay, that's about it for animals infected by ⊙ coronavirus.

'But there is an additional scenario to consider ... ⟿

♀ - I thought 'species' was always lower case like the poems of e e cummings?
♂ - The rules are a bit different for virus taxonomy.
- Alpha/Beta/Gamma/Delta (page 113) are the 4 choices for the coronavirus Genus.
- But the species name is so long that the first word tends to be Capitalized.
- And a 'strain' is kind of like a sub-species.
                              e.g. Spotted hyena coronavirus

[3] Has a human transmitted ⊙ coronavirus to an animal in the current pandemic? [4] And did that animal transmit it back to humans?

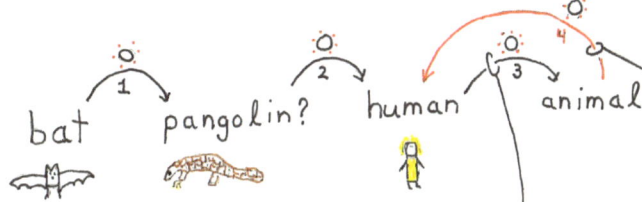

bat →1 pangolin? →2 human →3 animal →4 ⊙

This has happened

This has not happened as far as anyone knows

- The following 13 animals have tested POSITIVE for ⊙ SARS-CoronaVirus-2.

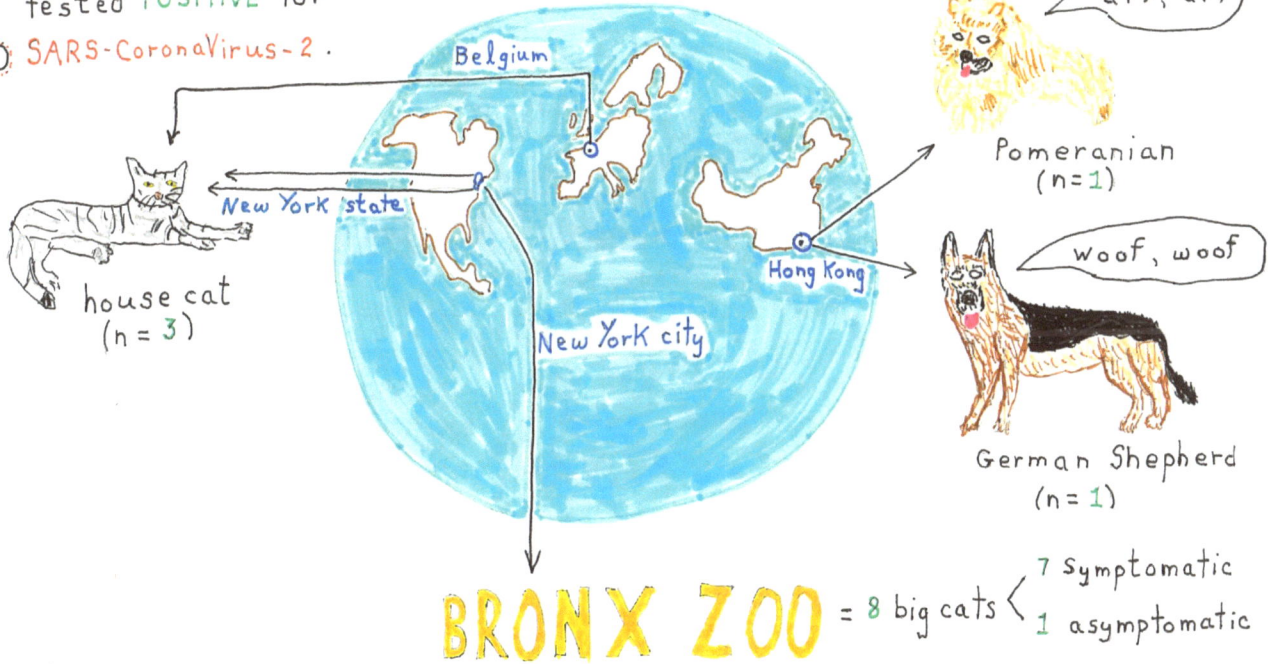

Belgium

New York state

house cat (n = 3)

Hong Kong

New York city

arf, arf

Pomeranian (n = 1)

woof, woof

German Shepherd (n = 1)

BRONX ZOO = 8 big cats ⟨ 7 symptomatic / 1 asymptomatic

lioness

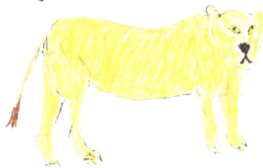

African lion (n = 3)
· Adamma
· Nala   ⟩ triplet sisters
· Shani

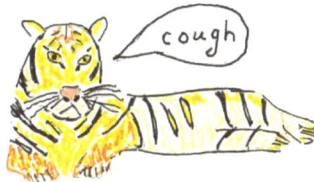

cough

Malayan tiger (n = 3)
· Nadia ⟩ sisters
· Azul
· Bumi ♂

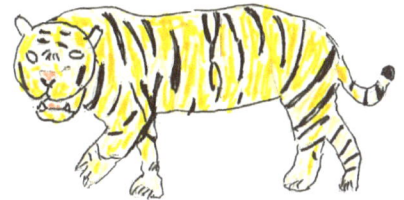

Siberian tiger (n = 2)
· Bashuta ♂
· Julian ♂

INVESTIGATION 2 April 2020
· Nadia (4 years old) has a cough and ↓ appetite → swabs taken from ⟨ nose / mouth / trachea (windpipe)
· The other 7 big cats → fecal (poop) samples

This requires being put to sleep with General Anesthetic

RESULTS All 8 big cats are ⊙ SARS-CoronaVirus-2 POSITIVE. They all recover.

CONCLUSION An asymptomatic zookeeper (identity unknown) probably infected them.

ACTION As punishment, a random zookeeper is chosen by drawing straws and fed to the lions.
Just Kidding.

- The mammal called a 'human' is infected by 7 different coronaviruses.

#1

Human

Homo   sapiens

↑   ↑

Genus   species

☼ Human CoronaVirus 229E (HCoV-229E)

· Found in humans and bats.

This virus is pretty mild. You get the Common Cold.

droplet → ZOOM →

AAACHOO

Coronavirus in nasal passages

· Inhales droplet
· Or touches it

This is a "droplet infection," meaning it was spread (transmitted) by droplets.

- What is a cold?
- I'll rephrase your question: Which body parts get infected by cold viruses?

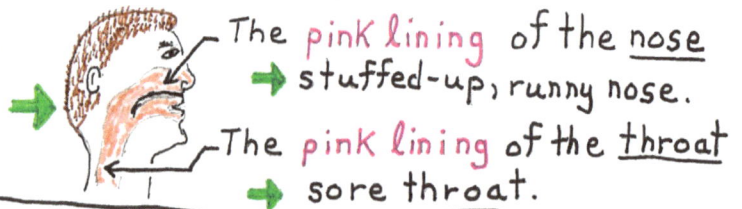

→ The pink lining of the nose
   ⇒ stuffed-up, runny nose.

→ The pink lining of the throat
   ⇒ sore throat.

- Time for a history lesson. The Common Cold Unit (CCU) was a research facility that studied colds in England from 1946 - 1989.

I say, old chap, I'll give you sixpence if you allow me to infect you with a cold virus.

virologist

Blimey, that sounds jolly good.

volunteer

Stonehenge

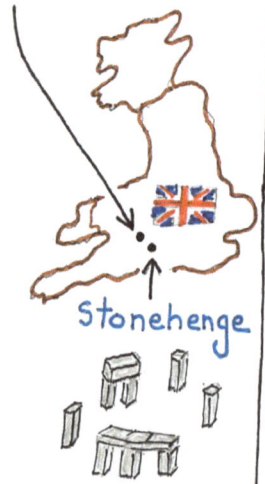

- Here's what they found out:
  ✿ Rhino-viruses cause 50% of colds.
  ☼ Corona-viruses cause 10% of colds.
  · In fact, the CCU discovered the coronavirus in 1965 and published that in **The British Medical Journal**:
  Cultivation of a novel type of common-cold virus in organ cultures

  · Then in 1968 they created the name 'coronaviruses'. That was in the science journal called **Nature**.

- By the way, 229E was from a student volunteer at a biology lab at the University of Chicago.

#2

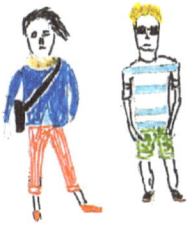

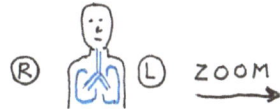

Homo sapiens

○ Human CoronaVirus NL63 (HCoV-NL63)

• This virus was first identified in a 7-month old child in the Netherlands.

• The infection was Bronchiolitis. What?

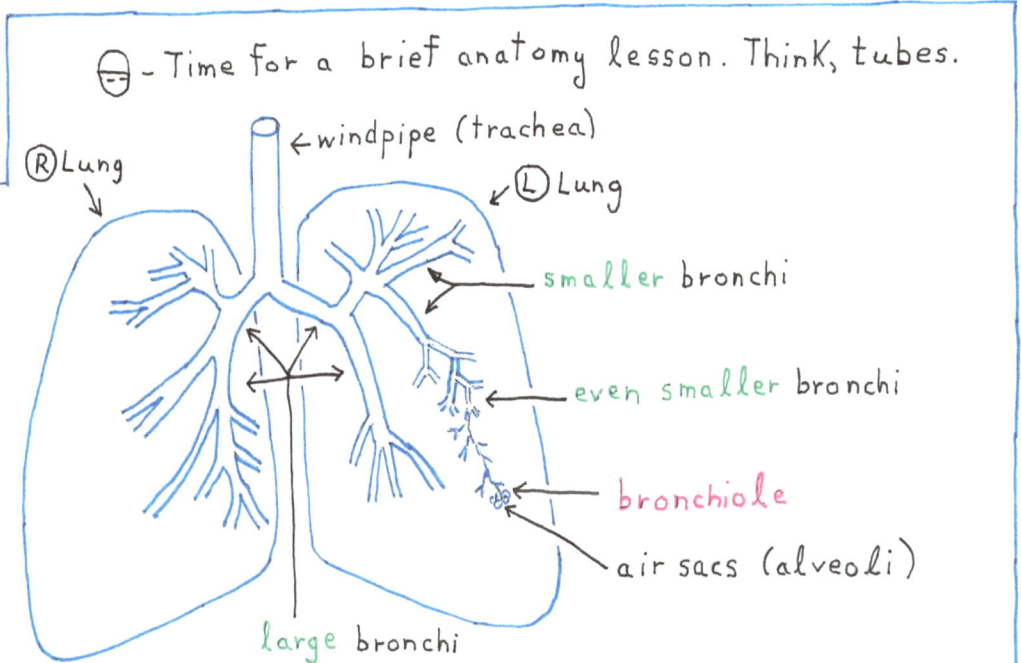

😑 - Time for a brief anatomy lesson. Think, tubes.

← windpipe (trachea)

Ⓡ Lung

↙ Ⓛ Lung

smaller bronchi

even smaller bronchi

bronchiole

air sacs (alveoli)

large bronchi

Ⓡ 🧍 Ⓛ ZOOM →

😑 - The default in anatomy drawings is that you are facing the patient. Their Ⓡ is your Ⓛ.

Airflow goes like this:

air → nose/mouth → windpipe (trachea) → bronchi → bronchioles → air sacs

These are the 'airways.'
They are tubes.

😑 - The airway divides many times.
  When the tube diameter is less than 1mm (1/25th ") , that's a bronchiole.
  The ○ CoronaVirus NL63 infects and irritates the bronchioles, and that's called bronchiolitis.

😑 - When you have a standard chest cough, it's usually bronchitis (in the bronchi).
  Can ○ coronavirus cause that? Yes. So can Influenza A virus.

  Heavy smokers 🚬 may cough every day (which to them is normal but actually isn't). The smoke irritates the bronchi. This is called Chronic Bronchitis.

Chronic Bronchitis plus Emphysema is COPD (Chronic Obstructive Pulmonary Disease).

😑 SOMPOO SAYS
  「 "brong key ole" ━━ rhymes with hole
  「 "brong key ole eye tiss"

#3

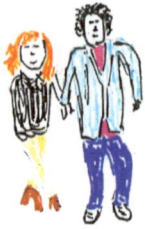

Human

Homo sapiens

⭕ Human CoronaVirus HKU1 (HCoV-HKU1)

- The first identified case was a 71-year-old man in Hong Kong.
  - He had Pneumonia in both lungs which patients call 'double pneumonia' but doctors call it bi-lateral pneumonia.

  2 sides

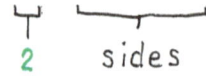

- It also causes { Common Cold
                   Bronchiolitis

😐 - The sample from the man was renamed 'Hong Kong University, sample 1.'

∴ HKU1

#4

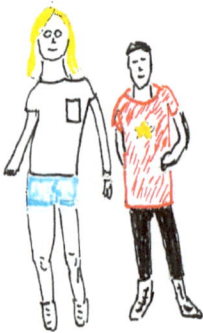

Human

Homo sapiens

Latin for 'man' Latin for 'wise'

⭕ Human CoronaVirus OC43 (HCoV-OC43)

↑ That's a letter 'O' as in Oscar

- Common Cold

- It has similarity to the
  ⭕ Canine Respiratory Coronavirus that causes Kennel cough in dogs.

😐 - This was 'Organ Culture 43' at the Common Cold Unit.

∴ OC43

Interestingly, in an algebra book in 1659 the Swiss mathematican Johann Rahn created the symbols ∴ (therefore) and ÷ (divide).

♀ - Are all those humans wearing clothes from The Gap?

♀ - I was wondering that myself.

- The next 3 coronaviruses (#5, #6, #7) have caused pandemics and death [RIP]
  SARS   MERS   COVID-19

#5

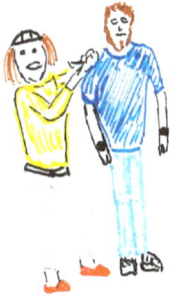
Human
Homo sapiens

○ Severe Acute Respiratory Syndrome CoronaVirus (SARS-CoV)(SARS-CoV-1)
• It's called "SARS" to refer to the illness.

• Pneumonia→ Acute Respiratory Distress Syndrome (ARDS)→ death
  Does everyone progress to this? No.   Everyone? No.

$$\frac{774 \text{ deaths [RIP]}}{8098 \text{ cases}} = 10\% \text{ Case Fatality Rate (CFR)}$$

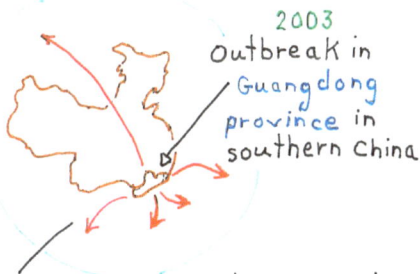
2003
Outbreak in Guangdong province in southern China

Pandemic: spreads to 25 countries
• Last reported case in 2004.

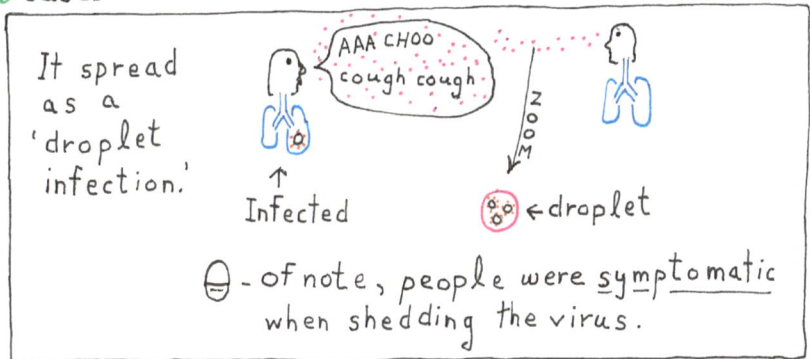
It spread as a 'droplet infection.'
AAA CHOO cough cough
ZOOM
Infected   ←droplet
- of note, people were symptomatic when shedding the virus.

SOMPOO SAYS - "A,R,D,S" (each letter is said aloud)

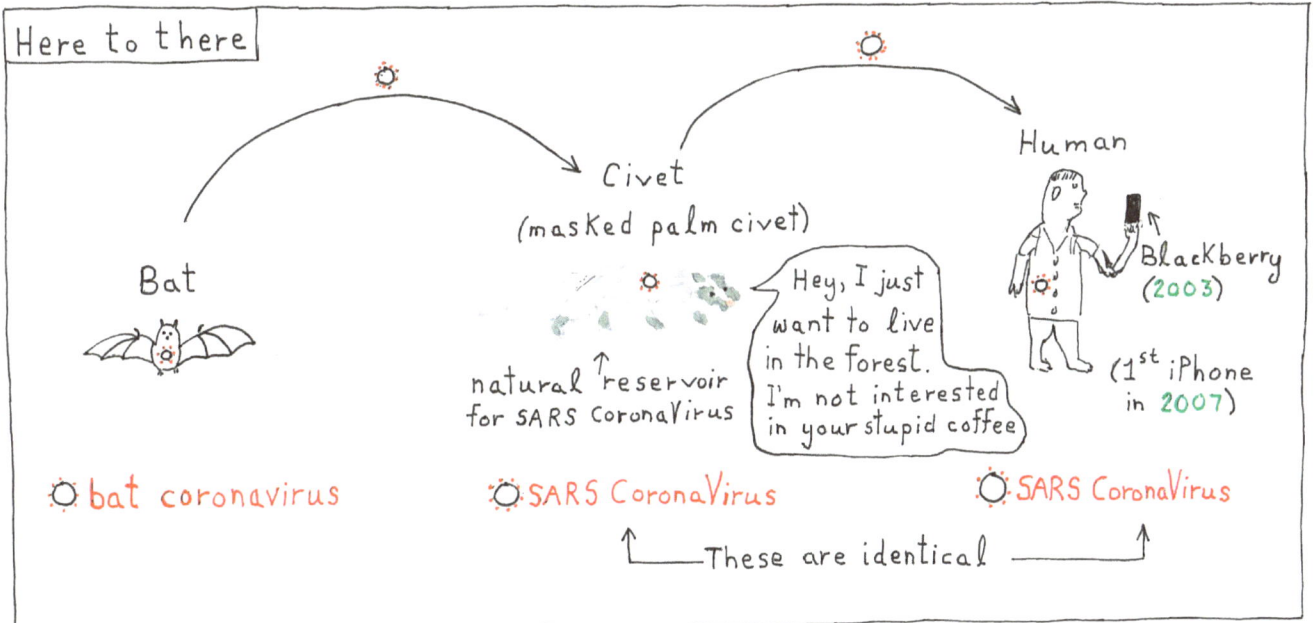
Here to there
Bat
○ bat coronavirus
Civet (masked palm civet)
natural ↑ reservoir for SARS CoronaVirus
Hey, I just want to live in the forest. I'm not interested in your stupid coffee
○ SARS CoronaVirus
Human
Blackberry (2003)
(1st iPhone in 2007)
○ SARS CoronaVirus
These are identical

- China - well, someone in China - Kills 10,000 civets to ↓ spread to humans.

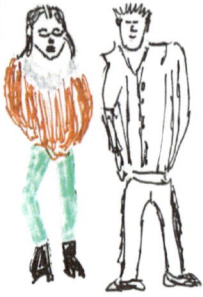

Human

Homo sapiens

☼ Middle East Respiratory Syndrome CoronaVirus (MERS-CoV)(MERS-HCoV)
• Sometimes called 2012-nCoV
  └ n = novel (as in, new).
  └ The year the pandemic started.

┐ for
H for
Human

• It's just called "MERS" to refer to the illness.

• Pneumonia ─┌→ Acute Respiratory Distress Syndrome (ARDS) ─┌→ death
                                    ↑   Everyone? No.
  Everyone? No.   details later   34%, yes.

SOMPOO SAYS "MERS" rhymes with hers

☼ Saudi Arabia 2012
• Outbreak (= epidemic in a limited geographical area)

Spread to other countries, hence a pandemic.
• 27 countries in total, as of 2020

858 deaths [RIP]
────────── = 34% Case Fatality Rate
2494 cases
      ↑
This data from the WHO
as of November 2019

- The ☼ MERS Coronavirus is still spreading!
  ... just very (very) slowly. You'd have to
  go to Saudi Arabia and kiss a camel's nose.
- People with MERS died/die of lung problems
  just like people with our current COVID-19.
  But far fewer.
- Even if these went unrecognized and there were
  1000 new MERS deaths (a generous overestimate)
  it would cause only a tiny distortion of COVID deaths
  (661,000 as of 29 July 2020).
       1000/661,000 = 0.15% MERS
  Restated, 99.85% of deaths by COVID.

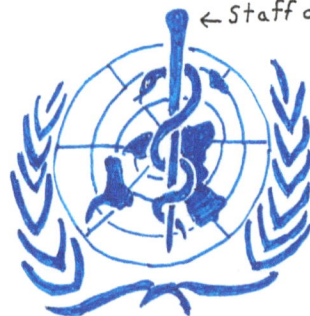

← Staff of Asclepius (the God of Medicine)

← WHO logo

World Health Organization

HQ in
Geneva,
Switzerland

Here to there

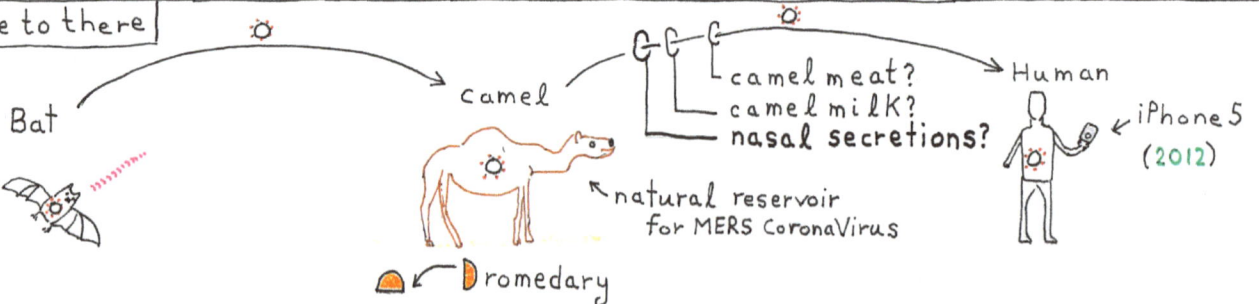

Bat

camel ─┌┌┌ camel meat?
              camel milk?
              nasal secretions? → Human
                                     ← iPhone 5
                                        (2012)
      ↖ natural reservoir
        for MERS CoronaVirus

[Dromedary]

☼ Pipistrellus bat coronavirus   ☼ MERS CoronaVirus   ☼ MERS CoronaVirus
☼ Tylonycteris bat coronavirus
                                    └── These are identical ──┘
        └──────────────── These are related ────────────────┘

#7

○ Severe Acute Respiratory Syndrome CoronaVirus-2

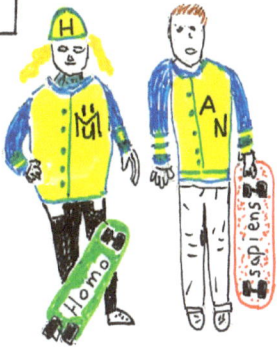

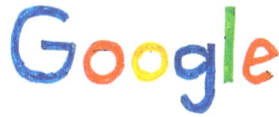

Google

🔍 Is Best Buy open during COVID-19? ✕

😐 -In case you arrived late, this coronavirus is the one currently wreaking havoc on our lives.

| Same, same |

😐 -You may encounter different names for the virus.
-They all mean the same thing.

◆ 2019-nCoV
　CoronaVirus
　n = novel (new)
　Year of discovery

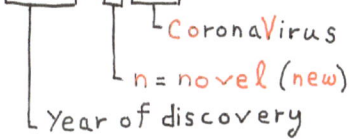

😐 - This was the original name assigned to the virus in the **New England Journal of Medicine** (one of the top journals in medicine) on 24 January 2020 in an article titled:

A novel coronavirus from patients with pneumonia in China

◆ Wuhan Human 1 Coronavirus
　. This name was assigned in the journal **Nature** (a top-tier science journal) on 3 February 2020 in an article titled:

　　A pneumonia outbreak associated with a new coronavirus of probable bat origin

◆ WHCV

◆ Severe Acute Respiratory Syndrome CoronaVirus-2
　.This is the official name as of 11 February 2020.
　.It was assigned by the Coronavirus Study Group of the International Committee on Taxonomy of Viruses (ICTV).
　.The CDC and WHO use this name.

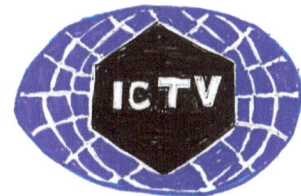

◆ SARS-CoV-2

◆ CoV-2
　😐 - "Kow vee 2"
　SOMPOO　rhymes with low
　SAYS

ICTV

We met them before. They have assigned an official name to 6590 viruses.

◆ COVID-19 virus
◆ COVID Coronavirus
◆ Coronavirus
　.If you hear this, 99.999% chance it means this particular coronavirus.

Here to there

Intermediate horseshoe bat
- Natural reservoir for
⊙ SARS-CoronaVirus-2 ?

Pangolin?

⊙ Pangolin coronavirus

iPhone 11 (2019)
← Samsung Galaxy Fold (2019)
↖ Google Pixel 4 (2019)

Human

~ SARS-CoronaVirus-2 (COVID-19)

spike 99% similar
Genetic code 92% similar

└ Not close enough to say with certainty that the pangolin is the middle man.

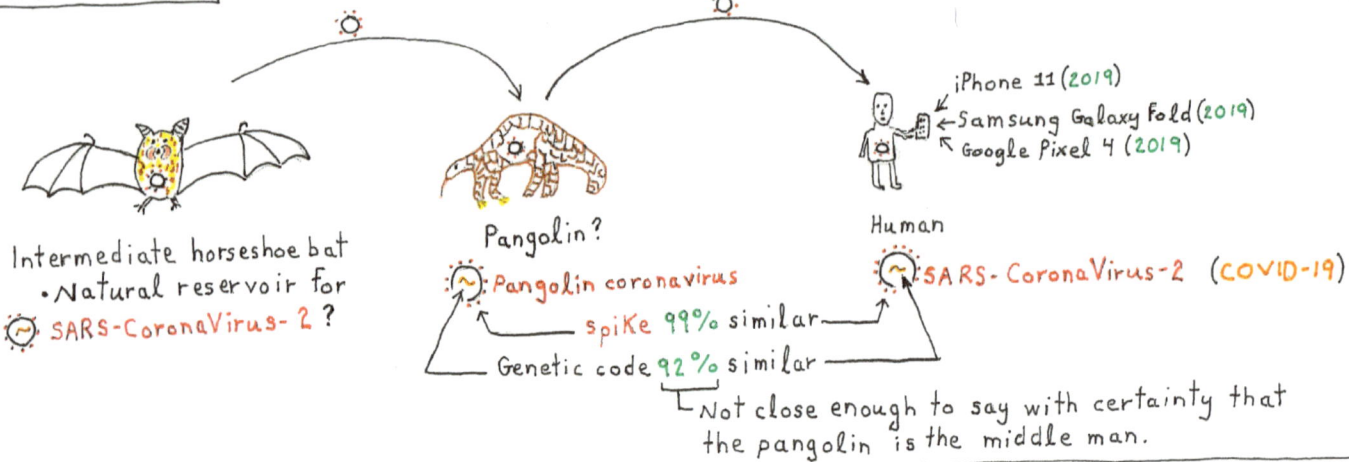

☺ - Let's compare Case Fatality Rates

SARS (2003) $\dfrac{774 \text{ deaths}}{8098 \text{ cases}}$ 🪦 = 10% Case Fatality Rate (CFR)

⊙ SARS-CoronaVirus-1

MERS (2012) $\dfrac{858 \text{ deaths}}{2494 \text{ cases}}$ 🪦 = 34% Case Fatality Rate (CFR)

⊙ MERS-CoronaVirus

COVID (2019) $\dfrac{6,881,995 \text{ deaths}}{676,169,955 \text{ cases}}$ 🪦 = 1% Case Fatality Rate (CFR)
↖ 10 March 2023

⊙ SARS-CoronaVirus-2
(I'm silent but deadly, like a nasty fart from Mother Nature)

⚥ - That's no way to talk about Mother Nature.
⚥ - She also releases super-volcanoes. She's not always motherly

---

☺ - What's special about COVID?

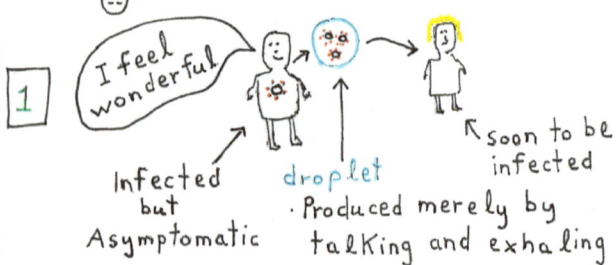

1 (I feel wonderful)

Infected but Asymptomatic

droplet
- Produced merely by talking and exhaling

↖ soon to be infected

☺ - People infected with the COVID coronavirus spread it to others even when they feel perfectly fine (asymptomatic).

‵ Whereas with the SARS coronavirus-1 people shed the virus only when they were coughing and sneezing (symptomatic).

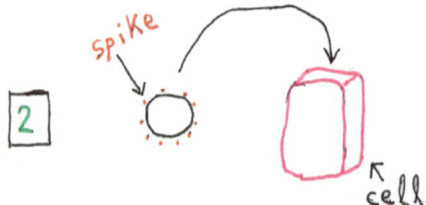

2 spike ↓

cell

☺ - A subtle mutation to the spike (a.k.a. S-protein) makes the COVID coronavirus more efficient at entering our cells.

⊖ - Let's collect our thoughts.

· There's a virus. It gets into us. It makes copies of itself
(or rather we do that for it, thank you very much). Then
it leaves without saying goodbye and infects someone else.

· Where <u>exactly</u> does it get <u>into</u> us? We need to learn some
anatomy. Actually, a lot of anatomy, because wherever the
virus goes, badness tends to follow.

· Somebody is generating the droplets the virus travels in.
That somebody is bats, pangolins (yes, a ? as usual) and humans.
And since we cannot put masks on bats and pangolins, we
need to understand masks and droplets in nitty gritty detail.

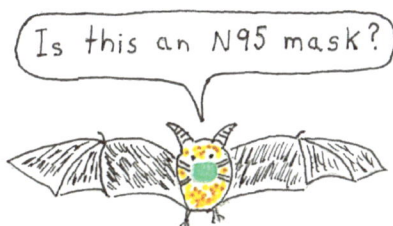

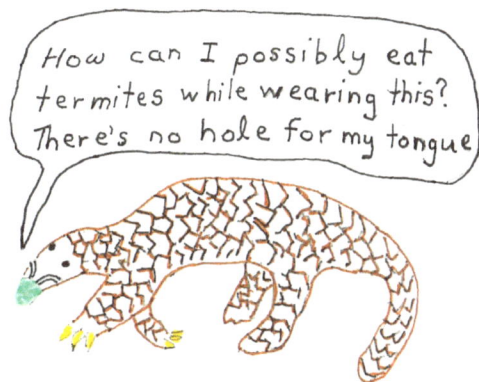

Is this an N95 mask?

How can I possibly eat
termites while wearing this?
There's no hole for my tongue

Location, Location, Location
Anatomy, Anatomy, Anatomy

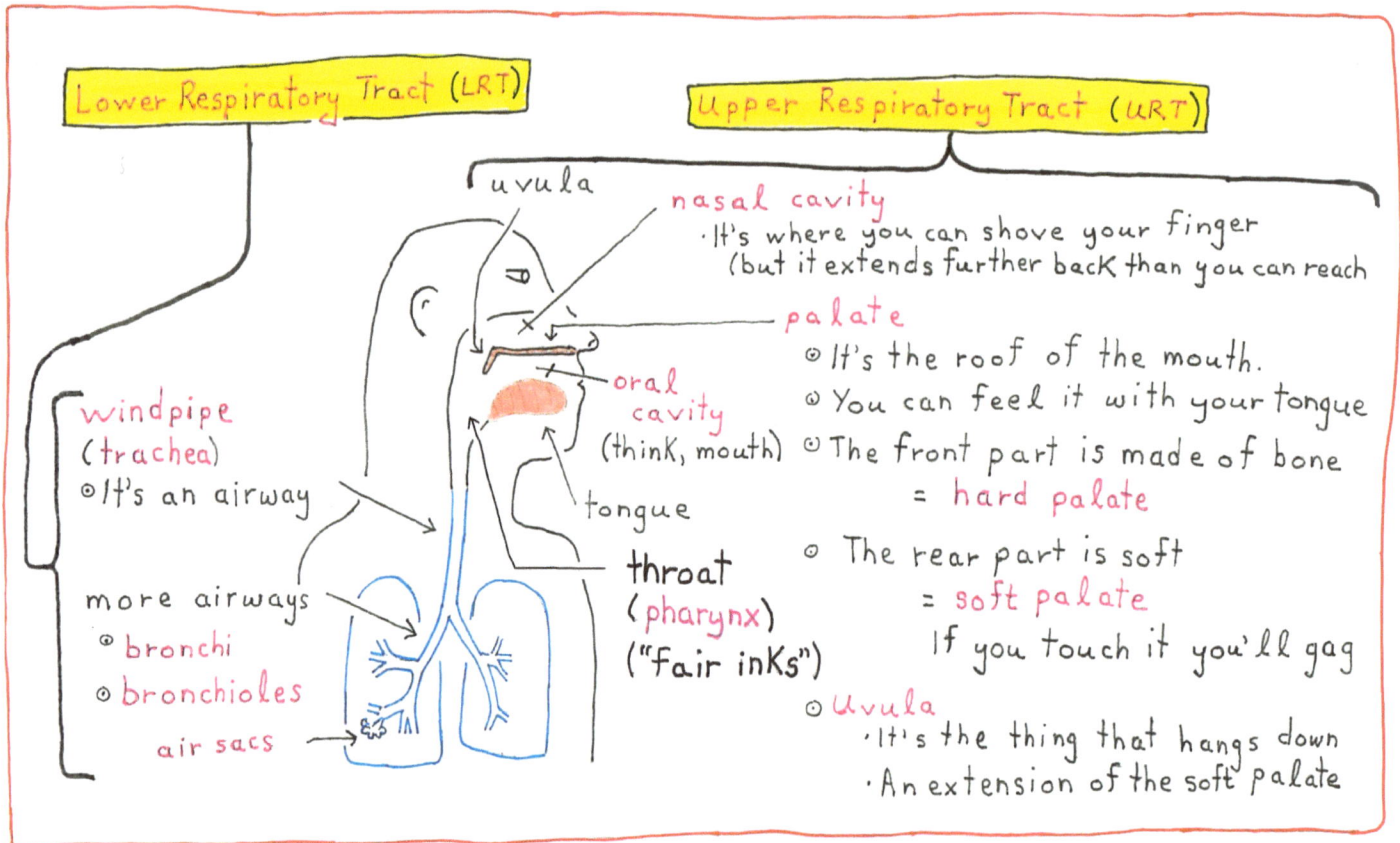

Lower Respiratory Tract (LRT)

Upper Respiratory Tract (URT)

uvula

nasal cavity
· It's where you can shove your finger
   (but it extends further back than you can reach

palate
◎ It's the roof of the mouth.
◎ You can feel it with your tongue
◎ The front part is made of bone
          = hard palate
◎ The rear part is soft
          = soft palate
       If you touch it you'll gag

oral cavity
(think, mouth)

tongue

windpipe
(trachea)
◎ It's an airway

more airways
 ◎ bronchi
 ◎ bronchioles
  air sacs

throat
(pharynx)
("Fair inKs")

◎ uvula
· It's the thing that hangs down
· An extension of the soft palate

- In the grand scheme of things, you have a < URT
                                              LRT
` And if they get infected, whether by bacteria or viruses,

it's a < URTI
         LRTI ← I for Infection

` Plot Spoiler:

      ⦿ Coronavirus has a preference for certain
      cells in the URT ... it multiplies there...
      then spreads to the LRT ... potentially ruining your day
                                                    (or life)
      : Could ⦿ coronavirus be inhaled directly
        into the LRT? Yes, if it's in a small droplet.

- That man up there looks rather
  brutish with his thick neck.

~ Maybe it's a self-portrait.

SOMPOO's SOLILOQUY

⊖ - Let's back up. How do we actually know this stuff like URT and LRT? It all started with ancient physicians like Hippocrates and Galen; then knowledge and technology were added over the centuries.

'To understand what a 'human being' is, you need 2 things:

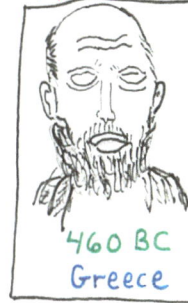

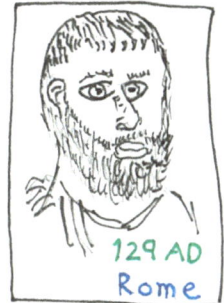

460 BC
Greece

129 AD
Rome

① Gross anatomy = What you can see with the naked eye. 👁

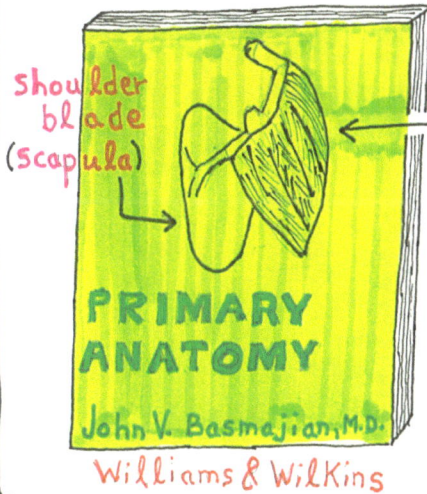

shoulder blade (scapula)

PRIMARY ANATOMY

John V. Basmajian, M.D.

Williams & Wilkins

— Deltoid muscle : It is shaped like the Greek letter delta △. It allows you to lift your arm to shoulder level.

⊖ - I absolutely ❤ this book. It has the Goldilocks amount of information and is easy to read.

② Microscopic anatomy = All that is invisible.

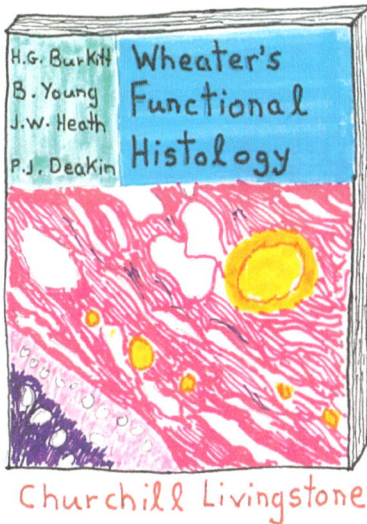

H.G. Burkitt
B. Young
J.W. Heath
P.J. Deakin

Wheater's Functional Histology

Churchill Livingstone

⊖ - I ❤ this book even more.

It is God's recipe book and fills me with awe and wonder.

What is Histology? You take human tissue, slice it really thin, then 'stain' it with dyes, now cells can be seen with a microscope.

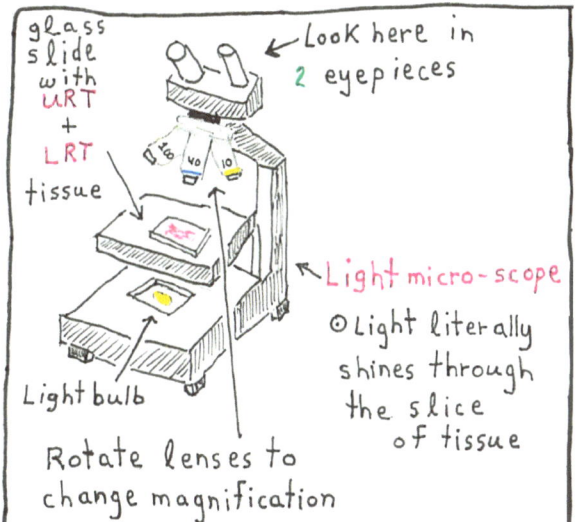

glass slide with URT + LRT tissue

Look here in 2 eyepieces

Light micro-scope

⊙ Light literally shines through the slice of tissue

Light bulb

Rotate lenses to change magnification

⊖ - "Hiss tall aw jee"

SOMPOO SAYS

- All the tubes and cavities in the human body have a lining called epithelium.

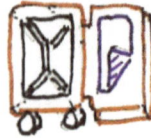

Think of it as the lining of a suitcase.

There are 3 basic options for the lining:

nucleus (because all cells contain DNA telling them what to do)
flat cells
1) Squamous Epithelium

cube-shaped cells
2) Cuboid Epithelium

Tall cells shaped like a column a.k.a. columnar cells
3) Columnar Epithelium

- Coronavirus likes to invade and replicate in this lining!

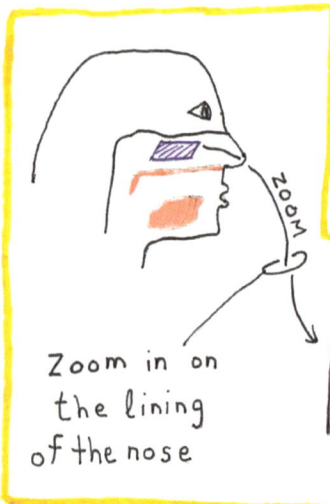

"eppa theel ee um"
SOMPOO SAYS
th like in thistle

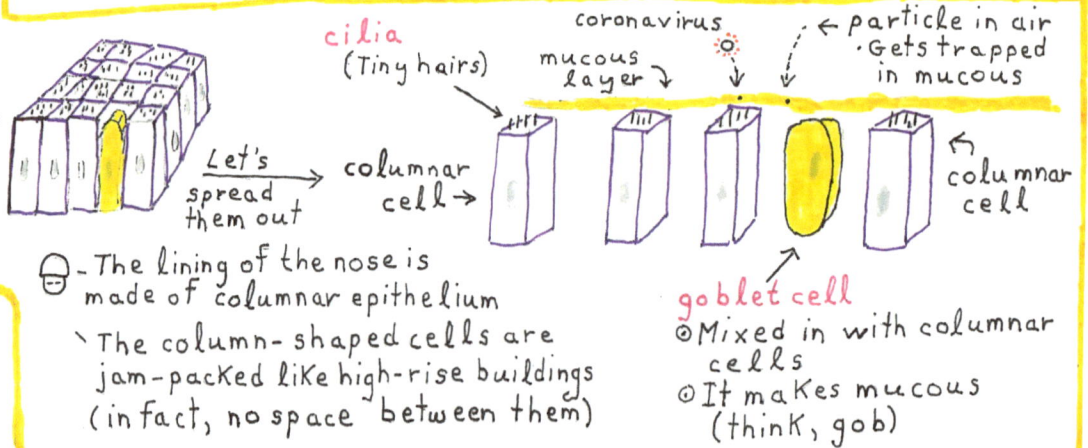

Zoom in on the lining of the nose

cilia (tiny hairs)
coronavirus
mucous layer
particle in air. Gets trapped in mucous

Let's spread them out
columnar cell →

← columnar cell

goblet cell
⊙ Mixed in with columnar cells
⊙ It makes mucous (think, gob)

- The lining of the nose is made of columnar epithelium
  ` The column-shaped cells are jam-packed like high-rise buildings (in fact, no space between them)

- Get it?
⊙ The goblet cells produce a layer of mucous to trap particles/virus/bacteria.

⊙ The columnar cells have microscopic hairs (300 per cell) that beat and propel the mucous (along with trapped stuff) to the back of your throat → you swallow the mucous (which is usually pretty watery and thin) → stomach acid kills most bacteria and viruses.

Keep exploring your nose. Gently put the tip of your index finger up your nostril to convince yourself it's a moist suitcase lining.

🙍 - I feel silly.   🙍 - All in the name of science.

Now let's pretend there's a microscope on the tip of your finger.

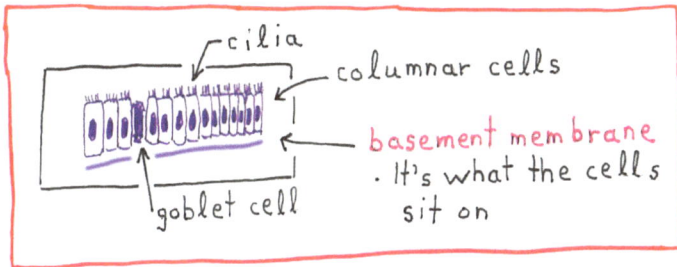

---

cilia
columnar cells
basement membrane
· It's what the cells sit on
goblet cell

Doctorspeak:

"The nasal epithelium is composed of ciliated columnar epithelium."

This is the 2-dimensional view of the pink lining of your nose, magnified about 400 x.

! hairs (cilia)
· Do not confuse with hairs on your arm. Cilia are waaaay smaller. Need a microscope to see cilia

---

Now let's zoom in like 50,000 times with an electron microscope.

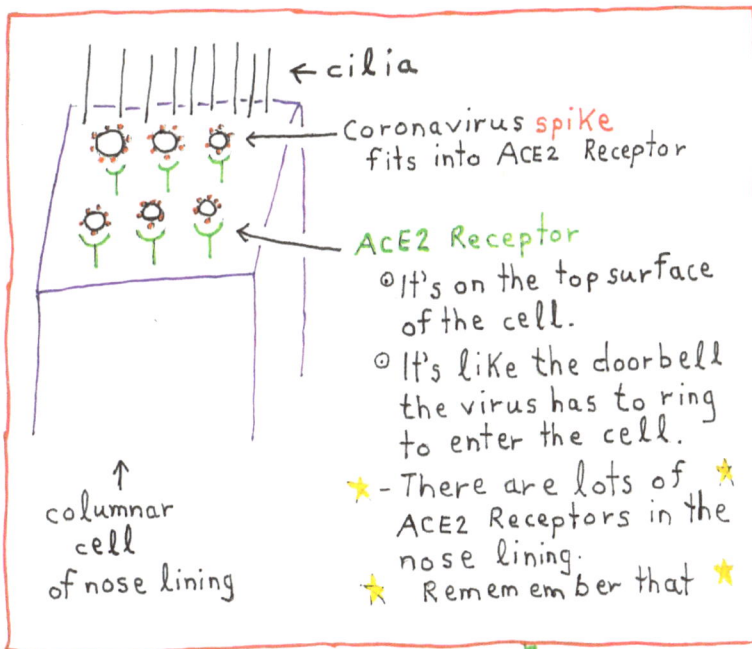

🙍 -An electron microscope is capable of 2-D or 3-D images.

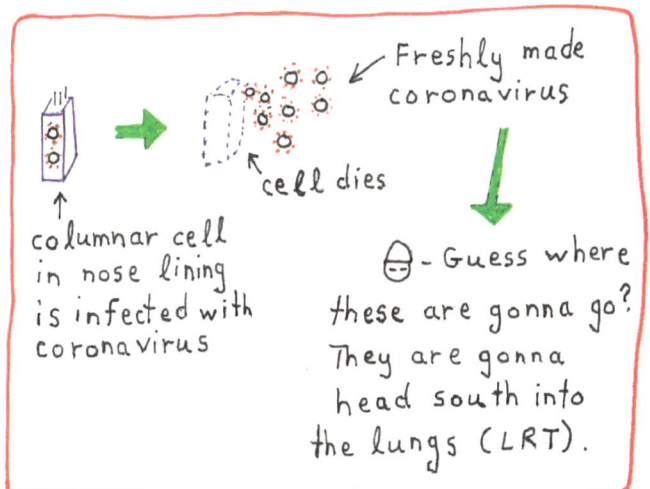

←cilia

Coronavirus spike fits into ACE2 Receptor

ACE2 Receptor
◉ It's on the top surface of the cell.
◉ It's like the doorbell the virus has to ring to enter the cell.
⭐ -There are lots of ACE2 Receptors in the nose lining.
⭐ Remember that

↑
columnar cell of nose lining

The virus enters the cell, hijacks the genetic machinery, and makes 100s to 1000s of copies of itself. So narcissistic!

Freshly made coronavirus

cell dies

↑
columnar cell in nose lining is infected with coronavirus

🙍 - Guess where these are gonna go? They are gonna head south into the lungs (LRT).

☺ - The ☼ coronavirus heads to the lungs.

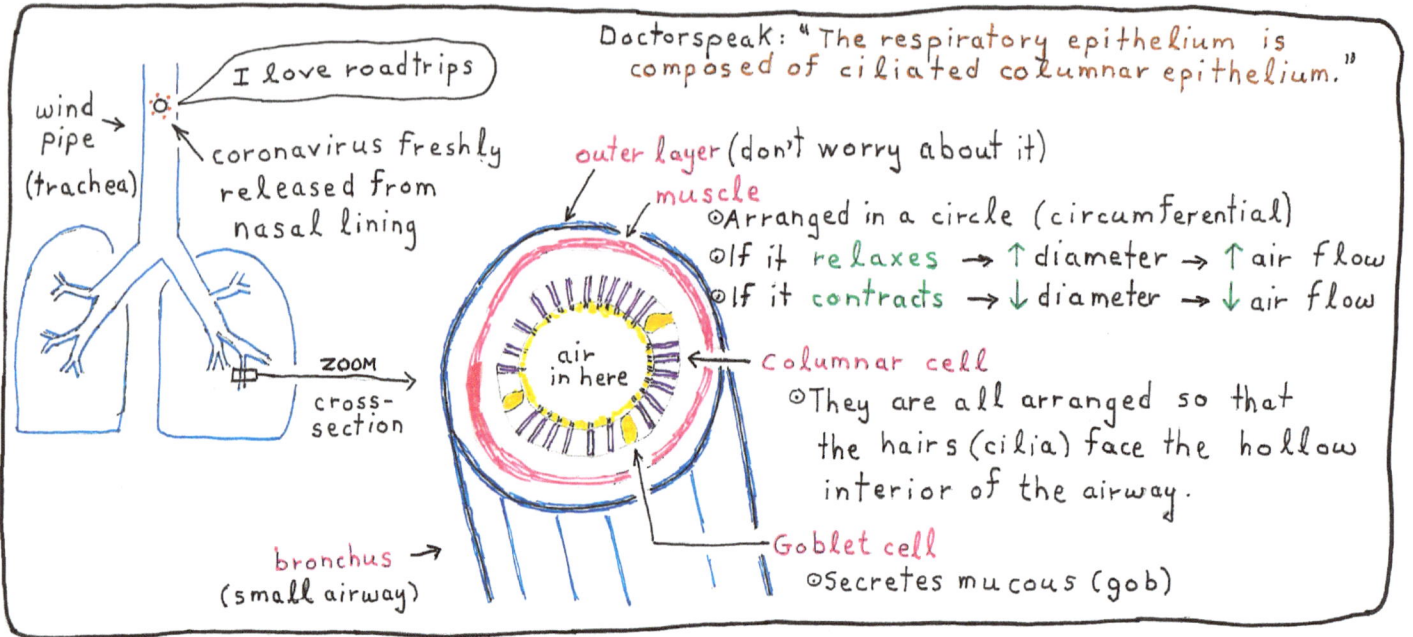

wind pipe (trachea)

I love roadtrips

coronavirus freshly released from nasal lining

Doctorspeak: "The respiratory epithelium is composed of ciliated columnar epithelium."

outer layer (don't worry about it)

muscle
◉ Arranged in a circle (circumferential)
◉ If it relaxes → ↑ diameter → ↑ air flow
◉ If it contracts → ↓ diameter → ↓ air flow

air in here

columnar cell
◉ They are all arranged so that the hairs (cilia) face the hollow interior of the airway.

ZOOM cross-section

bronchus → (small airway)

Goblet cell
◉ Secretes mucous (gob)

☺ - The arrangement is pretty similar to the nasal lining.
⟍ The goal here is to beat crap and corruption out of the lungs.
⟍ The cilia (hairs) beat upwards, pushing mucous to your throat
   → you swallow/spit out the mucous.
⟍ This combination of mucous + cilia + upwards movement is called the muco-ciliary escalator.

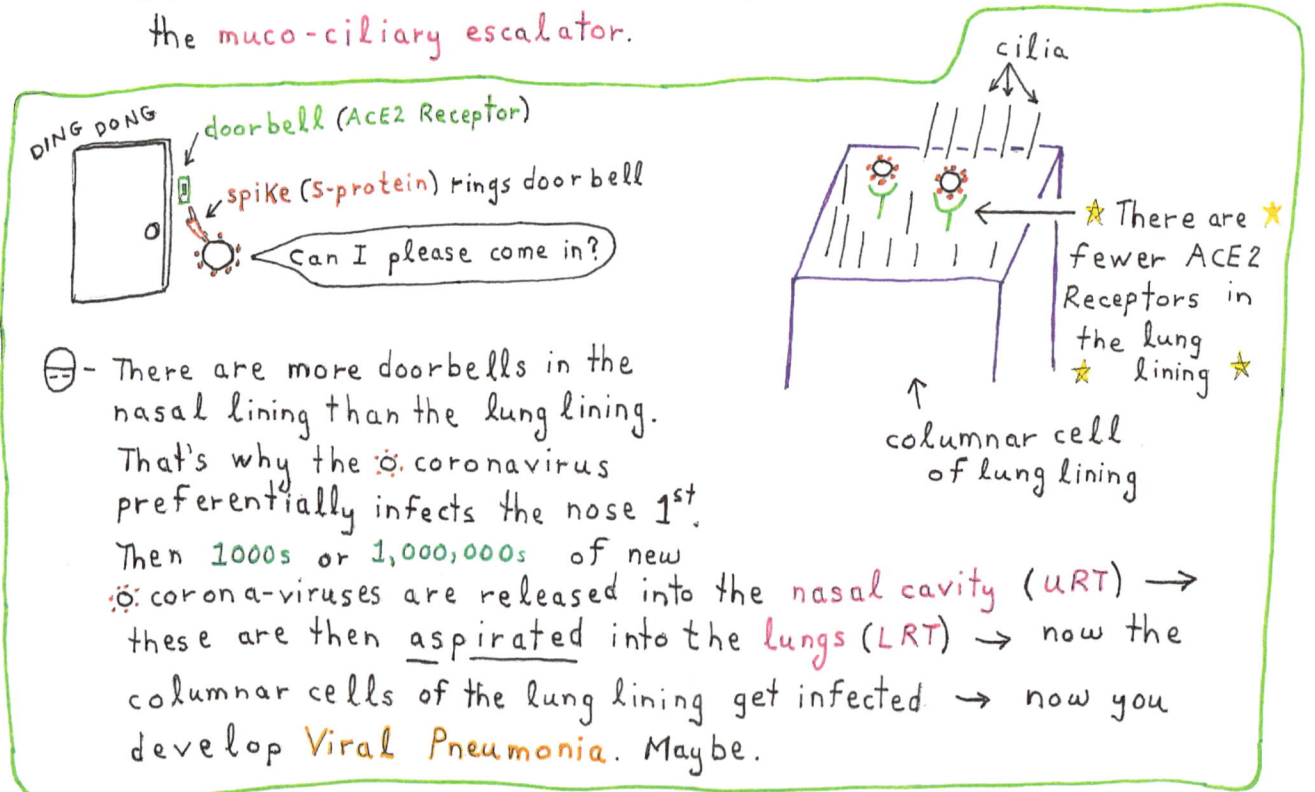

cilia

DING DONG

doorbell (ACE2 Receptor)

spike (S-protein) rings doorbell

Can I please come in?

☆ There are ☆ fewer ACE2 Receptors in the lung ☆ lining ☆

columnar cell of lung lining

☺ - There are more doorbells in the nasal lining than the lung lining. That's why the ☼ coronavirus preferentially infects the nose 1st. Then 1000s or 1,000,000s of new ☼ corona-viruses are released into the nasal cavity (uRT) → these are then aspirated into the lungs (LRT) → now the columnar cells of the lung lining get infected → now you develop Viral Pneumonia. Maybe.

☺ - If you recall from the Death Certificates, aspiration basically means you inhale something bad into the lungs. It usually refers to liquids or solids, not gases.

☺ - "mew Kow" "sill ee air ee"
SOMPOO SAYS   └ rhymes with low

😑 - Let's not forget about air sacs. There are 300 million in each lung.

← bronchiole
○ The smallest airway
○ As wide as an eye lash

ZOOM →

😑 - It takes 19 years to count to 600 million (at 1 number per second).

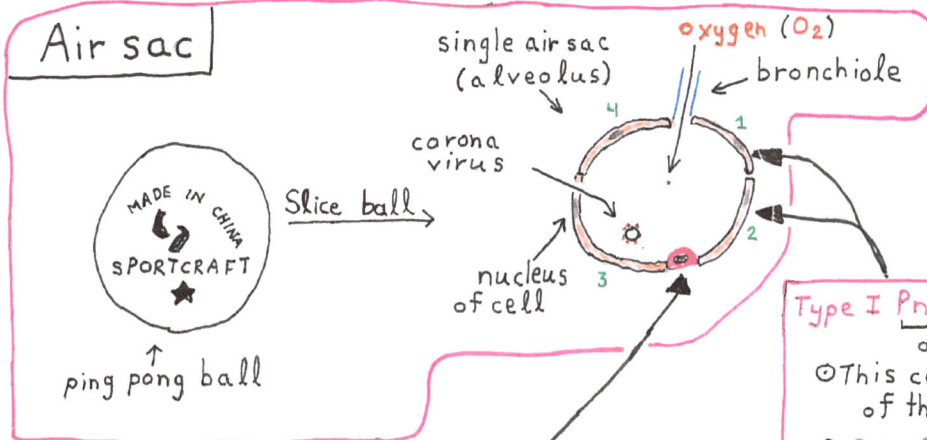

600 million air sacs (alveoli) That's really what our lungs are.

air sacs
○ Think of them as hollow ping pong balls.
○ Except not made of plastic, rather living cells.
○ And connected to a tube (bronchiole) delivering air.

Air sac

MADE IN CHINA SPORTCRAFT

↑ ping pong ball

Slice ball →

single air sac (alveolus)

oxygen (O₂)

bronchiole

corona virus

nucleus of cell

4
1
2
3

Type I Pneumo-cyte (4 of them in the drawing)
air   cell
○ This cell is flat and forms the wall of the (hollow) air sac.
○ oxygen passes through it, enroute to the blood.
○ 🦠 Coronavirus does not infect it.

This is how
COVID-19
(CoronaVirus Disease 2019)
kills people. ☆

😑 - The Type I Pneumo-cytes are squamous epithelium. 'Squamous' means 'scale', which is why snakes belong to Order Squamata in zoology. (page 86) In medicine, 'squamous' means flat and thin like a scale.

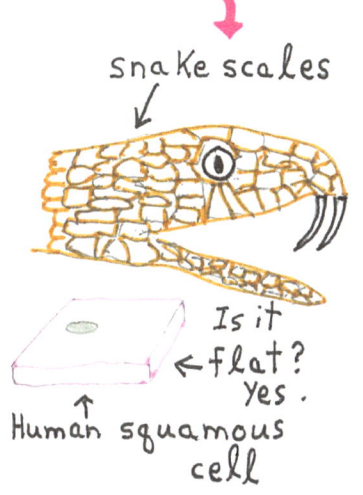

snake scales

Type II Pneumo-cyte
○ Its job in life is to make surfactant, which is a fluid coating the interior surface of the ping pong ball, preventing it from collapsing.
○ These cells are cube shaped a.k.a. cuboidal epithelium.
○ 🦠 Coronavirus infects it.
○ Does it have ACE2 Receptor doorbells? Yes.
○ When the infection is very bad in this cell, the whole air sac (ping pong ball) can fill with fluid and other gunk. This is what is called ARDS (Adult Respiratory Distress Syndrome). Now you can "drown in your own fluids"... but it's not technically Drowning (think 🐟 Fish and a lake).

Is it
← flat?
Yes.

↑ Human squamous cell

- We'll revisit air sacs in Volume 2 when ventilators are explained.

'For now, the take-home message is: coronavirus rings the doorbell (ACE2 Receptor) in the Upper Respiratory Tract (URT). Then those cells get infected and release more coronavirus that can now enter the Lower Respiratory Tract (LRT).

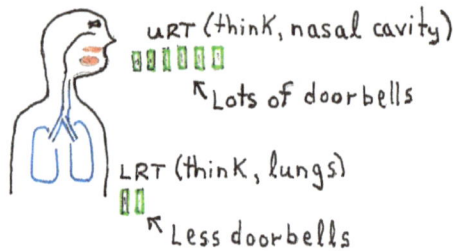

URT (think, nasal cavity)

↖ Lots of doorbells

LRT (think, lungs)

↖ Less doorbells

'You'll learn way more about the doorbell (ACE2 Receptor) in Volume 2. That's because you need to get up to speed in Genetics (all about DNA). As you'll discover everything about viruses ultimately reduces to understanding DNA — and that's not an easy topic to grasp. But you will.

- Nor should we forget the conjunctiva.

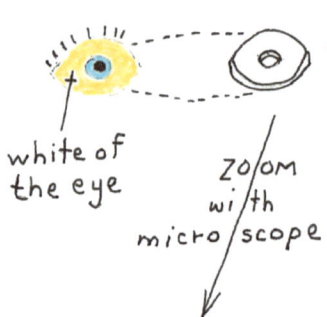

← conjunctiva (page 79)
◉ It's transparent.
◉ Sits on top of the white of the eye.
◉ Does coronavirus get into our body via the conjunctiva
  • That's debated.
  • A Chinese study found ACE2 Receptors (doorbells) in the conjunctival epithelium.
  • A German study found only "neglible" numbers of doorbells.

white of the eye

ZOOM with microscope

conjunctival epithelium

goblet cells
• Secrete mucous to protect the eye.
• It will get mixed into tears (next page).

columnar cells
• But without cilia (beating hairs)

- "con jung ty va
SOMPOO   or
SAYS
"con jung tih va"

- Well, let's assume the coronavirus infected a columnar cell of the conjunctiva. What next?
  'To answer that, you need to start crying.

😑 - Crying is surprisingly sophisticated so be proud of this the next time you're bawling your eyes out.

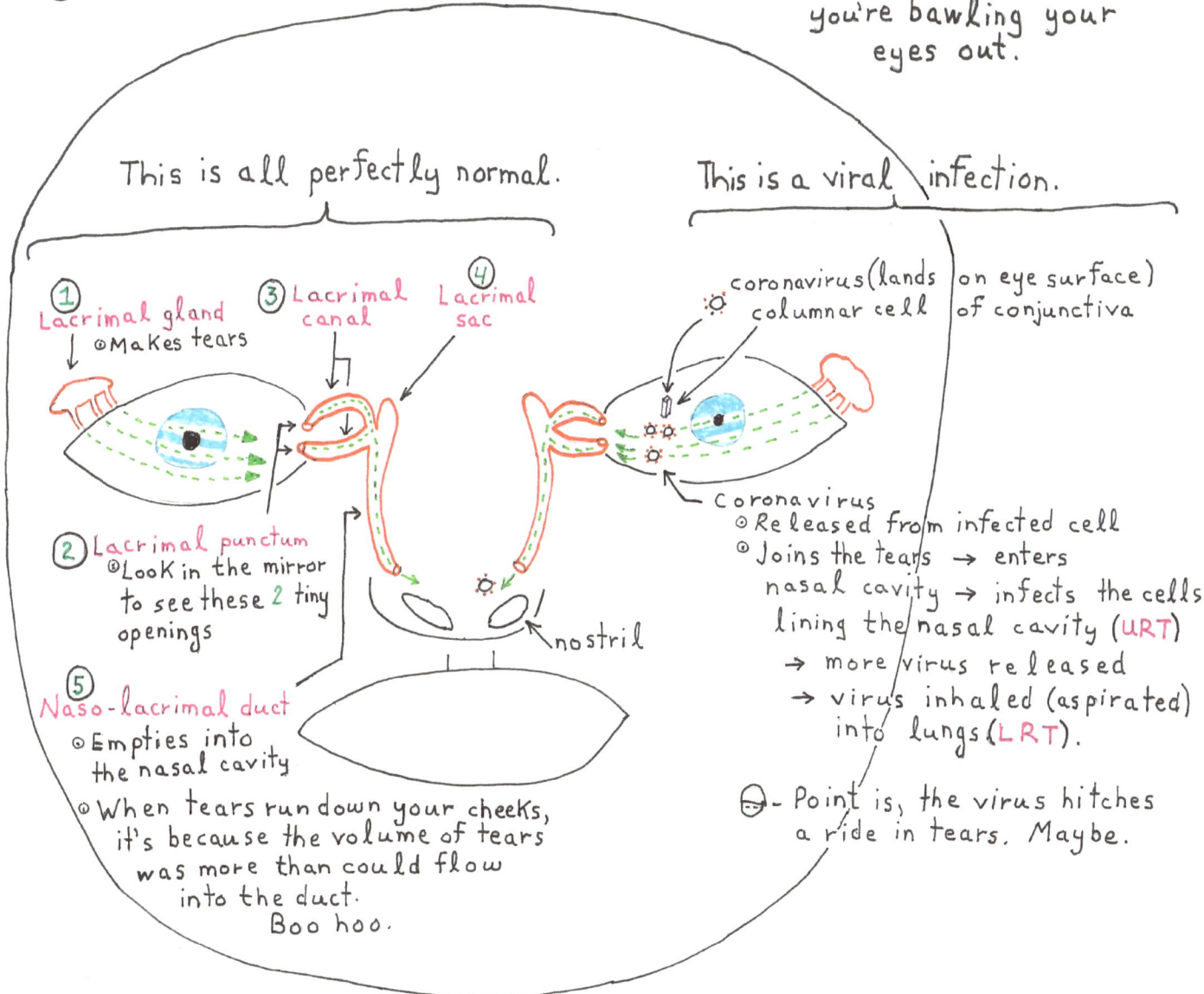

This is all perfectly normal. | This is a viral infection.

① Lacrimal gland
◎ Makes tears

③ Lacrimal canal ④ Lacrimal sac

coronavirus (lands on eye surface)
columnar cell | of conjunctiva

② Lacrimal punctum
◎ Look in the mirror to see these 2 tiny openings

Coronavirus
◎ Released from infected cell
◎ Joins the tears → enters nasal cavity → infects the cells lining the nasal cavity (URT)
→ more virus released
→ virus inhaled (aspirated) into lungs (LRT).

← nostril

⑤ Naso-lacrimal duct
◎ Empties into the nasal cavity
◎ When tears run down your cheeks, it's because the volume of tears was more than could flow into the duct.
Boo hoo.

😑 - Point is, the virus hitches a ride in tears. Maybe.

😑 - Okay, here's the deal. The Latin word 'Lachryma' means tear. Everything in the diagram above is the Lacrimal Apparatus
  ① The Lacrimal (tear) gland constantly produces tears that moisturize the surface of the eye (plus, kill bacteria) → we blink to spread the tears → the tears flow across the eye and enter the ② tiny holes called punctum → then flow through ③ canals into a ④ sac → and downwards in the ⑤ naso-lacrimal duct → and into the nasal cavity
  When you cry, it's tears coming out your nose.

😑 - "Lack rim ul"
SOMPOO SAYS

⚲ - What tearjerker movie should I watch to activate my lacrimal apparatus?
⚲ - The Lion King when Mufasa gets trampled by the stampeding wildebeest. Gets me every time.

😑 - And finally, let's not forget about the shag carpet.

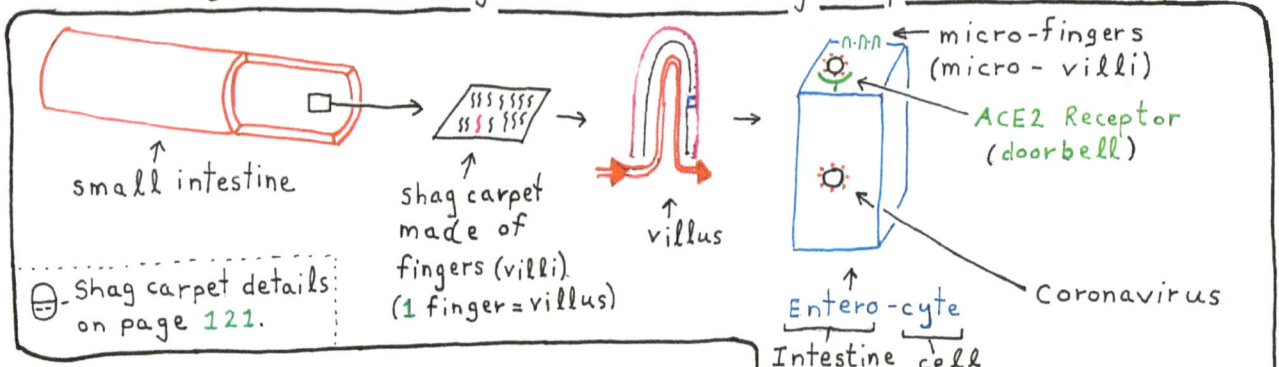

micro-fingers (micro-villi)

ACE2 Receptor (doorbell)

small intestine

Shag carpet made of fingers (villi). (1 finger = villus)

villus

Coronavirus

😑 - Shag carpet details on page 121.

Entero-cyte
Intestine cell

♀ - Is the entero-cyte shaped like a column?

☿ - Yes. The lining of the Small Intestine is Columnar Epithelium

😑 - How did 🦠 Coronavirus arrive at the shag carpet of the small intestine?

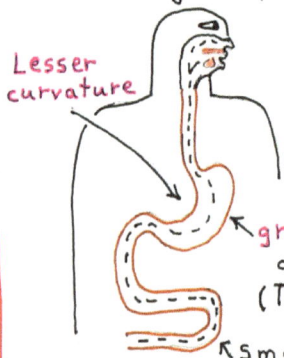

Stomach acid should kill any swallowed 🦠 coronavirus ... but saliva and secretions may protect the virus in some cases ... which may be why 10% of patients have "diarrhoea and nausea" 1-2 days before fever and respiratory symptoms.

Lesser curvature

greater curvature of stomach (This is just FYI)

← small Intestine

That's how the British doctors spell "diarrhea." They toss in an 'o' for good measure.

😑 - And yet, here are the last names of the 14 doctors who studied virus transmission:
Zhang, Kang, Gong, Xu, Wang, Li, Li, Cui, Xiao, Zhan, Meng, Zhou, Liu, Xu

◎ 12 are from China. 2 are from Australia.

◎ Well it turns out their research was published in June 2020 in the journal called **Gut** which is published by the British Society of Gastro-enterology, so British spelling ruled.
└ stomach └ intestines

◎ The article was called:
Digestive system is a potential route of COVID-19: an analysis of single-cell co-expression pattern of key proteins in viral entry process

😑 - So, to summarize how 🦠 Coronavirus enters us:

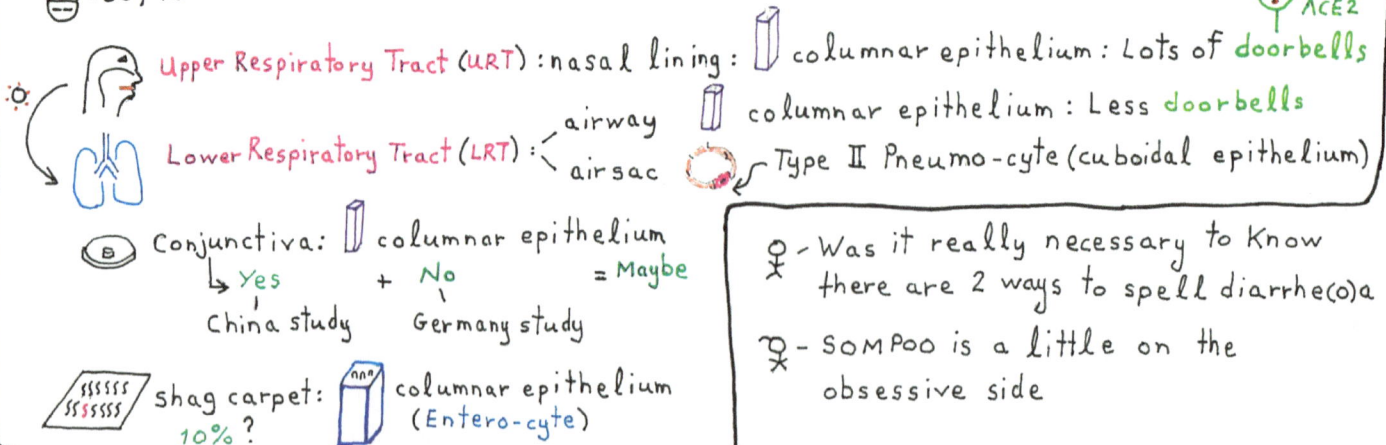

ACE2

Upper Respiratory Tract (URT): nasal lining: columnar epithelium: Lots of doorbells

Lower Respiratory Tract (LRT): < airway columnar epithelium: Less doorbells
                                   airsac Type II Pneumo-cyte (cuboidal epithelium)

Conjunctiva: columnar epithelium
↓ Yes + No = Maybe
China study Germany study

shag carpet: columnar epithelium (Entero-cyte)
10% ?

♀ - Was it really necessary to know there are 2 ways to spell diarrhe(o)a

☿ - SOMPOO is a little on the obsessive side

- Some germane concepts ...

Mucous Membranes

- As a generality, the linings of tubes and cavities are kept moist by mucous, so they are also known as **mucous membranes**.

in the **lungs**
in the **digestive tract**

♀ - Germane? Does that mean germs? Germans? German germs?

⚥ - No. Germane means relevant.

- Don't think of this mucous as the thick snot when you have a cold (although that is mucous, just an abundance of it).

- It's slick and watery, precisely why your nasal cavity feels moist.

The moist lining does 2 things < **humidifies** the air / helps **trap** crap and corruption

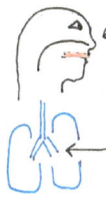

The moist lining here is critical for trapping bacteria (who like nothing better than to colonize the ping pong balls (air sacs)) and viruses.

- So ... these moisture-laden surfaces are great at what? Producing secretions ... which, if you ...   cough ...
   sneeze
   talk   ... create **droplets**
   sing
   exhale

- You already know the answer to this, but will the **Coronavirus** be present in those **droplets**?

Yes

Excretion + Secretion

- In medicine, we make a (not-too-rigidly enforced) distinction between **excretion** and **secretion**.

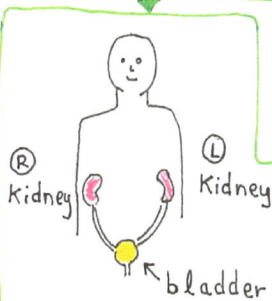

Many substances are secreted

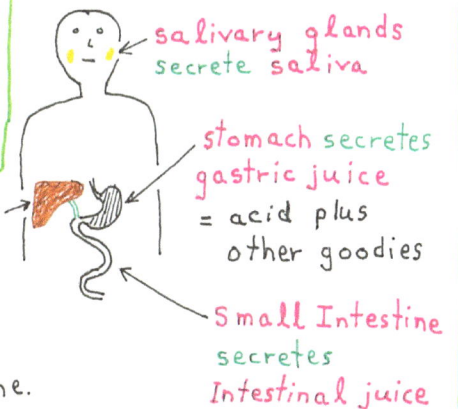

feces a.k.a. excrement

Ⓡ Kidney   Ⓛ Kidney

↖ bladder

⊙ The kidneys **excrete** waste into the urine.

⊙ But this gets complex because sodium and potassium can be excreted then recovered. Whatever.

salivary glands secrete **saliva**

stomach secretes **gastric juice** = acid plus other goodies

Liver secretes **bile** to help digest fats.
⊙ Bile enters the small intestine.

Small Intestine secretes **Intestinal juice**

- We can also speak of:
  - nasal secretions
  - oral secretions
  - Respiratory secretions

} Source of droplets

Broncho-what?

Sarin gas is a deadly chemical warfare agent.
- It is an organo-phosphate (also used in pesticides).
- One of the things it causes is excessive secretions in the bronchi (airways) ... and that, interestingly, is called:

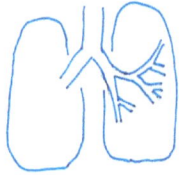

Broncho - rrhea
air way   flow

- See a similarity to these words?

dia - rrhea
through   Flow

rhino - rrhea
nose   flow

- That means you have a runny nose.

- The use of Sarin gas is prohibited by the 1997 Chemical Weapons Convention. 193 countries have signed it.

"Project 112" is the ominous name for Sarin gas tests in the 1960s. A bad time to be a bird, rabbit, or goat - they die in 4 minutes.

SOMPOO SAYS - "brong Kow ree ah"
    └ rhymes with low

Cystic Fibrosis (CF)

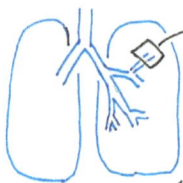

ZOOM

columnar cells

Thick mucous

→ There can be so much that it blocks the airway. That's called a mucous plug.

air in here

bronchus (cross-section)

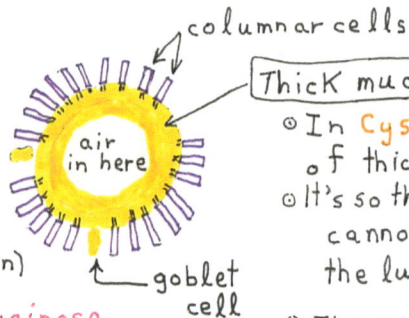

goblet cell

← Pseudomonas aeruginosa
- This is the #1 bacteria in CF patients.
- It's hard to treat because it is hardy (as in, resilient).

- In Cystic Fibrosis, there is secretion of thick mucous in the airways.
- It's so thick that the muco-ciliary escalator cannot properly move mucous out of the lungs.
- The cause is a mutation in the DNA, affecting fluid transport in the cells.
- Part of the treatment of CF involves thumping the chest wall. It's not a pounding as if it's Thor with his hammer. But it's of sufficient force to loosen the secretions so they can be coughed up.

SOMPOO SAYS - "Soo dow moan us" "air rooj in oh sa"
    rhymes with low

- Okay, let's head from germane back to specific and dive deep into masks and droplets.

CHAPTER 5

THE HORRENDOUSLY

CONFUSING 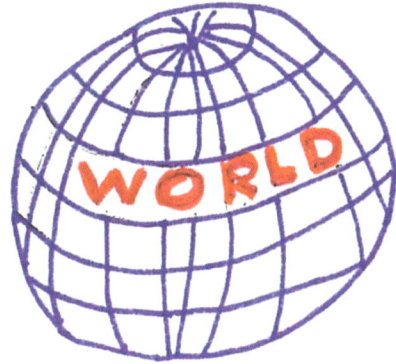 OF

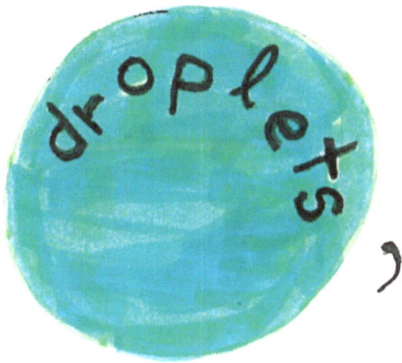 , aerosols,

P A R T I C L E S ,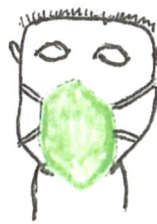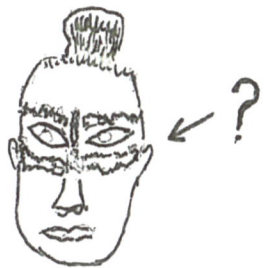

MASKS;

AND SOCIAL

DISTANCING.

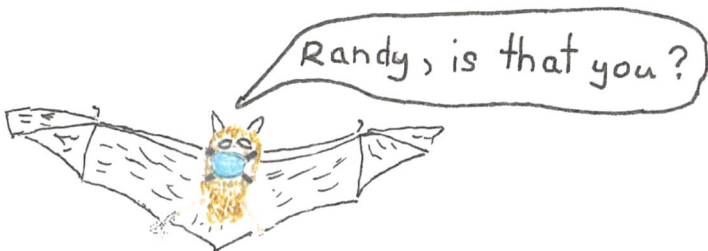

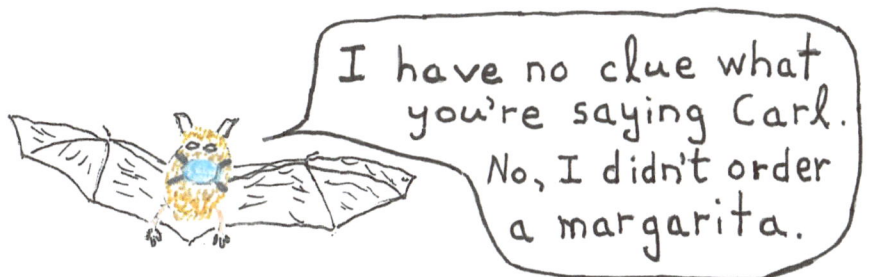

- 'Breathing' is the act of getting air into your lungs. Breathe in, breathe out.
- 'Respiration' means the oxygen in the air got delivered to cells in the body.
- A 'Respirator' is a device worn on the face to filter out crap and corruption.
- Here are 5 choices for Respirators.

1 Gas mask

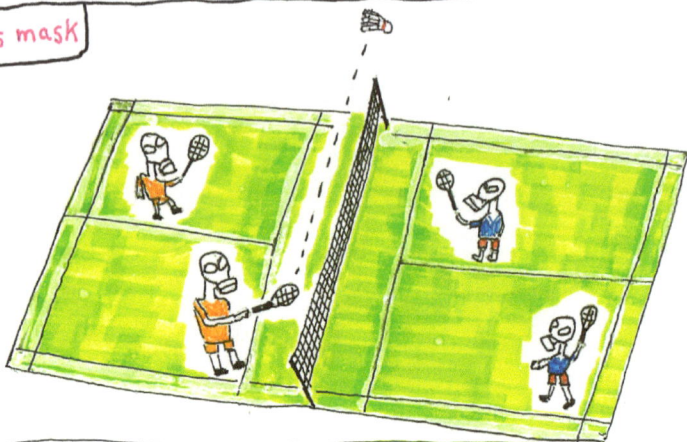

Badminton at the Gas Warfare Olympics

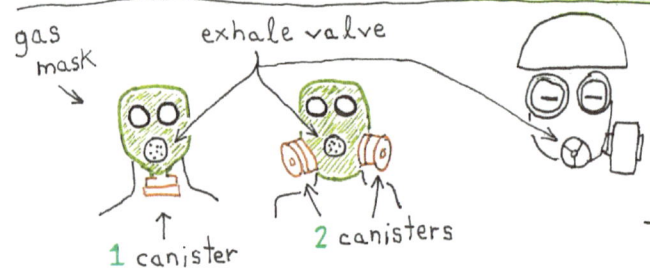

gas mask

exhale valve

1 canister

2 canisters

- Yes, it's me, SOMPOO. Thought I'd try on this British Army S10 gas mask.
- Notice that the canister is on the Left so as not to interfere with my rifle on my Right.

○ Canister screws into mask
○ Filter(s) inside canister
○ Filter blocks ⟨ gas particles
○ But!, there is no all-in-one gas mask that stops everything.
  · You choose the filter you think you'll need.

2 Escape respirator

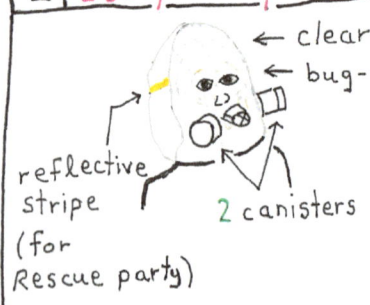

← clear hood (to ↓ claustrophobia)
← bug-eyed in terror

reflective stripe (for Rescue party)

2 canisters

- The escape respirator provides 30 minutes of protection
  `1-time use

ATTENTION! THIS IS COMMANDER VALIANT. THE EXPLOSIONS YOU ARE HEARING ARE THE HYDRAZINE TANKS. IF YOU ARE LATE ARRIVING AT THE EVACUATION POINT YOU CANNOT CLAIM OVERTIME PAY

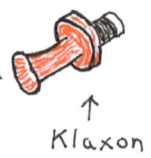

Klaxon

- Getting technical, there are 2 definitions of Respiration.
  ` The whole business of O_2/CO_2 pick-up and delivery is
  ① "Physiologic Respiration."
  ` Don't lose sleep over it.

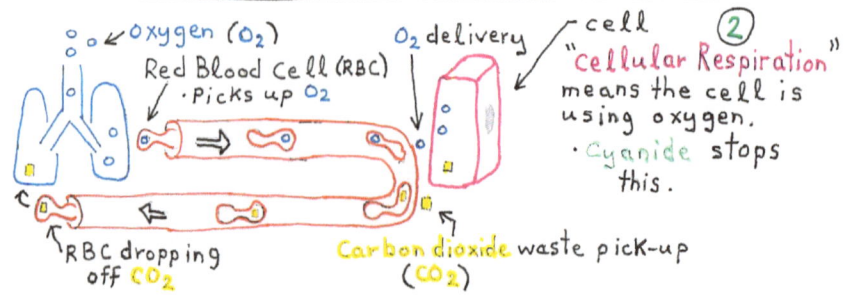

Oxygen (O_2)
Red Blood Cell (RBC)
· picks up O_2

O_2 delivery

cell ② "cellular Respiration" means the cell is using oxygen.
· Cyanide stops this.

RBC dropping off CO_2

Carbon dioxide waste pick-up (CO_2)

3 Self-Contained Breathing Apparatus (SCBA)

⊙ There are 3 parts:

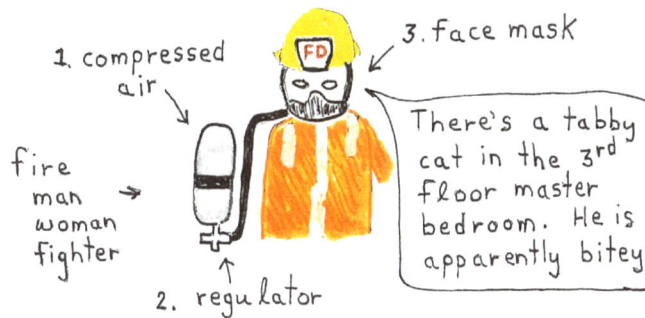

1. compressed air
3. face mask

fire man woman fighter →
2. regulator

There's a tabby cat in the 3rd floor master bedroom. He is apparently bitey

– You have your own tank so you breathe in clean air.

If that tank is used Underwater then SCBA → SCUBA. And you use a mouthpiece instead of a facemask (and have to use hand signals).

You insist on avoiding terra firma!   OK →

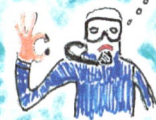

4 Powered Air Purifying Respirator (PAPR)

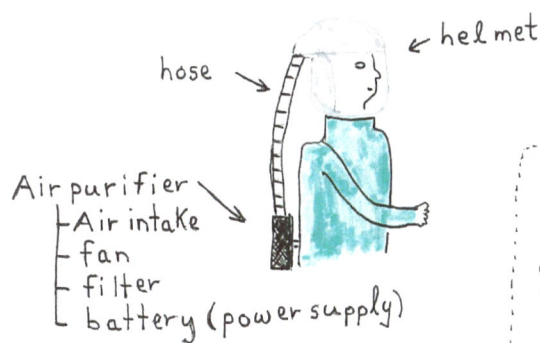

hose   ← helmet

Air purifier
├ Air intake
├ fan
├ filter
└ battery (power supply)

SOMPOO SAYS – "pap er"
└ rhymes with tap

doctor (sterile)

operating table

– It's easier to breathe because of the fan.

There are other designs where the fan and filter are built into the helmet.

These are popular in the ICU
Intensive Care Unit

or in the OR (Operating Room)

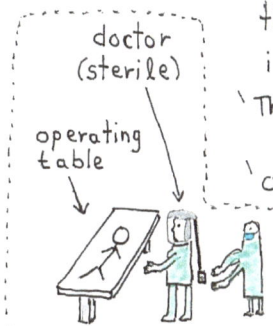

OR Nurse (not sterile) can change the battery, which is why it clips into waistband of pants

5 Particulate Respirator

N95 mask

N95 mask with exhale valve

manufacturer

model #

3M 1860S
NIOSH   N95 LOT #623

HEALTHCARE PARTICULATE RESPIRATOR AND SURGICAL MASK

– In this case, the mask is the filter.

NIOSH, which is an arm of the CDC, sets the standard for N95 (and all other) masks.

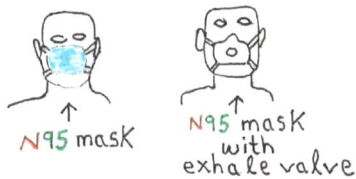

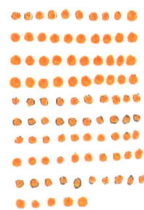

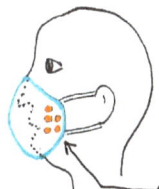

5 particles made it through the filter into your mouth or nose

95 particles blocked (filtered) = 95% efficiency = N95

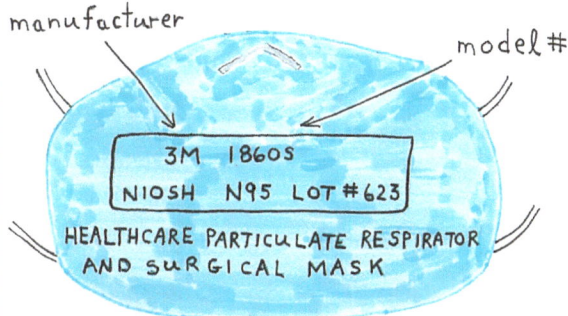

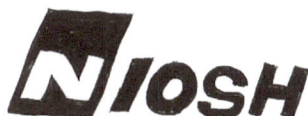

NIOSH National Institute for Occupational Safety and Health

♀ - So I just put the mask on and start doing heart surgery?

♂ - No. First you have to do a 'fit test' to ensure the N95 fits your face.
  ` Interestingly, the fit test is actually a _taste_ test.

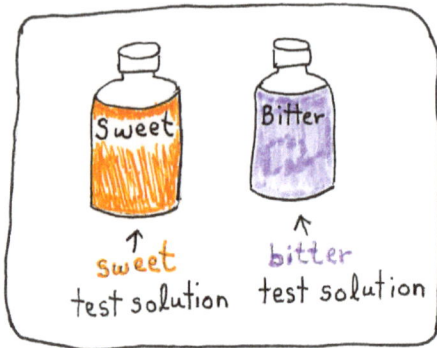

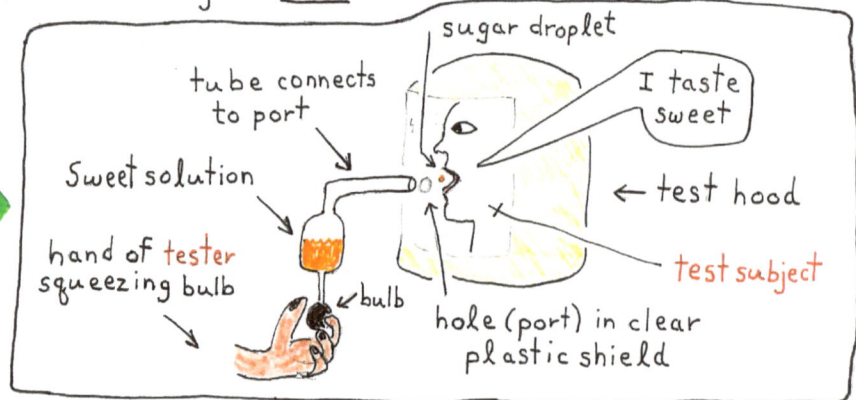

Sweet | Bitter

↑ sweet test solution

↑ bitter test solution

sugar droplet

tube connects to port

Sweet solution

hand of tester squeezing bulb

bulb

I taste sweet

← test hood

test subject

hole (port) in clear plastic shield

☺ - The fit test is quite a lot more involved than this and includes turning the head Left and Right to see if droplets can sneak in from the side.

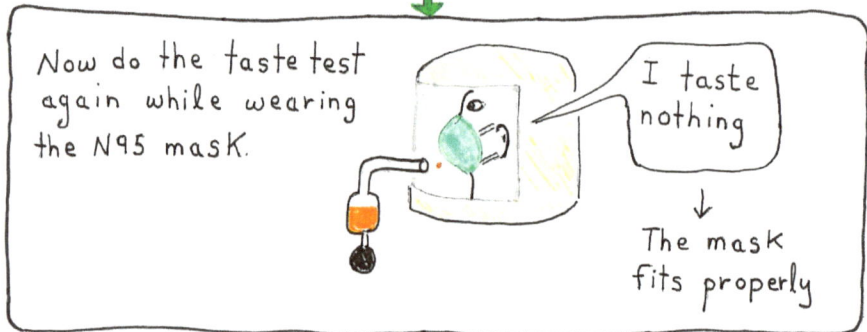

Now do the taste test again while wearing the N95 mask.

I taste nothing

↓

The mask fits properly

` You can watch a 12-minute video if you Google this:
  Medical Respirator N95 Fit Test Instructions 3M Health Care Respirator & Surgical Mask

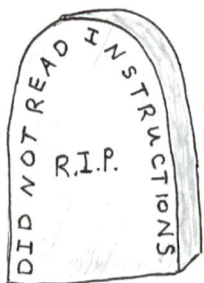

DID NOT READ INSTRUCTIONS

R.I.P.

☺ - The N95 mask does _not_ stop gas.
  - You could still die of Carbon Monoxide (CO) Poisoning

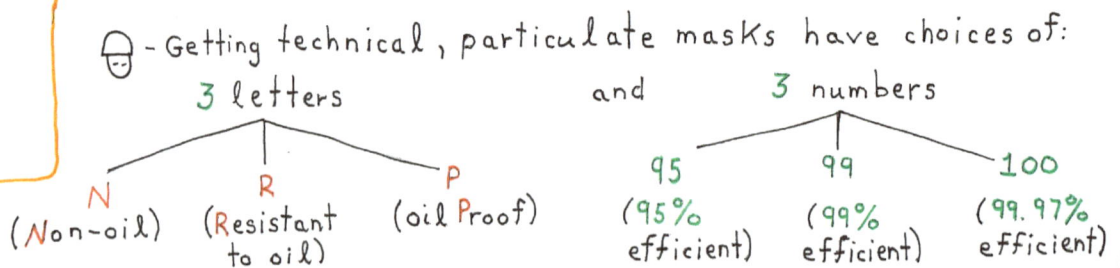

☺ - Getting technical, particulate masks have choices of:
  3 letters   and   3 numbers

N   R   P   95   99   100
(Non-oil)   (Resistant   (oil Proof)   (95%   (99%   (99.97%
              to oil)   efficient)   efficient)   efficient)

☺ - So that's why there could be
N 95   R 95   P 95
N 99   R 99   P 99
N 100   R 100   P 100

` And the model depends on the setting
— health care (blood splash)
  sandblasting
  petroleum
  whatever

Particle Respirators (continued)

😑 - It's time to make your large brain think of small things.

The quick brown fox jumps over the lazy dog.

This sentence contains all 26 letters a-z, from the 3 rows of the keyboard.

That's a period - a big one. ↙ 300 microns wide

That's about the size of a period in a book.

300 microns

300 microns

Keep thinking about periods. And the dot over the i. ↙ 300 microns
↖ 300 um

↑ 300 microns

Metric shorthand for micron

Now think of a droplet that is 1000 times smaller than this period!
This is what the N95 mask is 95% effective at stopping.
This droplet is 300 nano-meters (nm) in diameter.

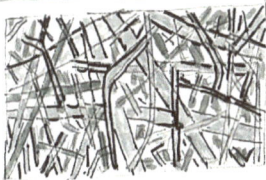

← Electron microscope view of N95 mask fibers

😑 - The fibers are randomly arranged, forming a mat, so there isn't a straight 'path' going through ...

😑 - ... but let's imagine an idealized mask perforated by tiny holes

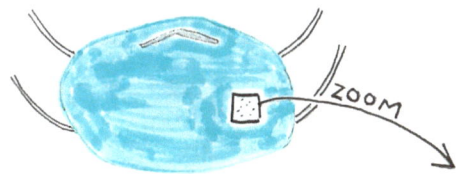

ZOOM

Too big to go through ⇒ that hole

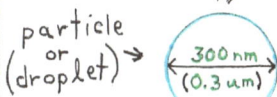

particle or (droplet) → 300 nm (0.3 um)

95% of these 300 nano-meter droplets are blocked by N95 mask.
· It is 1000 x smaller than a period.

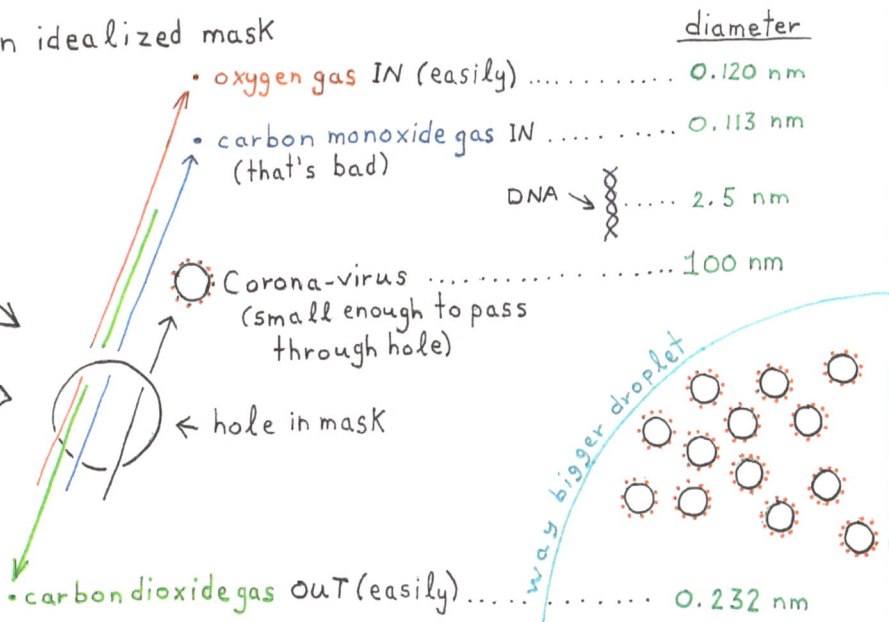

diameter

· oxygen gas IN (easily) .... 0.120 nm

· carbon monoxide gas IN .... 0.113 nm
(that's bad)

DNA ↘ ..... 2.5 nm

○ Corona-virus .... 100 nm
(small enough to pass through hole)

← hole in mask

way bigger droplet

· carbon dioxide gas OUT (easily) ... . 0.232 nm

😮 - So what use is a mask if Coronavirus can pass through it?
😮 - Well, 1st of all, the mask doesn't actually have holes.
- 2nd of all, the virus is carried in way bigger droplets.

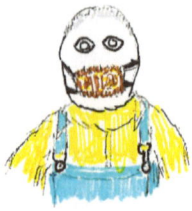

UNCLE WALTER'S SUPREMO MASK is made of spider silk, my scrap underwear, and graham crackers. It is ga-ron-teed to stop Ebola, croonervirus, and comet-hitching bacterions from outermost space.

$9.99 for 1
$99.99 for 5

AS SEEN ON TV

- Before this conversation goes off the rails, the whole concept of social distancing and masks (whether N95 or otherwise) is based on <u>droplets</u>.

' Coughing / sneezing / talking / breathing generate droplets of liquid — some are big and fall to the ground, and some are small and float in the air.

' Let's look at some seminal scientific experiments on droplets because they highly influenced the understanding of disease transmission.

- Seminal?
- An adjective for groundbreaking experiments that change how we think about a topic.

EXPERIMENT #1 - 1954

- ← Myco-bacterium tuberculosis (TB, for short)

- Remember this guy? It's the rod-shaped bacteria that causes the lung infection called TB.

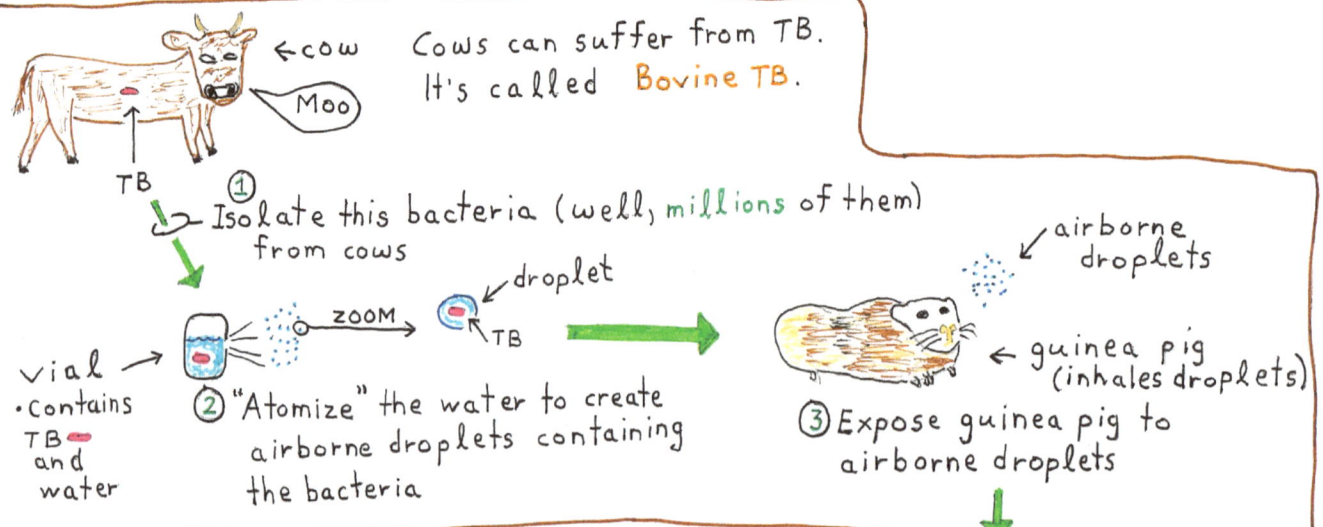

←cow   Cows can suffer from TB. It's called Bovine TB.
Moo

TB
① Isolate this bacteria (well, millions of them) from cows

vial →
•Contains TB and water

② "Atomize" the water to create airborne droplets containing the bacteria

ZOOM
←droplet
TB

←airborne droplets

←guinea pig (inhales droplets)

③ Expose guinea pig to airborne droplets

④ Guinea pig develops TB

- This experiment was performed by an "eccentric genius" named William Firth Wells.
  - Guess what? The guinea pigs were in hospital rooms (without patients) at the VA Hospital in Baltimore, Maryland.
  - And airborne droplets were released into the ventilation system.

Experiment # 2 - 1954

☺ - This time, humans instead of cows.

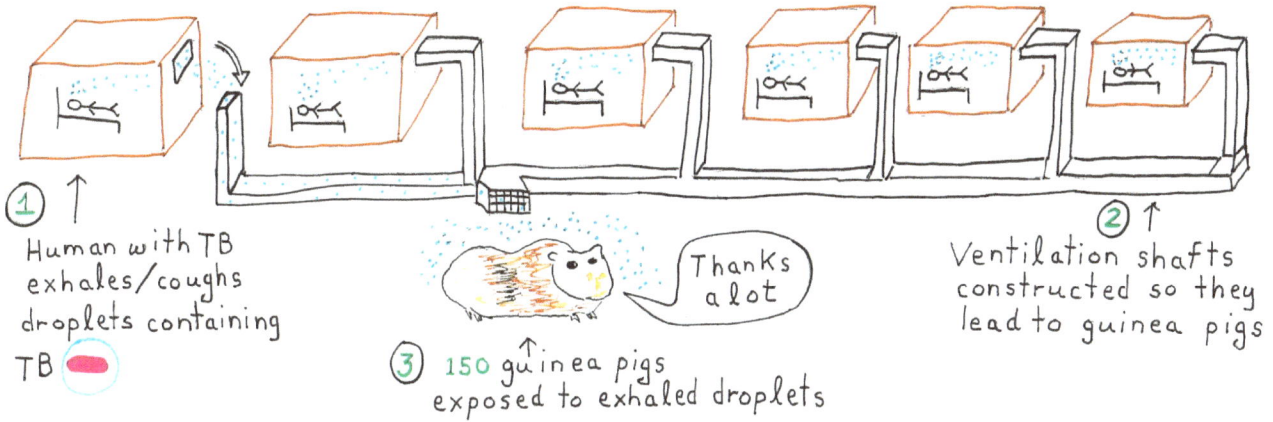

① ↑ Human with TB exhales/coughs droplets containing TB 🔴

③ 150 guinea pigs exposed to exhaled droplets

Thanks a lot

② ↑ Ventilation shafts constructed so they lead to guinea pigs

☺ - There were 6 human patients with TB, each in their own room.
- This was a 2-year experiment.
- 3 guinea pigs per month became infected. On average.
- The experiment proved that TB can spread in the air a.k.a. airborne transmission

Experiment #3 - 1954

☺ - The same experiment but the air is exposed to ultra-violet (uv) light, which is known to disinfect the air.

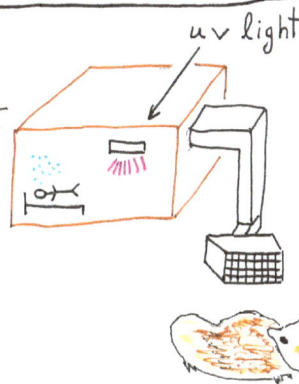

uv light

Thank you, uv

RESULT: No guinea pigs develop TB.

CONCLUSION: The TB must be airborne to transmit the infection. This is like a double-check to verify the data in Experiment # 2 That's good science.

☺ - Some more conclusions:

A.

visible light
uv light (invisible)

The amount of uv light emitted by the sun does not stop the airborne transmission of TB.

B.

← drone

My personal drone follows me, protecting me from airborne TB.

concentrated uv light with a wavelength of 294 nano-meters (nm) to kill TB 🔴

A reasonable conclusion ... except all that uv light causes skin cancer and Cataracts 👁. Plus, you can get TB by drinking unpasteurized milk if the cow has TB.

☺ - By the way, the light shone on premature babies is not ultra-violet. It's blue light in the visible range.

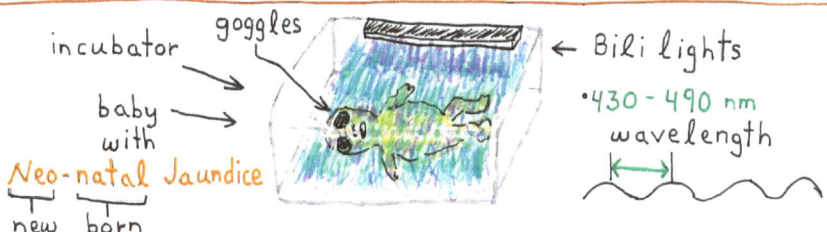

incubator

goggles

baby with Neo-natal Jaundice

new born

← Bili lights

·430 - 490 nm wavelength

- The application of those science experiments was to design **Negative Pressure Rooms** in hospitals.

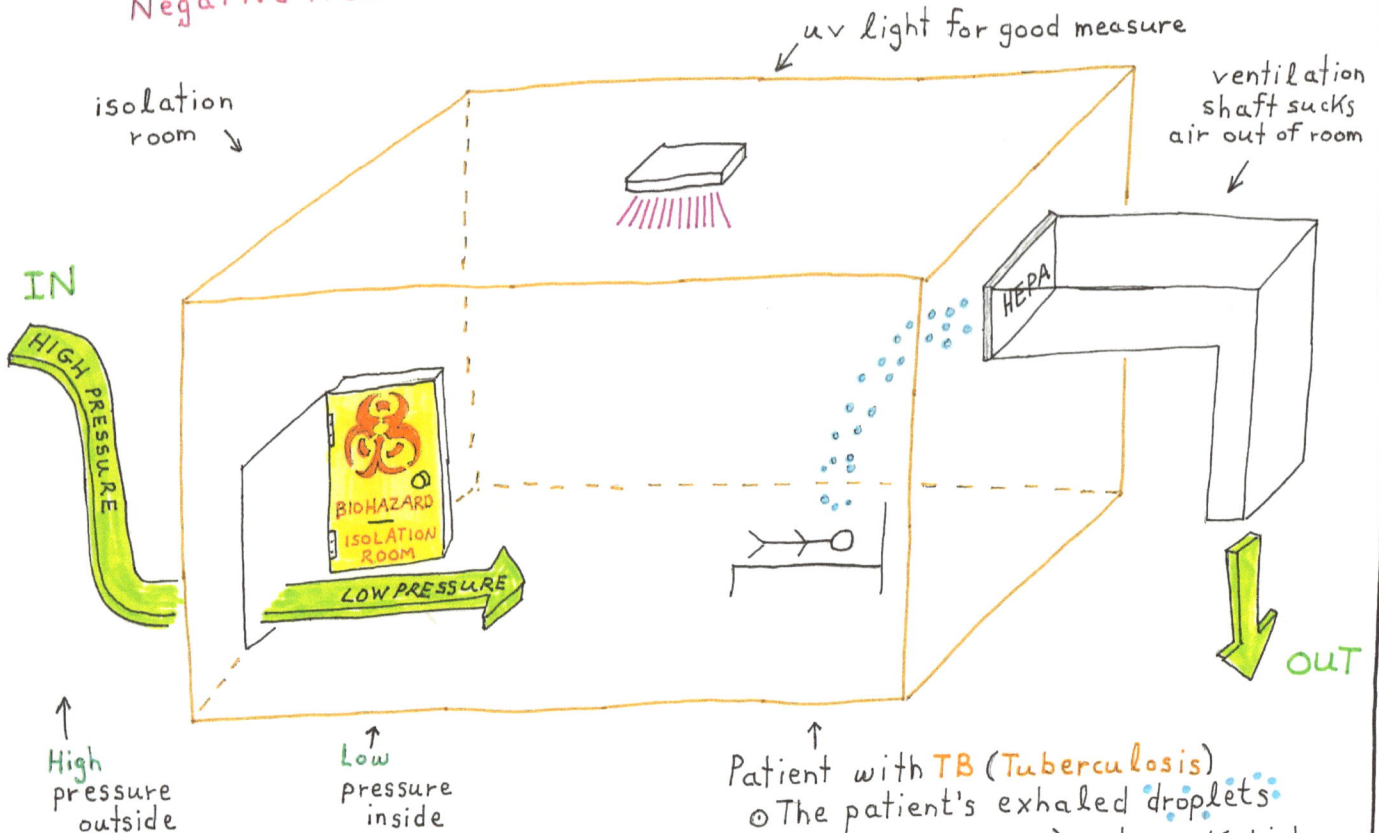

uv light for good measure

isolation room ↓

ventilation shaft sucks air out of room

IN

HIGH PRESSURE

HEPA

BIOHAZARD ISOLATION ROOM

LOW PRESSURE

OUT

↑ High pressure outside

↑ Low pressure inside

↑ Patient with **TB** (Tuberculosis)
  ○ The patient's exhaled droplets (containing TB ●) get sucked into a **HEPA** filter

○ When the door opens, air flows i_n_.
  . That's called a Negative Pressure Room.

○ The patient's exhaled droplets cannot escape into the hallway and infect everyone else in the hospital.

High **E**fficiency **P**articulate **A**ir filter
  ○ In simple terms, this is an **N 100** mask (99.97% efficient) turned into a

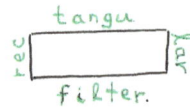

rec | tangu | lar
filter.

- Any discussion of 'droplets' is _horrendously_ _confusing_.

drop
droplet

aerosol
aerosol droplet

Is this a small drop or a large droplet?

droplet nuclei
condensation nuclei

particle
particulate

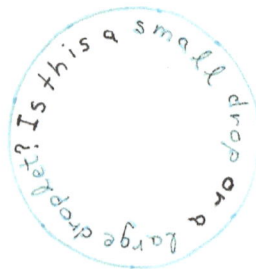

Air Borne
Jason Bourne

- stick with me, We'll get to the bottom of it and you'll feel much better.

☺ - The naming is all based on a **5-micron dividing line**
(in medicine)

← Droplets **larger** than 5 microns
in diameter (wide)

Droplets **smaller** than 5 microns →
in diameter

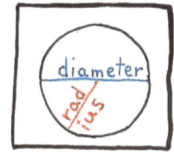

⟳ 5 micron (μm)
dividing line

diameter / radius

bigger ← → smaller

droplet → ○

aerosol · The droplet evaporates in the air → **droplet nuclei**

◇ Any droplet wider than **5 microns** is a "droplet."

Droplet follows an arc-shaped trajectory to the ground

Bacteria or virus can be present in the droplet.

This droplet is so heavy (well, relatively heavy compared to an aerosol) that it falls to the ground within **1-2 meters (3-6 feet).**

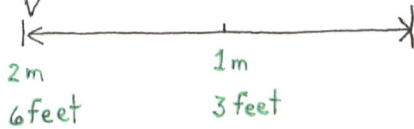

|← 2m 6feet ——— 1m 3feet →|

◇ If this droplet is less than **5 microns** in diameter it is called an "aerosol."

◇ It is made of **97% water + 3% solids.**

◇ The solids are the proteins in the mucous (since this drop was generated by a mucous membrane).

◇ Plus the solids could be bits of dead cells a.k.a. cellular debris

◇ Bacteria or virus can be inside the droplet.

◇ This can float in the air for **minutes to hours**

◇ What's left behind is called a "droplet nuclei."

◇ This is the **3% solids** that did not evaporate

◇ Bacteria or virus could be present.

◇ This is practically weightless. It can float for **hours to days**

◇ Depending on what you read, "aerosol" may also include "droplet nuclei."

DROPLET TRANSMISSION

○ This means an infection is transmitted by droplets (> 5um wide) at close range (1-2 m)(3-6 feet) to another person.
○ For sure, ☼Coronavirus is transmitted this way.

AIR-BORNE TRANSMISSION

○ This means an infection can be transmitted in the air by aerosols (<5um) or droplet nuclei.
○ It is an open question whether (or to what degree) ☼Coronavirus is transmitted this way.

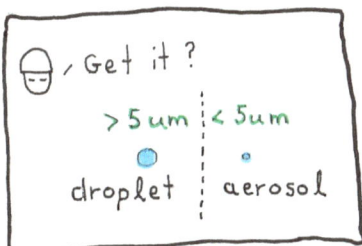

☺, Get it?
> 5um | < 5um
○   ·
droplet | aerosol

☿ - So if a droplet is less than 5 microns wide I'm not allowed to call it a droplet?
☿ - Correct. You have to call it an aerosol.

☿ - Even though an aerosol is actually a droplet?
☿ - Correct.

☿ - That's ridiculously confusing
☿ - Correct

Let's pretend a person infected with a bacteria or virus in their nasal cavity, oral cavity or lungs is like a bomb that explodes every time they sneeze or cough, sending 'shrapnel' everywhere.

Anyone inside a blast radius of 2 meters (6 feet) from the infected guy in the center will get blasted in the face by a droplet (larger than 5 μm wide).

○ We'll call it the BLAST ZONE

○ This is Droplet Transmission (by the way, the droplet could land on a surface and then be touched, then transferred by your fingers to your mouth or nose or conjunctiva).

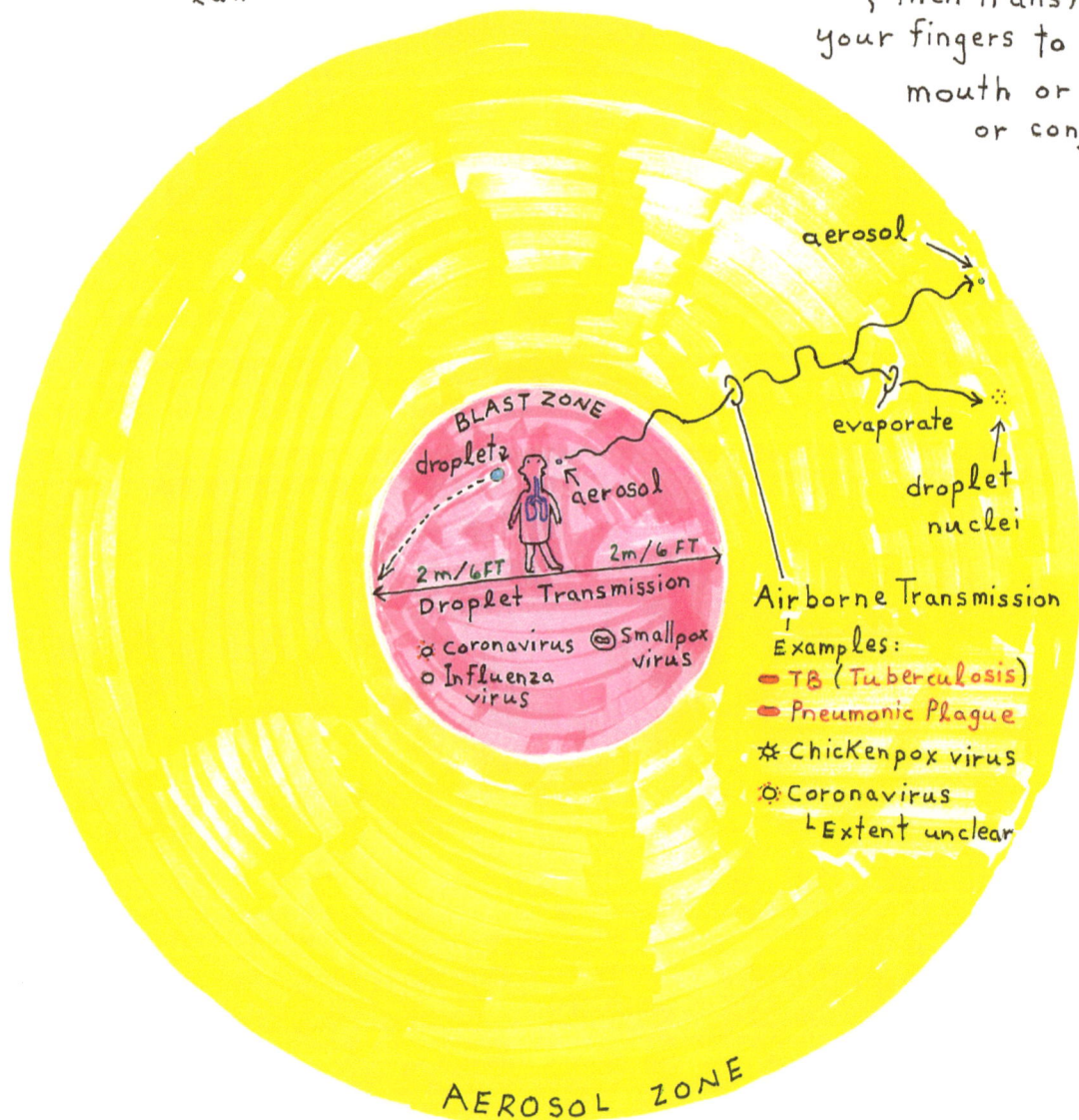

aerosol

BLAST ZONE

droplets

aerosol

2m/6FT   2m/6FT

Droplet Transmission

○ Coronavirus   ⊕ Smallpox virus
○ Influenza virus

evaporate

droplet nuclei

Airborne Transmission

Examples:
— TB (Tuberculosis)
— Pneumonic Plague
✳ Chickenpox virus
○ Coronavirus
  └ Extent unclear

AEROSOL ZONE

- Anyone in the Aerosol Zone (I made that term up) can inhale the aerosol (a droplet < 5 μm wide) or droplet nuclei.

  - This is Airborne Transmission
    ○ The classic example is ⬭ TB (Tuberculosis), which was the point of those experiments with guinea pigs.

    ○ This also includes Aspergillus fungal spores released into the air.

    ○ Some pathogens simply die in the air. They don't cause Airborne Transmission.

😐 - Location, Location, Location

Enclosed room →
  ⊙ 4 walls
  ⊙ 1 ceiling

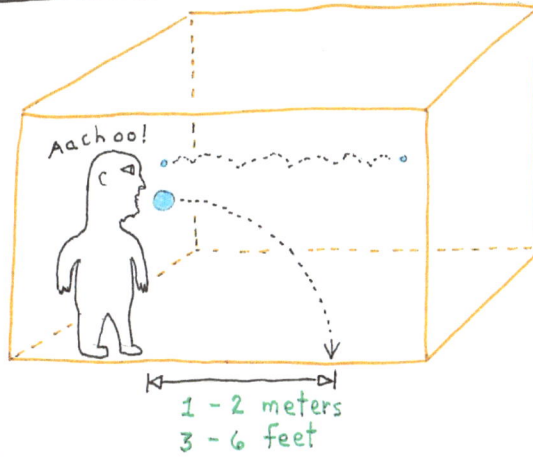

Aachoo!

1 - 2 meters
3 - 6 feet

Small droplet • ("aerosol")
  ⊙ Floats in the air for minutes to hours.
  ⊙ It is 'air-borne'.

Large droplet ◎ ("droplet")
  ⊙ Follows a curved path (trajectory) to the ground
  ⊙ Lands 1-2 m (3-6 FT) away.
  ⊙ Did it travel through the air? Yes.
  ⊙ Is it air-borne? No.
  ⊙ Can it get blasted into your face? Yes.

😐 - Are you more likely to inhale that small airborne droplet in an enclosed space? Yes.

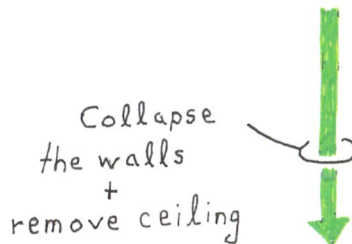

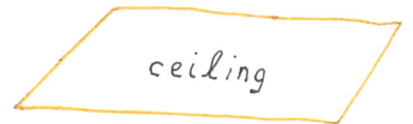

Collapse the walls + remove ceiling

ceiling

wind (maybe)

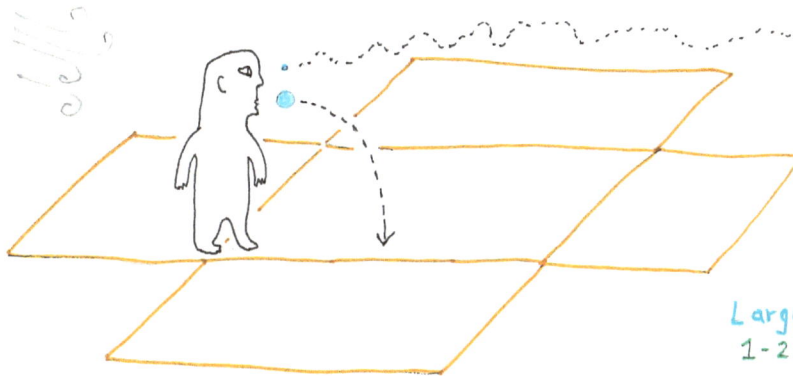

Small droplet still floating but the 'room' is now enormous (you're outside)

Large droplet still falls 1-2 m (3-6 FT) away.

😐 - Okay, that seems logical. Small droplets float. Large droplets drop to the ground.
- Could ⊛ coronavirus be present inside the small or large droplets? Yes, absolutely.

♀ - Isn't 1 m = 3 FT 3" ?

♂ - Yes. But 1 m = 3 FT is close enough.

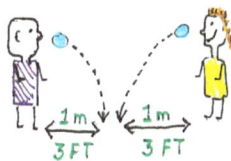

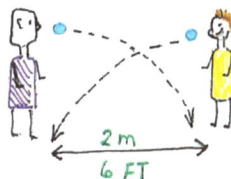

1m 3FT   1m 3FT

2 m 6 FT

⭐ This is precisely why we social distance at 2 meters (6 feet). We play it safe and assume a 2-meter (6-foot) trajectory for the large droplets

😐 - We've not finished with William Firth Wells.
He was obsessed with droplets.
Here is his droplet experiment from 20 years earlier, in 1934.

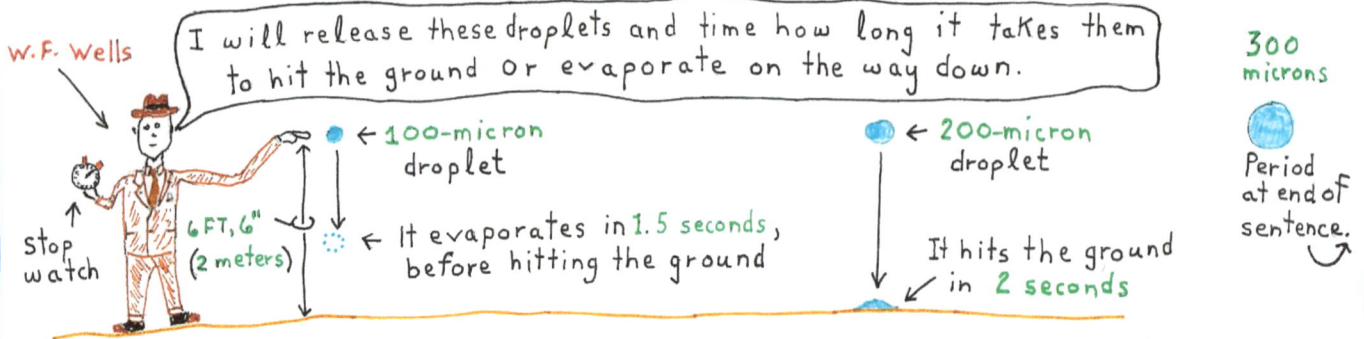

W.F. Wells →

I will release these droplets and time how long it takes them to hit the ground or evaporate on the way down.

stop watch

6 FT, 6" (2 meters)

← 100-micron droplet

← It evaporates in 1.5 seconds, before hitting the ground

← 200-micron droplet

It hits the ground in 2 seconds

300 microns

Period at end of sentence. ↷

😐 - Then he wrote a scientific paper in the American Journal of Epidemiology, 1934:
On air-borne droplets. Study II. Droplets and droplet nuclei
So that terminology has been around for 80+ years.

😐 - Notice how that 100-micron droplet is way bigger than a 5-micron aerosol?
Yet how tiny 100 microns actually is, considering a period is 300 microns. ↖ 300 μm
Which tells you just how small 5 microns is.

Today's Unsolicited Math Lesson

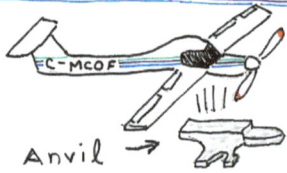

C-MCOF

Anvil →

😐 - How long does it take for an anvil dropped from
1 mile (5280 feet)(1609 meters)(1.609 km) to hit the ground?

Formula:
$d = \frac{1}{2} at^2$

Given:
d = distance = 1609 meters
a = acceleration due to gravity = 10 meters per second per second
(That means for every second you fall, you increase speed by 10 meters every second)
t = ? = time in seconds

$d = \frac{1}{2} \times a \times t^2$
$1609 = \frac{1}{2} \times 10 \times t^2$
$1609 = 5 \times t^2$
$\frac{1609}{5} = t^2$
$322 = t^2$
$\sqrt{322} = t$
18 seconds = t

😐 - "d equals one half a t squared"
SOMPOO SAYS

😐 - It takes 18 seconds for an anvil to fall 1 mile (1609 meters)

Now to Problem #2 →

😐 - Now let's drop the anvil from 2 meters, the height Wells released his droplets from.
$d = \frac{1}{2} at^2$
$2 = \frac{1}{2} \times 10 \times t^2$
$2 = 5 \times t^2$
$\frac{2}{5} = t^2$
$0.4 = t^2$
$\sqrt{0.4} = t$
0.6 seconds = t

😐 - It takes 0.6 seconds for an anvil to fall 6 FT, 6 inches (2 meters)

😐 - The point of that math lesson - and specifically Problem #2 - is that the anvil (0.6 seconds) falls faster than the 200 μm droplet (2 seconds). The anvil is not actually faster; it falls at the expected rate due to gravity. It is the droplet which is slower; it is so tiny that air currents significantly affect its descent.

- Time again for a sense of scale, looking specifically at liquid droplets and solid particles.
  Remember, micron shorthand is μm.

☼ Coronavirus
atmospheric dust
radioactive fallout
0.1 μm

100 nm
0.1 μm ← scale bar

0.2 μm · Cloud Condensation Nuclei (CCN) ← cloud
· This is the minute dust that water condenses on to form clouds.

0.3 μm · N95 mask filters 95% of 300 nm (0.3 μm) particles or droplets

1 μm — Small droplet ("aerosol") produced by cough/sneeze
tobacco smoke
Staph aureus ← single coccus in cluster is 1 μm in diameter

2 μm ● Fungal spore ← air-borne spore is 2 μm wide
Aspergillus

hair on scalp is 100 μm wide (diameter)

AAACHOO!
100 μm is a large droplet

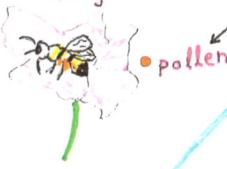

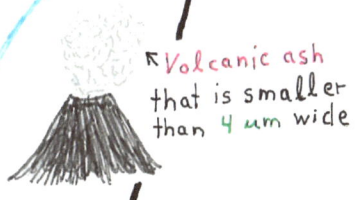

100 μm

· pollen

2.5 μm ● PM$_{2.5}$ = Particulate Matter small enough to be inhaled deep into the lungs (into the air sacs).
= Environmental Protection Agency (EPA) sets PM$_{2.5}$ as a hazardous size.

Volcanic ash that is smaller than 4 μm wide

4 μm capillary diameter is 4 μm
Red Blood Cell (RBC)

"aerosol"
5 μm dividing line
"droplet"

5 μm broncho-dilator particle size
eg, Ventolin
· We want these particles to land in the bronchi (airway) where they cause the muscle to relax → ↑ diameter → ↑ air flow

Fuel injection gasoline droplet

7 μm Red Blood Cell (RBC) squished flat on a glass microscope slide is 7 μm wide

9 μm Type II Pneumo-cyte that ☼ Coronavirus infects (okay, it's not a particle; it's a cell)

- Basically, everything on this page fits inside a period with ease.

20 μm
cloud droplet
· This is the water that condenses on the Cloud Condensation Nuclei (CCN)

1,000,000 of these 20 μm droplets make a raindrop.

The quick brown fox jumps over the lazy dog. ← 300 μm

The period is so big it cannot fit on this page

A raindrop is 2000 μm (2 mm) ($^2/_{25}$") wide. Relatively huge.
On the scale of this page, a raindrop is 4 m (12 feet) wide - probably about the size of the room you are in.

GERMANE DEFINITIONS

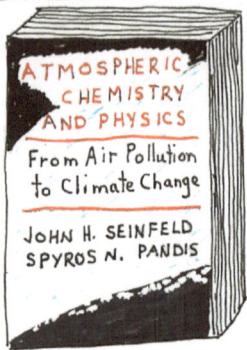

☺ - When in doubt, ask an atmospheric scientist.

— air molecules (oxygen, nitrogen, carbon dioxide)
O_2 N_2 CO_2

parcel of air →

particles or droplets

ATMOSPHERIC CHEMISTRY AND PHYSICS
From Air Pollution to Climate Change
JOHN H. SEINFELD
SPYROS N. PANDIS

1232 pages
1.9 Kg / 4.2 LB

⊙ This is reference no. 3 in Wikipedia - particulates
⊙ You can borrow it for 1 hour from archive.org

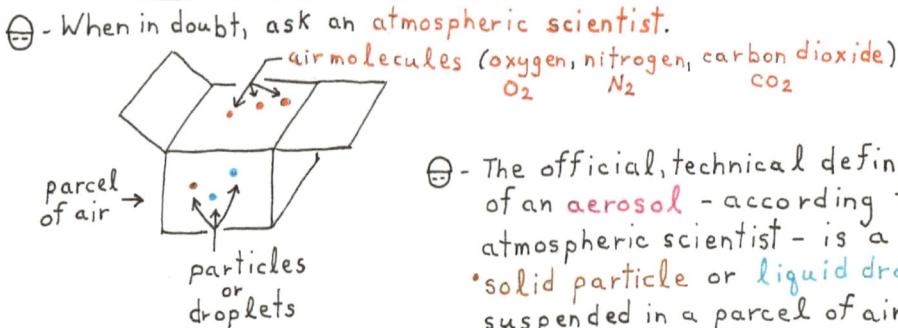

☺ - The official, technical definition of an aerosol - according to an atmospheric scientist - is a •solid particle or liquid droplet• suspended in a parcel of air.

The point is, it is so tiny that it is suspended / floating / hanging in the air.

· A "particulate" is a particle contributing to pollution/contamination of the atmosphere. But no one enforces that definition. So say whichever you please - particle or particulate.

5 LAYERS OF EARTH'S ATMOSPHERE

twinkle, twinkle little star

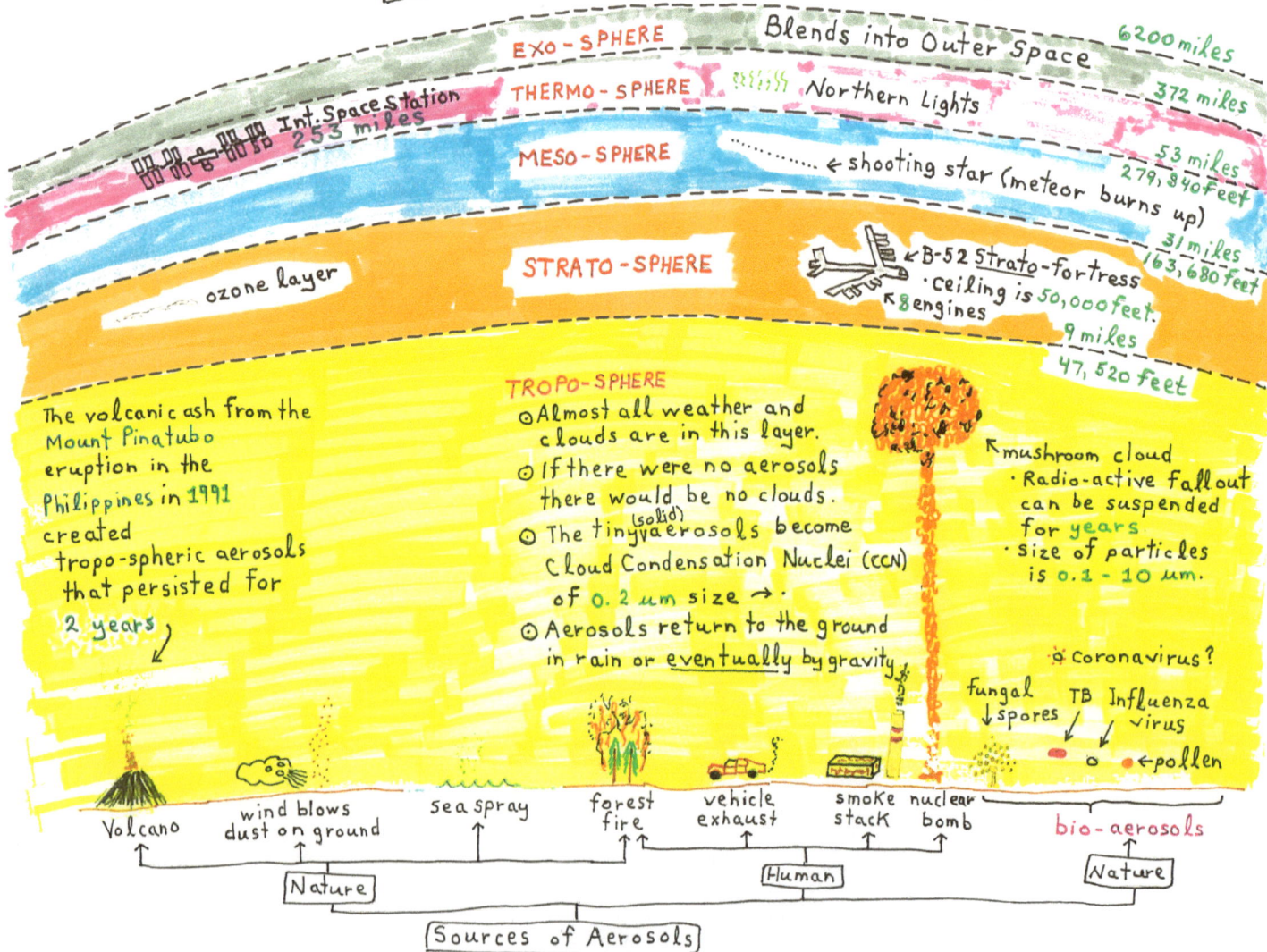

EXO - SPHERE   Blends into Outer Space   6200 miles

THERMO - SPHERE   Northern Lights   372 miles

Int. Space Station
253 miles

MESO - SPHERE   ← shooting star (meteor burns up)   53 miles
                                                          279,840 feet

                                                          31 miles
                                                          163,680 feet

STRATO - SPHERE   ←B-52 Strato-fortress
                     · ceiling is 50,000 feet
ozone layer   ←8 engines   9 miles
                                                          47,520 feet

TROPO-SPHERE

The volcanic ash from the Mount Pinatubo eruption in the Philippines in 1991 created tropo-spheric aerosols that persisted for 2 years

⊙ Almost all weather and clouds are in this layer.
⊙ If there were no aerosols there would be no clouds.
⊙ The tiny aerosols (solid) become Cloud Condensation Nuclei (CCN) of 0.2 um size →
⊙ Aerosols return to the ground in rain or eventually by gravity

←mushroom cloud
· Radio-active fallout can be suspended for years.
· size of particles is 0.1 - 10 um.

⊙ Coronavirus?

fungal ↓ spores   TB Influenza virus

                     ←pollen

Volcano   wind blows dust on ground   sea spray   forest fire   vehicle exhaust   smoke stack   nuclear bomb   bio-aerosols

Nature   Human   Nature

Sources of Aerosols

☺ -Our lives are surrounded by droplets and particles, so here are some more definitions.

← liquid droplets

↑ aerosol spray can

⊙ There are 2 things inside the can:
1. **Payload** - for example, red spray paint
2. **Propellant** - it blasts out the payload

← puffer (inhaler)(broncho-dilator) eg. Ventolin for *Asthma*

← What ends up in your lungs are solid particles of a drug

↑ "**atomization**"

⊙ This means a substance is separated into fine droplets (size is not specified) or particles.
⊙ The goal is not to produce atoms, so it's a confusing word.

☺ -The propellants called **CFC**s (**C**hloro-**F**luoro-**C**arbons) were banned because they cause *ozone holes*.

Lung penetration

← volcanic ash

⊙ Volcanic ash is <u>not</u> ash like in a fireplace.

⊙ Volcanic ash is { rock fragments / glass } → Into your lungs
↳ The result of lava (molten rock) rapidly cooling in the air

← 100 μm **volcanic ash** deposited into windpipe (trachea)
⊙ Could also be a 100 μm droplet containing
☼ Coronavirus.

← 4-10 μm ash into smaller airways (bronchi)
⊙ Could also be a droplet containing
☼ Coronavirus.
⊙ Could also be 5 μm Asthma drug particle. That's a good thing.

ZOOM

← air sac (hollow ping pong ball)

PM$_{2.5}$
2.5 μm particle

↓

Environmental Protection Agency (EPA) monitors Particulate Matter (PM) that, if inhaled, may be harmful.

Volcanic ash < 4 μm deposits in air sac

↓

"Restrictive Lung Disease" (lungs cannot easily expand)

Aspergillus 2 μm spore

↓

Fungus ball (maybe)

Coronavirus 0.1 μm

Invades Type II Pneumo-cyte

— electron
nucleus { protons / neutrons

atom

} "Particle Physics" is all about sub-atomic particles.

♀ - Is this on the Coronavirus final exam?

♂ - No

Nitty gritty definitions

← salt (NaCl) (sodium chloride) dissolves in H$_2$O

↑ sea water

Salt (sea) water is a <u>solution</u>.

time passes →

sand grains suspended in H$_2$O

☺ -Sand does not dissolve in water.
← sand has settled on bottom

This is called a "Suspension" so long as the sand has not settled.

☺ -Neither does fat or oil.
← invisible milk fat globules are suspended in H$_2$O for a <u>long time</u>.

↑ milk

This is called a "colloidal suspension" or "colloid".

☺ -Point is { Particles can be suspended in <u>water</u> (a liquid).
Tiny particles or tiny droplets ("aerosols") can be suspended in <u>air</u> (a gas).
↳ ☼ ← Maybe Coronavirus is in the droplet

← dead horse (*Equus ferus*)

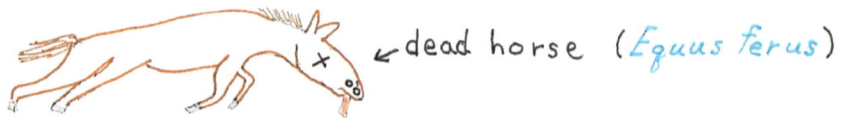

- Okay, we beat that to death.
  - I didn't say you'd feel <u>completely</u> better. I said you'd feel <u>much</u> better.
  - Because droplets, aerosols, and particles can be S/M/L/XL, confusion results. The most accurate descriptor is simply the diameter in microns (μm); however, as with most things in life, definitions become entrenched due to tradition.

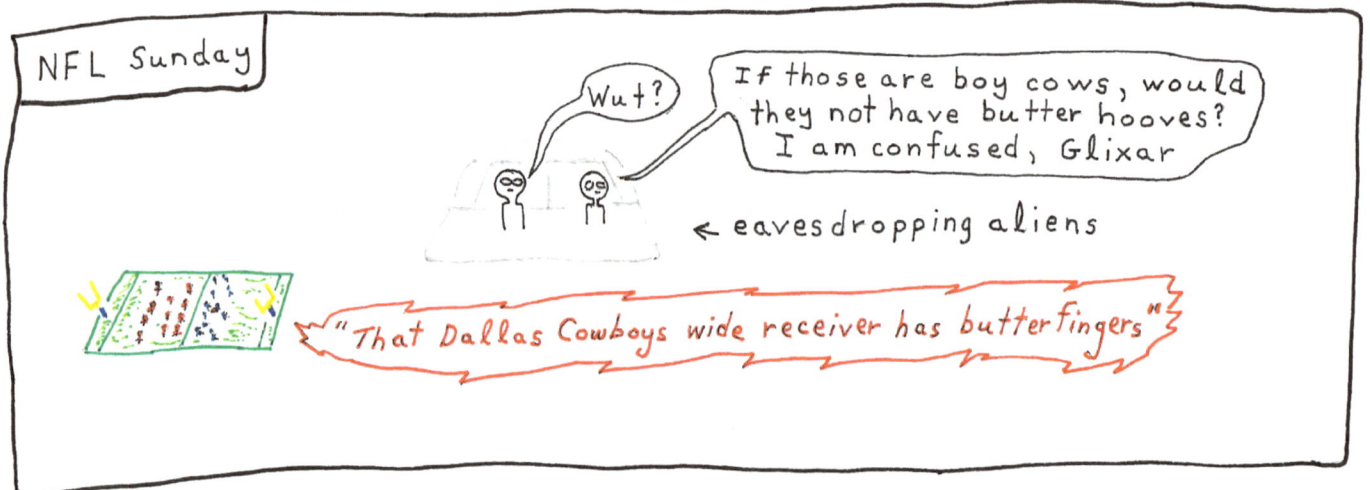

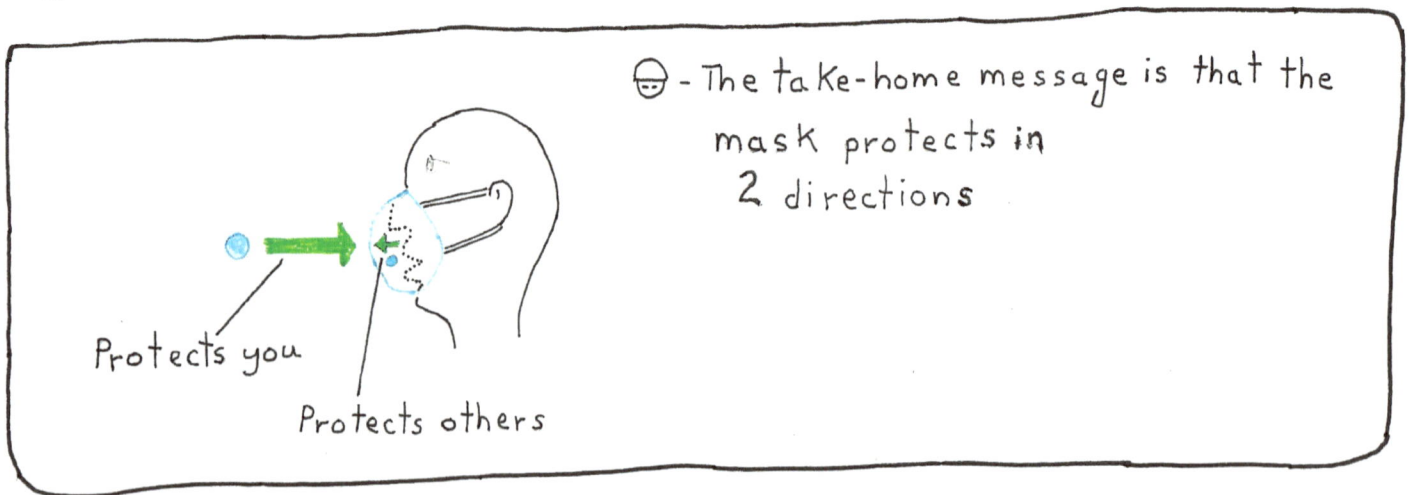

NFL Sunday

Wut?

If those are boy cows, would they not have butter hooves? I am confused, Glixar

← eavesdropping aliens

"That Dallas Cowboys wide receiver has butterfingers"

- The take-home message is that the mask protects in 2 directions

Protects you

Protects others

CHAPTER 6
OMG WHAT A DISASTER

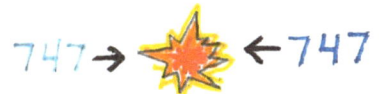

WHAT CAN THE TITANIC,
A NUCLEAR ACCIDENT,
A PLANE CRASH,
AND COW INTESTINES
TEACH US ABOUT MANAGING
A PANDEMIC?

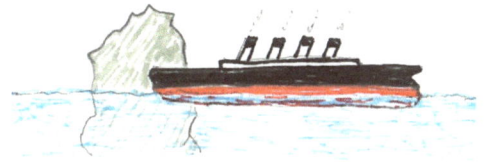

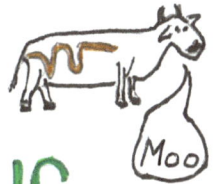

☺ - Oh, silly me, I almost forgot that we first met at the Titanic. There are 4 reasons why she sank.

#1 CALM WEATHER, ironically.

☆ ☆ ← Moonless night
☆   Iceberg not visible by reflected moonlight.

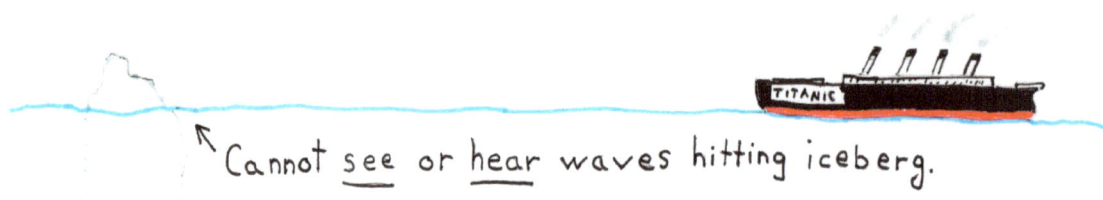

← Cannot see or hear waves hitting iceberg.

... impact at 11:40 p.m., 14 April 1912
... 20 knots (1 knot = 1.15 miles per hour)
   ↳ 23 miles per hour
... sinks (as in, disappears) 2:20 a.m., 15 April

#2 A PAPERWEIGHT, bizarrely.

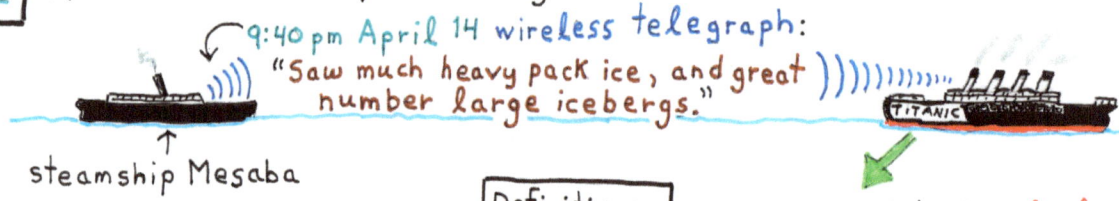

9:40 pm April 14 wireless telegraph:
"Saw much heavy pack ice, and great number large icebergs."

steamship Mesaba

Titanic wireless operator Jack Phillips (25 years old)
"I'm gonna put that vital iceberg telegram under a paperweight."

Definitions

16 feet or higher Above Sea Level (ASL)
3-16 feet ASL
0-3 feet ASL

5382 square feet
1076-3299 sq.ft.
215 sq. ft

'bergy bit'
'growler' (size of a grand piano)

iceberg

← paper weight

wireless telegraph

Printed telegram from steamship Mesaba

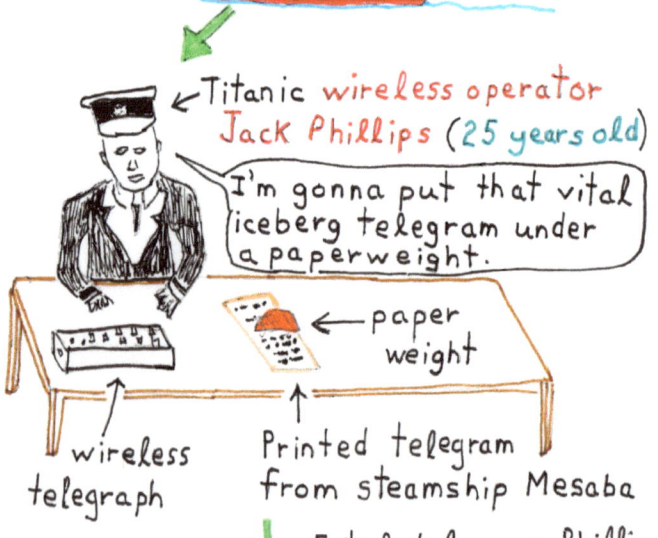

Fatal delay as Phillips continues to send passenger messages to Cape Race, Newfoundland

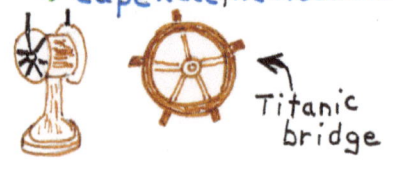

Money Talks

1896 - Guglielmo Marconi invents wireless telegraph.
1903 - Marconi wireless telegraphs installed on ships.
  ↳ Ship-to-ship message $
  ↳ Passenger-to-land message $$$
     10-word 'Marconigram' is $82 (if 2023).

Titanic bridge

#3 The Titanic was a gigantic, floating ICE CUBE TRAY.

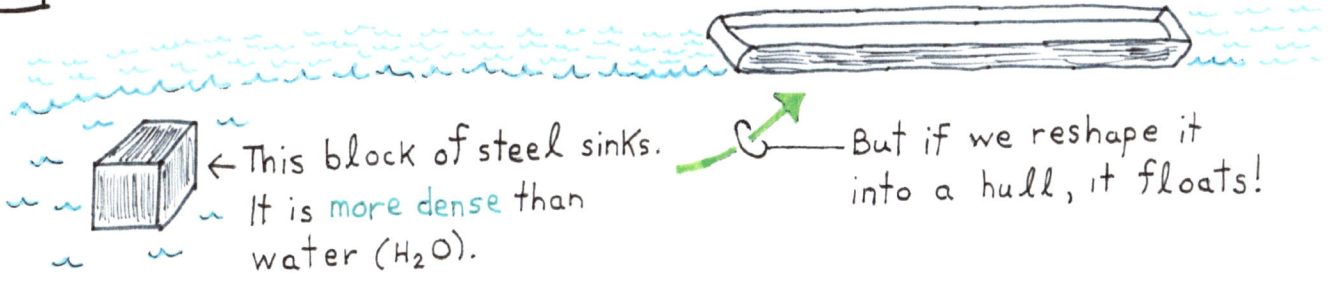

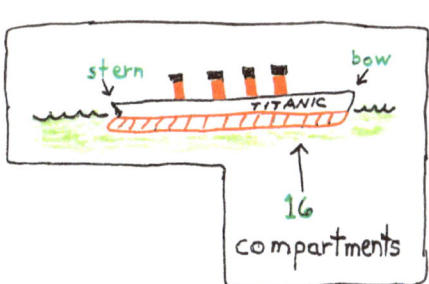

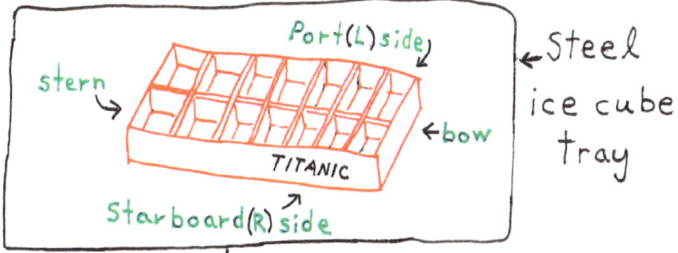

← This block of steel sinks.
It is more dense than
water (H_2O).

→ But if we reshape it
into a hull, it floats!

stern   bow
TITANIC
16 compartments

stern
Port(L) side
bow
TITANIC
Starboard(R) side

← Steel ice cube tray

Except it's empty! ←
That's why it floats, even though it's made of steel.
The hull displaces 46,000 tons of water.
That's called Archimedes' Principle.

Archimedes also derived the value of
π (pi) (3.14) without a calculator in ~250 B.C.

... But if water floods into an ice cube tray ➡ the water spills
over from one 'compartment' to the next (just hold an ice
cube tray under a slow stream of water to prove this to yourself).

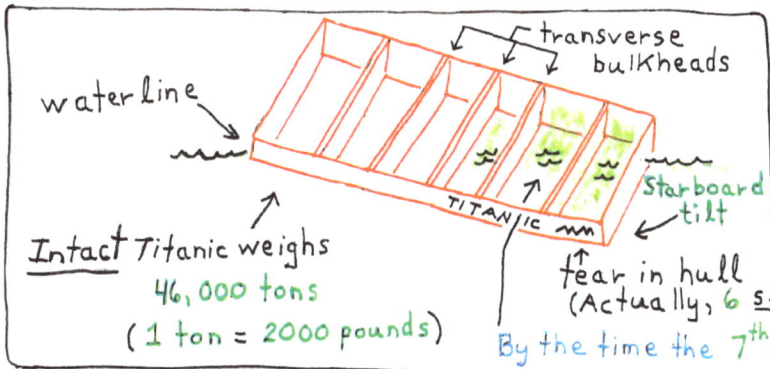

waterline
transverse bulkheads
TITANIC
Starboard tilt

Intact Titanic weighs
46,000 tons
(1 ton = 2000 pounds)

◆ The Titanic, more accurately,
is an ice cube tray with
16 compartments and no
central divider.
← (But only 6 compartments
drawn here)

tear in hull
(Actually, 6 slits in hull where plates separate)

By the time the 7th (of 16) compartment has flooded,
there is 34,970 tons of water onboard ... when
it gets to 46,000 ... she is going down in 1 piece
... but she breaks in $\frac{1}{2}$ before that happens
... she's a goner

Now she weighs:
46,000 ship
+ 34,970 water
──────────
80,970 tons
Not good for floating

#4 RIVETS, RIVETS, RIVETS

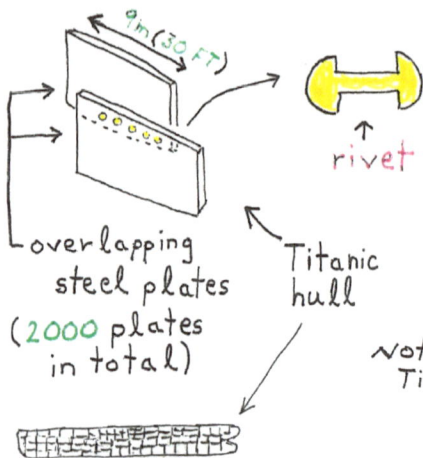

9m (30 FT)

overlapping steel plates (2000 plates in total)

rivet

Titanic hull

- ⊙ 600 rivets per steel plate.
- ⊙ 3,000,000 rivets in total.
- ⊙ Manually pounded into holes with a rivet hammer.
- ⊙ Made of steel.
  - ⊙ Iron + 1% Carbon = Steel
  - ⊙ steel is stronger than iron alone.

Not the Titanic [
  - ⊙ Chromium is added to make Stainless Steel (like a Japanese knife to chop credit cards).
  - ⊙ Sulfur is added to increase the 'machinability' of steel (which is how easy it is to cut).

★ The steel rivets of the Titanic had a <u>high</u> Sulfur content, ★ causing them to be brittle in cold water, which when combined with the high impact forces with the iceberg, caused the steel plates of the hull to separate, allowing ★ water to enter the ship.

😑 — What was the point of that Titanic trivia?
- ·The Titanic was a state-of-the-art ship in 1912.
  - ·It had more rivets than the Eiffel Tower.
  - ·It had motors to lower the bulkhead between compartments.

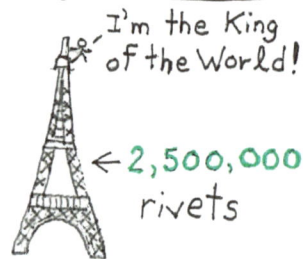

I'm the King of the World!

← 2,500,000 rivets

`After the Titanic sank ~ 👤 there were changes to ship design.

This water is freezing! Where's global warming when you need it?

① ↓ sulfur in rivets

② ← The 5-sided compartments (think, ice cube tray) of new ships became 6-sided. Basically a lid was added ∴ ∅ H_2O spill-over if a single compartment floods. Alternatively, a taller bulkhead.

😑 — Disasters reveal the flaws in 'state-of-the-art' technology and prompt change and innovation. State-of-the-art during the 1918 Influenza Pandemic was basically subpar cloth masks. No vaccine existed. And no one had ever even seen a virus (the electron microscope was invented in 1931).
`Let's explore some disasters to gain context on how to manage a pandemic.

☺ - Ever heard of the **Three Mile Island accident** ?

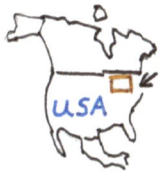

USA → Pennsylvania → Susquehana River → Three Mile Island (TMI)

Nuclear reactor — cooling tower — Hot / Cold — coolant pipes (contain radioactive water)

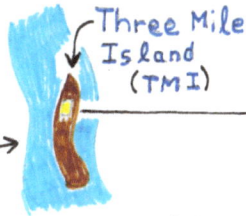

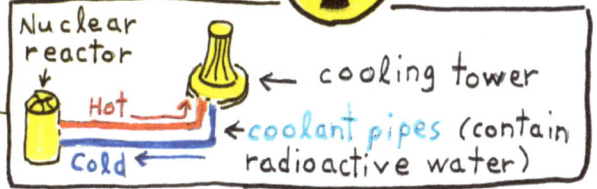

Event: 1979 March 28: nuclear reactor meltdown, TMI nuclear plant, Pennsylvania.

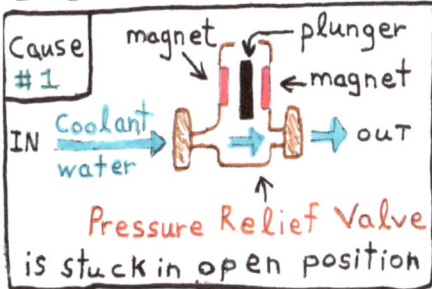

Cause #1

magnet — plunger — magnet

IN Coolant water → OUT

Pressure Relief Valve is stuck in open position

Cause #2

SOLENOID
ACTIVE   WARNING

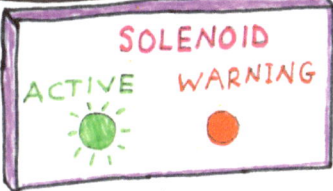

↑
solenoid status

☺ - The **solenoid** is the magnet that raises or lowers the plunger.

N   S

The control room lights only indicate if the solenoid is worKing.

The **Control Room operators** do not Know if the **Pressure Relief Valve** is OPEN or CLOSED

The loss of pressure is not noticed for hours

☺ - That was a **design flaw** in **the way information is presented**.

☺ - A **Pressure Relief Valve** remained in the OPEN position (the plunger stayed up)

↻ bad
↓
Constant **coolant water** outflow
↻ bad
↓
Loss of pressure a.K.a. **Loss Of Coolant Accident** (LOCA)
↻ bad
↓
Top of reactor core exposed
↻ bad
↓
reactor core
½ the uranium melts
↓
Core Temperature **2000°C** (partial ↗ meltdown)
↻ bad
coolant water evaporating
↻ very bad
↓
Total core meltdown imminent
↪ Exceedingly bad for **Pittsburgh Steelers fans**
↓
The **state of Pennsylvania** is about to get irradiated
↪ YiKes!
↓
Emergency Core Cooling System (ECCS) is activated
↻ good
↓
New source of **water** is pumped into core
↻ good
↓
Disaster is avoided

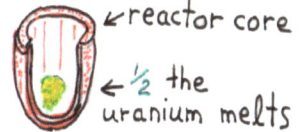

bad ↺

♀ - Is this how the **HULK** got created?

♀ - I dunno

⊝ - After the nuclear accident, a sociologist named Charles Perrow wrote a book with an oxymoron title: **Normal Accidents.**

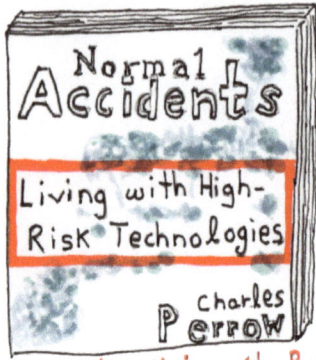

Normal **Accidents**

Living with High-Risk Technologies

Charles P errow

Princeton University Press

♀ - What's a sociologist?

⚥ - Someone who studies sociology, which is basically how individuals, groups, and organizations interact in a society.

♀ - What's an oxymoron?

⚥ - A phrase with words that contradict each other, like 'normal accidents' or 'generous pharmaceutical company'.

⊝ - Charles Perrow argued that accidents are inevitable in 'tightly-coupled systems.'

♀ - What's a tightly-coupled system?

⚥ - One example is buses and taxis.

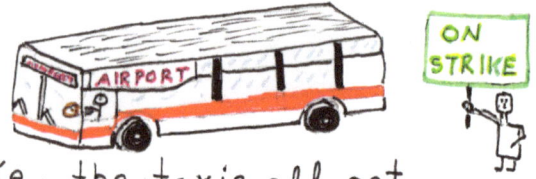

When there's a transit strike, the taxis all get used up. The buses and taxis are tightly coupled, though when things are functioning fine (no strike) we don't notice they are tightly coupled.

ON STRIKE

AIRPORT

TAXI

⊝ - He concluded that the Three Mile Island nuclear plant was a tightly-coupled system.

The accident that occurred was:

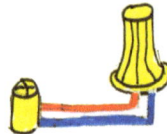

"unexpected, incomprehensible, uncontrollable and unavoidable."

5 μm

I'm a mammal?

⊝ - Let's compare that to the ☼ coronavirus pandemic.

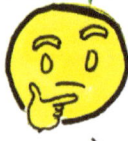

No one had a crystal ball.

Certainly Yes at the beginning, especially regarding transmission.

Government tried semi-successfully to control society because they only semi-agreed on what the goals were.

Bats are mammals that transmit viruses to humans who are mammals.

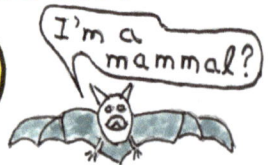

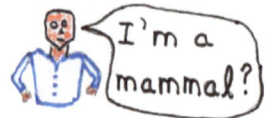

? I'm a mammal?

⊝ - A nuclear meltdown and a spreading virus are not exactly the same but they are food 🍔🍟🥤 for thought.

- Let's think some more about failure and disaster.

Worst Aviation Disaster in History

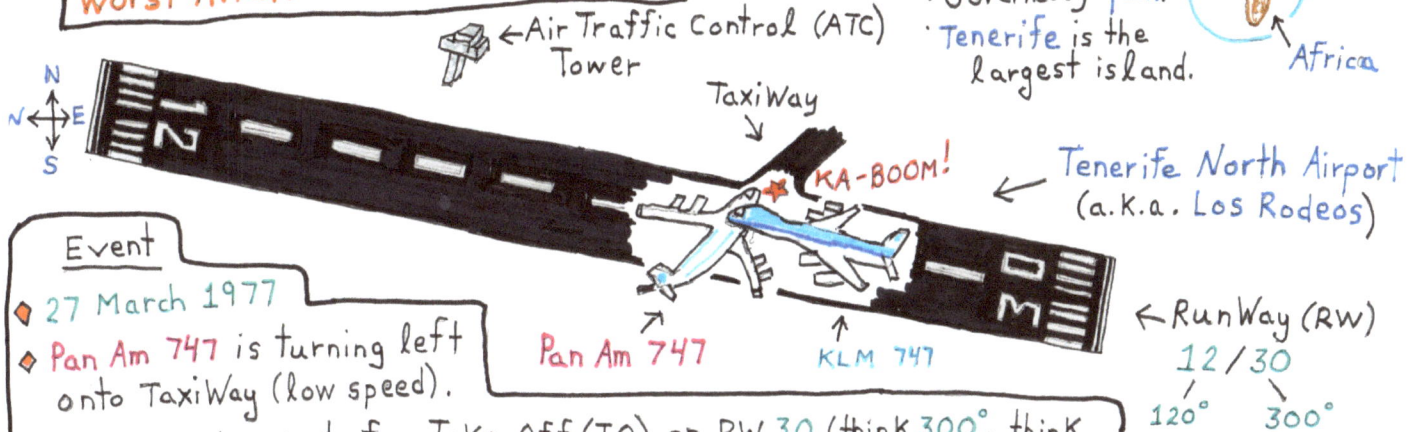

←Air Traffic Control (ATC) Tower

TaxiWay

KA-BOOM!

→ Tenerife North Airport (a.k.a. Los Rodeos)

Canary Islands → Africa
· Governed by Spain.
· Tenerife is the largest island.

N / E / S / W compass

Pan Am 747

KLM 747

←RunWay (RW) 12 / 30
120° 300°

Event

- 27 March 1977
- Pan Am 747 is turning left onto TaxiWay (low speed).
- KLM 747 is ready for Take-Off (TO) on RW 30 (think 300°, think moving West) but it must wait for CLEARANCE from ATC that Pan Am 747 has cleared the RunWay. It's also foggy.
- KLM Flight Engineer is unsure if ATC has given CLEARANCE.
- KLM Captain (much senior) ignores Flight Engineer and begins Take-Off without explicit CLEARANCE from ATC.
- PanAm 747 pilots look in horror as they see KLM 747 coming towards them.
- IMPACT! ➡ 583 Dead

R.I.P.

KLM ⟨ 14 crew / 234 passengers ⟩ Everyone on board dies

Pan Am ⟨ 9 of 16 crew (pilots spared because past point of impact.) / 326 of 380 passengers ⟩

- Of course, there's a big investigation, and the findings are:
  1. Foggy
  2. Vague command from ATC to KLM Flight Engineer.
  3. Pilot error, specifically the KLM Captain.

`One way of thinking about pilot error is 'Hazardous Attitudes.'
  1. Macho ➡ "I am Maverick."
  2. Impulsivity ➡ "I just have to try this!"
  3. Invulnerability ➡ "Accidents happen to other people, not me."
  4. Anti-authority ➡ "Don't tell me what to do."
  5. Resignation (during a flight emergency) ➡ "What's the use in trying?"
  6. Complacency ➡ "No need to practice my emergency drills."

- That wasn't good.
- Nope.

😐 – Here is an example of Complacency leading to disaster.

Walkerton E. coli outbreak

♀ – Are we going to talk about feces again?
⚥ – It's looking that way.

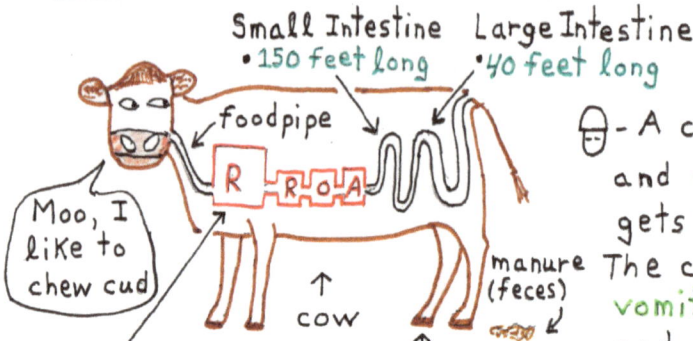

Small Intestine
• 150 feet long
Large Intestine
• 40 feet long

Rumen – Reticulum – Omasum – Abomasum

😐 – A cow has **4 stomachs**. Grass is swallowed and enters the rumen ("room in") where it gets turned into a paste called cud. The cud is regurgitated (not the same as vomiting) into the mouth, chewed more, and swallowed again into the rumen.

foodpipe

R R–O–A

Moo, I like to chew cud

manure (feces)

↑ cow

Hoof made of 2 toes (Order Artio-dactyla)(page 87).

Rumen
• Largest stomach.
• Capacity 25 gallons (100 liters).
• It's on the left side. It contracts 1-2 times per minute.
• Grass is mixed with swallowed saliva (100-150 liters produced daily).
• It contains 50 billion bacteria and 1 million protozoa (think, amoebas).

How did I end up in a cow?

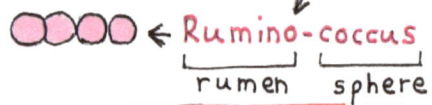

⬤⬤⬤⬤ ← Rumino-coccus
rumen   sphere

😐 – The most important bacteria in the rumen is Ruminococcus. Its job in life is to break down grass. And what is grass made of? Cellulose, which is a sugar.

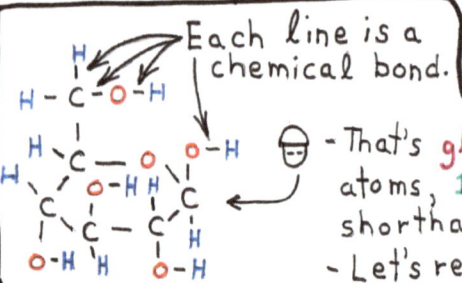

Each line is a chemical bond.

H–C–O–H

😐 – That's glucose (sugar). If you count them up, there are 6 Carbon (C) atoms, 12 Hydrogen (H) atoms, and 6 Oxygen (O) atoms. The chemistry shorthand for that is $C_6H_{12}O_6$.
– Let's reduce the clutter and stick to the important stuff.

Cellulose 😐 – The C atoms are numbered 1 to 6.

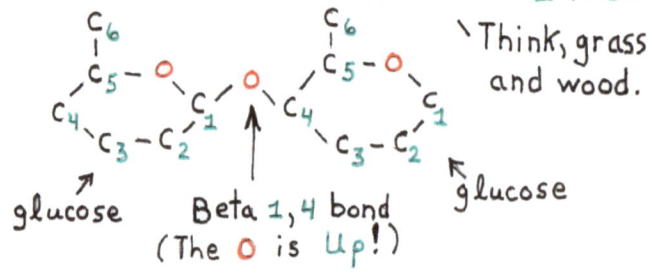

` Think, grass and wood.

C_6
C_5 – O
C_4 C_1 O C_4 C_1
C_3 – C_2 C_3 – C_2
↑   ↖ glucose
glucose   Beta 1,4 bond
(The O is Up!)

😐 – Rumino-coccus ⬤⬤⬤⬤ can split the bond and convert cellulose into individual glucose units. A similar process occurs in termites →

` I remember this as, "Mr. Termite, you Beta wake up."

Starch 😐 – Think, pasta and potatoes.

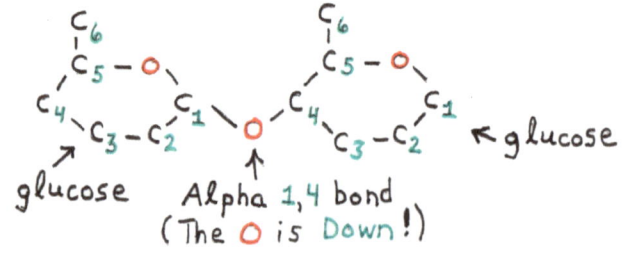

C_6
C_5 – O
C_4 C_1 O C_4 C_1
C_3 – C_2 C_3 – C_2 ← glucose
↑   ↑
glucose   Alpha 1,4 bond
(The O is Down!)

😐 – Humans can split this bond and turn starch into individual glucose units. Glucose is our energy source.

` Starch and Cellulose are actually chains of 100's or 1000's of glucose units.

- Okay, we're getting to Walkerton soon.
`Switch your brain to a totally different bacteria.

Human →

5 feet long
Large Intestine (colon)
It is considered to be a picture frame. And the 'painting' is the Small Intestine enclosed by it.

Small Intestine (10 feet long)

← E.coli

- You already met this guy on page 59
- It's a rod bacteria.
- It lives in our Colon.
- ← Sugar cube of human feces contains 5,000,000,000 E.coli

SOMPOO SAYS — "ee" "Kow lie" rhymes with low

← E. coli O157:H7
That's called a sero-type.

Large Intestine (colon)
• E.coli O157:H7 lives in the cow's large intestine. And in the cow's feces (manure).

Moo boo hoo

feces (manure)

w ← Toxin

• The toxin is harmful to humans, which is why great lengths are taken to keep cow feces out of our food and water.

O157:H7
↑   ↑
Those are letters.

• The toxin also harms Vero cells from the Green monkey.
  • Remember 'green' from the Wuhan Institute of Virology experiments.
  • For that reason it may be called a vero-toxin. (page 116)
• The official name is Shiga Toxin. That's because it's similar or identical to toxins made by a bacteria called Shigella. Therefore E. coli O157:H7 may also go by the name ShigaToxin-producing E. coli (STEC).

← Shigella

w ← Shiga Toxin (ST)

- Shigella is a rod bacteria Known for causing bloody diarrhea. The blood comes from the damaged lining of the intestines.

- Amazingly, a phage (virus of bacteria) introduced the genetic code for Shiga Toxin into E. coli O157:H7.
`The bacteria does not die in this scenario, rather it is enhanced!

phage

- The take-home message is that Rumino-coccus in the cow's rumen breaks down grass (basically, cellulose). And E. coli O157:H7 in the cow's Large Intestine produces ShigaToxin that's harmful to humans.

😐 - Welcome to Walkerton. The year is 2000.

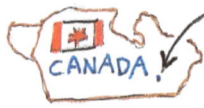

Walkerton, population 5000.

◊ The drinking water is supplied by an aquifer (water trapped by rock layers).

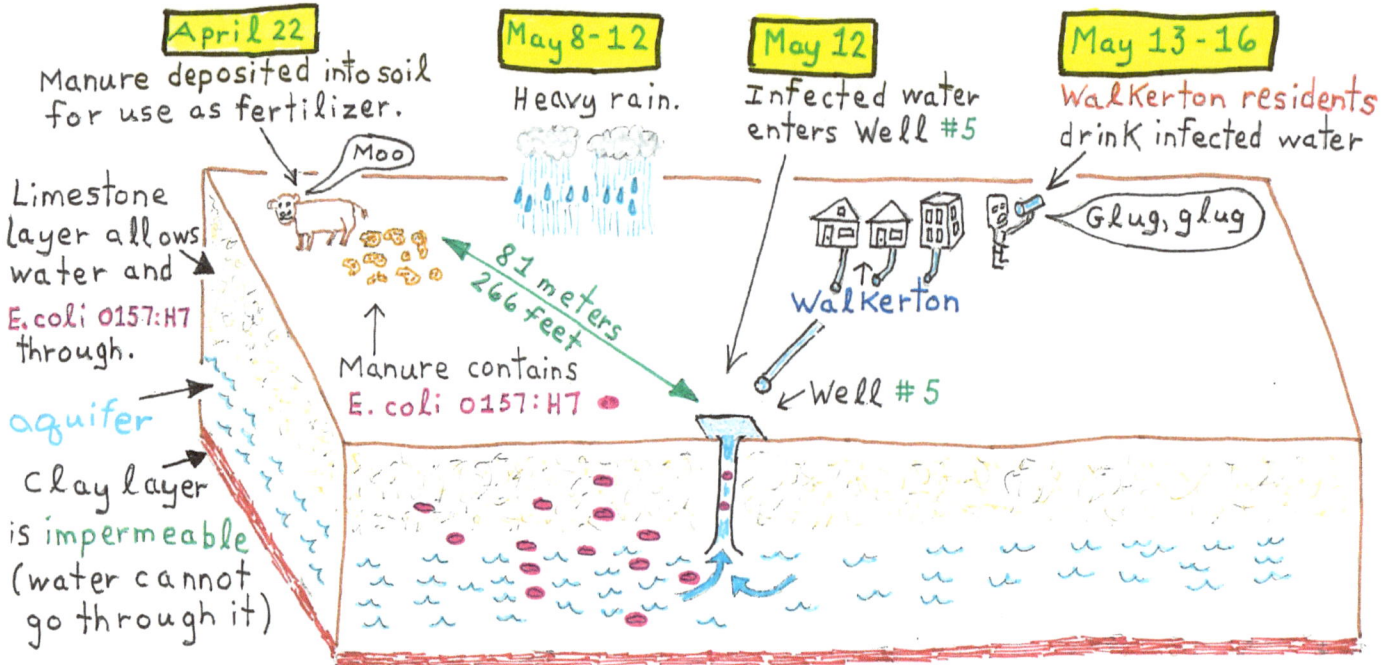

CANADA

April 22

Manure deposited into soil for use as fertilizer.

May 8-12

Heavy rain.

May 12

Infected water enters Well #5

May 13-16

Walkerton residents drink infected water

Moo

Limestone layer allows water and E. coli 0157:H7 through.

aquifer

Clay layer is impermeable (water cannot go through it)

81 meters 266 feet

Manure contains E. coli 0157:H7

Walkerton

Well #5

Glug, glug

😐 - This was a tightly-coupled system. The heavy rains were like a transit strike revealing flaws in the system.

① The Walkerton Public Utilities Commission (PUC) employees knew very little about water safety, nevertheless the government certified them as qualified. That's double complacency.

↳ Chlorine is added to water to kill E. coli 0157:H7.
  0.5 mg Chlorine per 1 ml of water **was** the standard.
  0.27 mg/ml was what the PUC maintained.

↳ Water samples were carelessly taken.

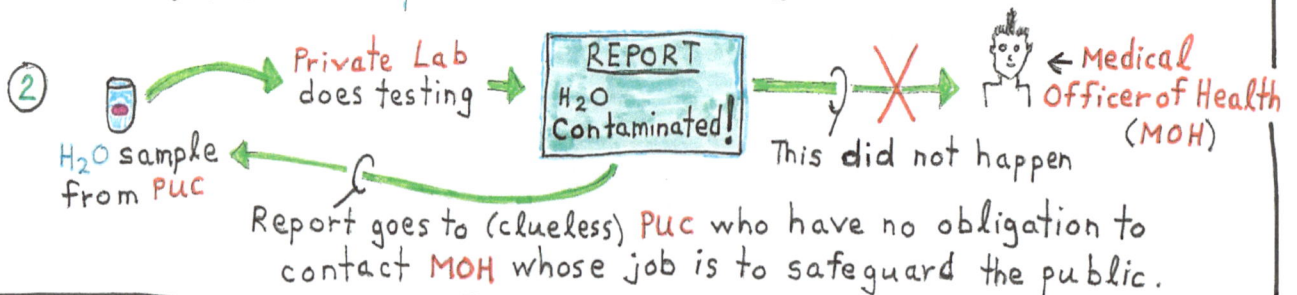

② H₂O sample from PUC

Private Lab does testing

REPORT H₂O Contaminated!

This **did** not happen

Medical Officer of Health (MOH)

Report goes to (clueless) PUC who have no obligation to contact MOH whose job is to safeguard the public.

What happened?

Shiga Toxin → 2000 cases of Gastro-Enteritis (diarrhea or bloody diarrhea).
  ↳ 6 deaths ΩΩΩΩΩΩ in children from Hemo-lytic Uremic Syndrome where Red Blood Cells fragment and there is sudden Kidney Failure.

☺ -Let's recap those disastrous information failures.

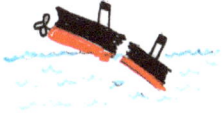

Titanic was a human delay in passing on vital information.

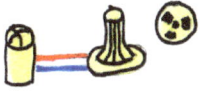

Three Mile Island was a design flaw in how information is displayed.

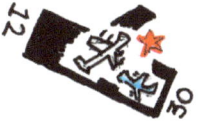

747's crashing in Tenerife was a failure to wait for information that it was safe to TakeOff.

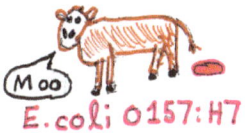

Walkerton was not even knowing what information was important despite other people knowing it was.

E.coli O157:H7

♀ - I can't even remember what I packed in my suitcase. Never put me in charge of anything.

⚥ - How about making a smoothie? Do you think you can handle that?

☺ -What about the ☉ Corona-virus pandemic? Was it a failure of information? Or simply the inevitable fact that Mother Nature creates viruses in her mighty, steaming cauldron?

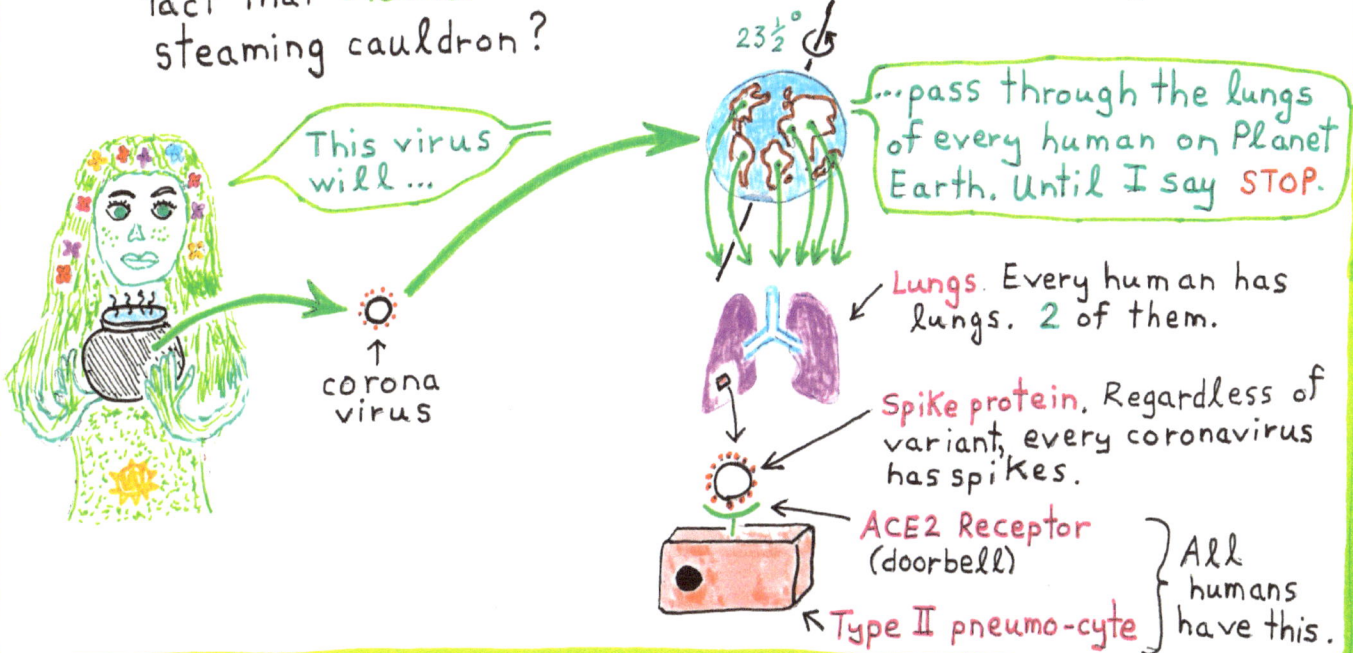

This virus will...

$23\frac{1}{2}°$

...pass through the lungs of every human on Planet Earth. Until I say STOP.

corona virus

Lungs. Every human has lungs. 2 of them.

Spike protein. Regardless of variant, every coronavirus has spikes.

ACE2 Receptor (doorbell)

Type II pneumo-cyte

All humans have this.

😐 - Mother Nature leaves it up to humans to solve their problems. And humans, of course, have a fondness for organization and governing bodies.

IMO	ICAO	IAEA	WHO	CDC
International Maritime Organization	International Civil Aviation Organization	International Atomic Energy Agency	World Health Organization	Centers for Disease Control and Prevention

WHO collaborates with CDC

😐 - Regarding Infectious Disease ( ), a huge, multi-layered organization exists in the U.S.A. Information flows between the layers.

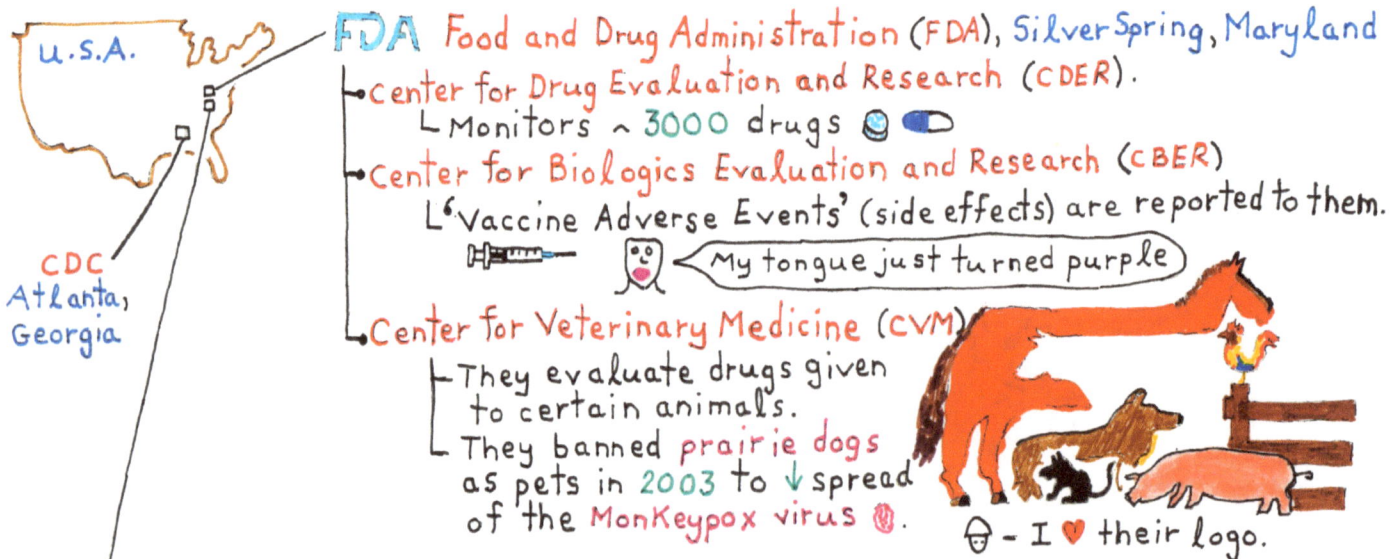

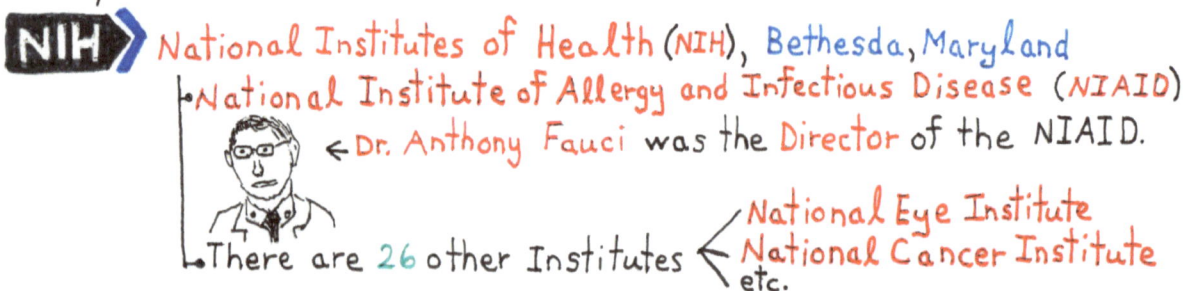

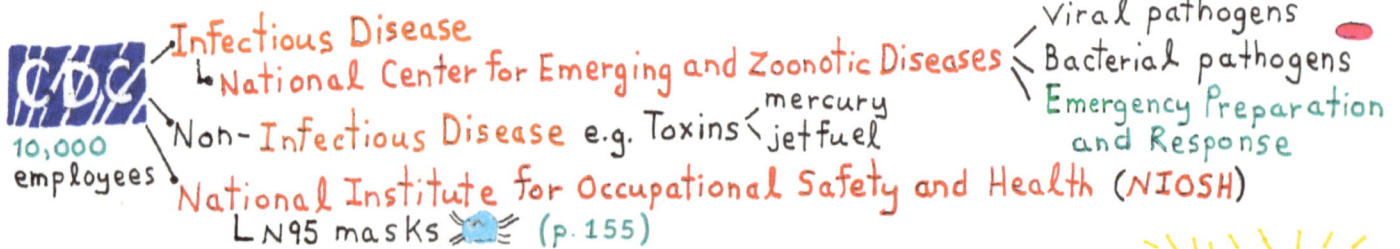

U.S.A.

CDC Atlanta, Georgia

FDA Food and Drug Administration (FDA), Silver Spring, Maryland
- Center for Drug Evaluation and Research (CDER).
  - Monitors ~3000 drugs
- Center for Biologics Evaluation and Research (CBER)
  - 'Vaccine Adverse Events' (side effects) are reported to them.

My tongue just turned purple

- Center for Veterinary Medicine (CVM)
  - They evaluate drugs given to certain animals.
  - They banned prairie dogs as pets in 2003 to ↓ spread of the Monkeypox virus.

😐 - I ♥ their logo.

NIH National Institutes of Health (NIH), Bethesda, Maryland
- National Institute of Allergy and Infectious Disease (NIAID)
  - Dr. Anthony Fauci was the Director of the NIAID.
- There are 26 other Institutes
  - National Eye Institute
  - National Cancer Institute
  - etc.

Viral pathogens
Bacterial pathogens
Emergency Preparation and Response

CDC
10,000 employees
- Infectious Disease
  - National Center for Emerging and Zoonotic Diseases
- Non-Infectious Disease e.g. Toxins < mercury / jet fuel
- National Institute for Occupational Safety and Health (NIOSH)
  - N95 masks (p. 155)

😐 - Point is, boatloads of experts exchange information devoted to Your Health.

- In an ideal world, there would be no disease and we'd all have a pet unicorn. In the real world, the best we can do is prevent disease.

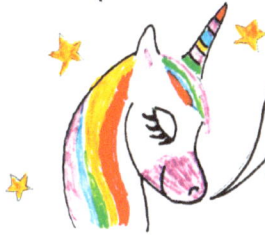

There are 2 kinds of prevention.

Primary (1°) Prevention = Prevent disease or injury from occurring.

1°

Seat belt

IGNORE ADVICE

Ejected through windshield

Uh oh

brain bleed   skull fracture

Ooooh, that smarts. Next time I'll wear my seat belt

1°

WARNING
Your momma will cry at your funeral

Cigarette warning label

- How do doctors measure the amount of smoking?

- Pack years

1 Pack Per Day × 20 years = 20 Pack years

2 PPD × 20 years = 40 Pack years

IGNORE ADVICE

Lung Cancer

If a surgeon has to cut out a lobe of the lung, that's called a lobectomy. ("lobe eK tuh me").

There are 4 kinds of lung cancer. 2 of them are highly correlated with smoking cigarettes.

1°

Clean Water Act
- 1972 legislation

EPA

- The Environmental Protection Agency (EPA) is another layer devoted to your health.
- The Act basically regulates the discharge of pollutants into water.

FACTORY IGNORES THE ACT

scary chemicals

river

MUTANT TOAD CONSUMES UNICORN

Burp

HELP

1° (continued)

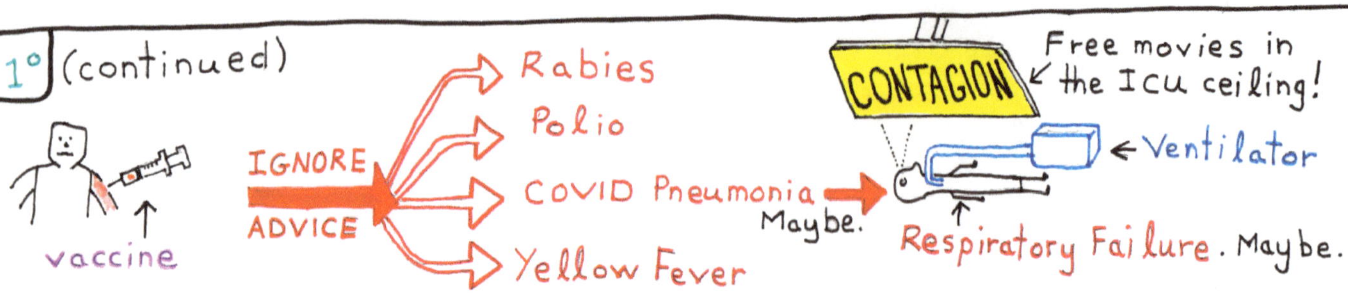

vaccine

IGNORE ADVICE →
→ Rabies
→ Polio
→ COVID Pneumonia Maybe. → Respiratory Failure. Maybe.
→ Yellow Fever

CONTAGION
Free movies in the ICU ceiling!
← Ventilator

☿ ~ A vaccine takes advantage of the fact that our immune system has a memory. So when exposed to the real pathogen (often a virus) at a *later date*, it reacts very strongly.

Secondary (2°) Prevention = Screening to detect disease that is already present. But the goal is *early detection*.

2° 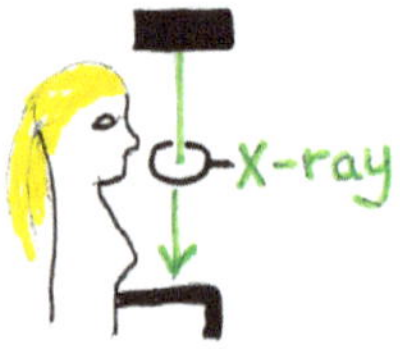
—X-ray
Mammo-gram to detect Breast Cancer

2° 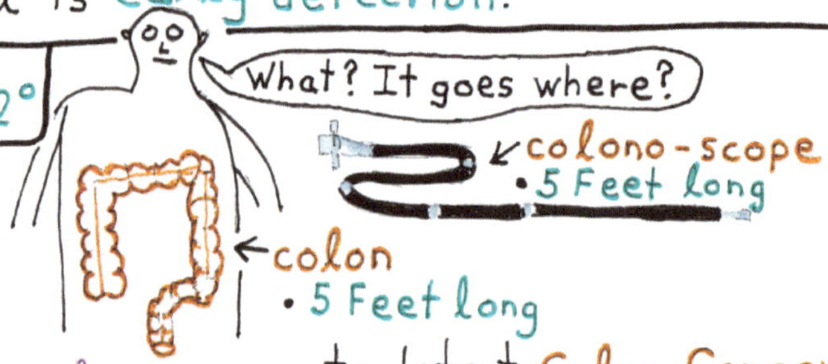
What? It goes where?
← colono-scope
• 5 Feet long
← colon
• 5 Feet long
Colon-oscopy to detect Colon Cancer

2° 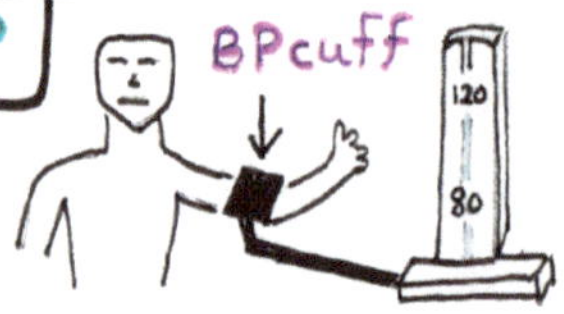
BP cuff
120 ← Blood Pressure when ♥ *contracts*.
—————
80 ← Blood Pressure when ♥ relaxes.

♀ - What does "120 over 80" actually mean?
☿ - It means that *mercury*, which is a *liquid metal*, rises 120 milli-meters (4.7 inches) in a glass tube. Then 80 milli-meters (3.1 inches).

♀ - Gee, that really helps.
☿ - It's physics. The important thing is that high blood pressure is a major Risk Factor for ♥ Attack or Stroke

☻ - The unicorn lied. There is also Tertiary (3°)("terr sherry") Prevention. = Basically, damage control after illness has occurred.

3° 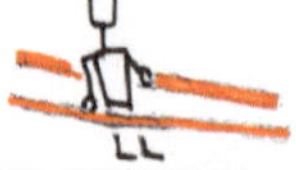
← Rehab(ilitation) exercises after a Stroke

- The stuff on this page is obscure but incredibly important. *So important that my hat fell off.*

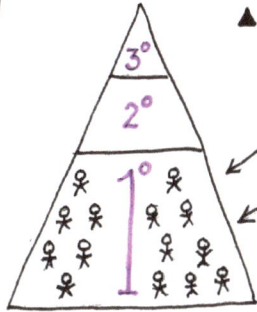

▲ Now you know how **doctors** and **epidemiologists** (who notice patterns of disease) look at $1°$, $2°$, and $3°$ **Prevention**.

$1°$ is the biggest bang for the buck.

It is far more cost-effective to print **cigarette warning labels** that 200 million people can read rather than pay **surgeons** $$$ to remove a lobe of the lung from smokers who develop Lung Cancer.

YOU WILL DIE. IT'S A PROMISE

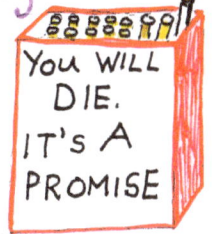

- Not to mention $$ **chemo-therapy** or $$ **radiation therapy**.

γ **gamma rays**

` Or $$ **hospital beds**.
` This is called **Health Economics**.

Lung Cancer treatment →

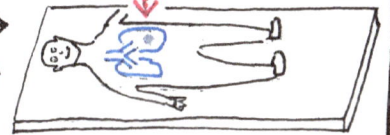

- What's the difference between X-rays and Gamma rays?

- Ahem, **X-rays** are emitted by **orbiting electrons**.
Gamma (γ) rays are emitted by the **nucleus**.

` Gamma (γ) is the 3rd letter in the Greek alphabet. →

∝ alpha
β beta
γ gamma
} → "alphabet"

More Health Economics **QALY**

- "Qually" rhymes with "Golly."
SOMPOO SAYS

- How do we measure how effective a drug (or intervention) is?

- 1. **Quality Of Life (QOL)**
  - How much did the drug improve QOL?
  - **Health economists** measure this in units of '**utility**.'

` 2. **Length Of Life (LOL)**
  - How long did the drug extend life? **Days? Years?**

QALY = Quality Adjusted Life Year
1 = Perfect health ☺ (Utility 1) × 1 year
0.5 = Perfect health ☺ (Utility 1) × 0.5 years
0.5 = So-so health ☹ (Utility 0.5) × 1 year
bed-ridden →

0 = Dead.
You can even get a negative score of "Worse than dead." Wow.

- **Doctors** are conservative and responsible. They are trained to err on the side of caution. They also consider $1°/2°/3°$ and **QALY**. This is important for the decisions made during a pandemic.

- Can a PANDEMIC actually be prevented?

'In a world of planes,

Singapore, here we come!

automobiles,

Road Trip!

ships,

S.S. CROWDED

AAACHOO!

trains,

All aboard!

droplets, aerosols,
>5μm   <5μm

and vectors

I have 1,000,000 followers in my cave. #dontblameme

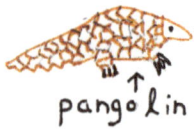

pangolin

Really? I'm a vector?

I transmit the Black Death. And I jump like a champ.

flea (Class Insecta: 6 legs)

... that's a challenge.

- The World Health Organization (WHO) divvies up the world into 6 regions, each with a Regional Director (usually a Medical Doctor).

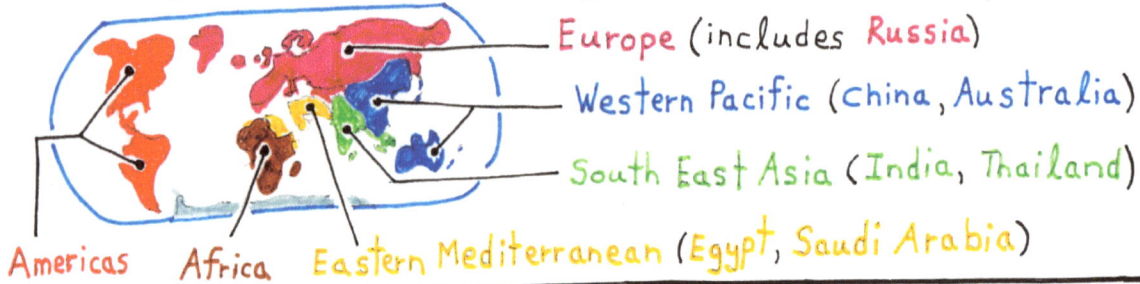

Europe (includes Russia)

Western Pacific (China, Australia)

South East Asia (India, Thailand)

Eastern Mediterranean (Egypt, Saudi Arabia)

Americas   Africa

Aspergillus

- Is there a regional director in Antarctica?
- Nope. But maybe they should send a vet down there because the nasty fungus Aspergillus can infect penguins.

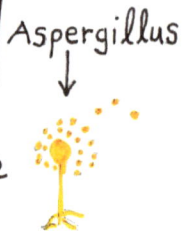

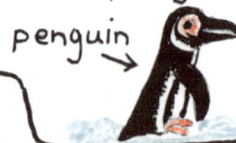

penguin

Call the vet on my sat phone

- Within each WHO region, every country has a Medical Officer of Health (MOH) to implement pandemic guidelines. But the MOH does not work for the WHO, necessarily.

I'm me
- What are the biggest obstacles to cooperation?

You're you
- Sovereign states do not have to comply with the WHO.
Lack of 'metrics' that measure how many people are infected.
Inability to cope with a surge in cases.
War, famine.

⊖ – Ultimately, a whole wack of experts assess the risk.

CONTINUUM OF BADNESS

↑? ↑? ↑?

Common Cold
(AAACHOO)
Sneezing, stuffed-up nose. Feel blah for a few days.
←rhino-virus

↑ Rather insignificant

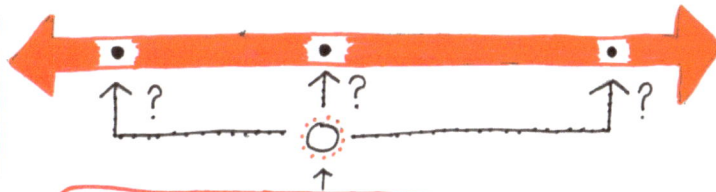

Corona-virus
- Where did it sit in the continuum?
- This was the question basically in January 2020.
- It had already caused SARS in 2003 and MERS in 2012.

Smallpox RIP
Bubonic Plague
Ebola
Influenza TypeA H1N1 1918 virus

↑ Severe consequences

◯–Decision Tree

Do nothing (∅)

Do something

Best Case Scenario
- It's all good.
- The virus passes over us like a harmless morning fog.

Worst Case Scenario
- 100 million dead? RIP
- All the ICU doctors die.
⊖ – Do you have any idea how bad that is?
`They are part of a tightly coupled system
`If they die, you die.

Best Case Scenario
- Massive global Primary (1°) Prevention efforts.
  - ←masks
  - 6 FEET social distancing
  - Hand washing to kill virus
  - vaccine
- The goal is ↓R_0 (spread).

Worst Case Scenario
- No one Listens ↓ RIP

Bergamo
- In Italy, the pandemic started here.
- The doctors died here, mostly.

- 61 doctors in Italy had died by March 2020. Doctors are not supposed to die. Or nurses. That really scared doctors. Things looked way worse than SARS or MERS.

☿ → ∅		$R_0 = 0$
☿ → ☿ → ☿		$R_0 = 1$
☿ → ☿ ☿ / ☿ ☿		$R_0 = 2$

Don't want this.

INFORMATION

⊖ - Medical Doctors (MDs), who made pandemic decisions, are taught in layers that resemble a Geographic Information System (GIS).

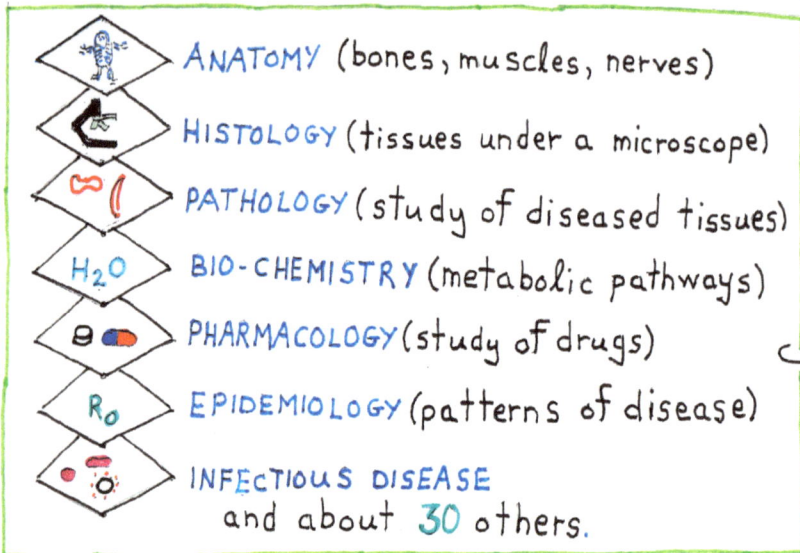

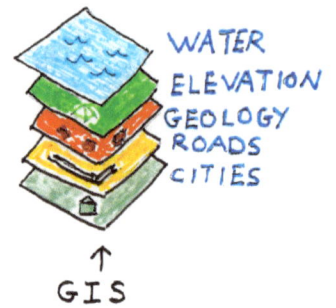

ANATOMY (bones, muscles, nerves)

HISTOLOGY (tissues under a microscope)

PATHOLOGY (study of diseased tissues)

H_2O BIO-CHEMISTRY (metabolic pathways)

PHARMACOLOGY (study of drugs)

R_o EPIDEMIOLOGY (patterns of disease)

INFECTIOUS DISEASE and about 30 others.

↪ Medical school courses

WATER
ELEVATION
GEOLOGY
ROADS
CITIES

↑ GIS

↪ ⊖ - By the end of 4 years of medical school, at which point the "M.D." title is granted, a kind of dogma (set of beliefs) is strongly learned. A kind of faith. This is not necessarily bad; it creates trust and predictability between doctors.

↪ ⊖ - What you get after everyone trains 5 more years (on average) to become a specialist is a faith-based community.

The ♥ is enlarged

Radiologist ('reads' X-rays, CT, MRI, ultrasound)

The surgery can wait.

Cardiac ♥ Surgeon (lots of sharp tools)

I have faith in those words

Other doctors

↪ ⊖ - But if you were not baptized in these layers, you might not share that faith.

I trust doctors. I'll do whatever they suggest.

I'm reluctantly masking up and getting the vaccine.

I'm not against the vaccine. I just don't have enough information. So I'm not getting it.

I don't have faith in you. I'm never getting the vaccine. You can't tell me what to put in my body.

- Well, I'm a fan of doctors, obviously, but I will readily admit that the 'INFORMATION' was heavily focused on COMMANDS:

Do this.
Do that.
Or else.

- What if I manage to get my hands on useful information but I can't read it because it's medical gobbledegook?

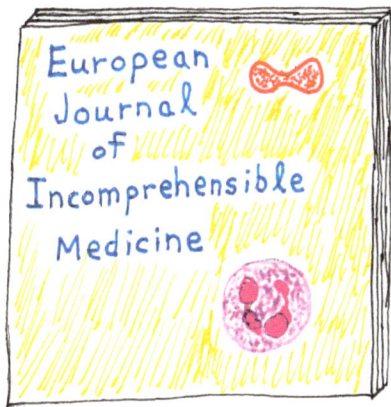

European Journal of Incomprehensible Medicine

→ "Histopathologic findings included exudative Diffuse Alveolar Damage (DAD), hyaline membranes, and interstitial fibrosis."

Hymie Van Strudel, M.D.

- Talk to your doctor.

- You mean talk to my doctor who took early retirement?

- Um, yeah. That one. Listen, it's probably easier to just play soccer and draw icosa-hedrons.

So everything worked out in the end?

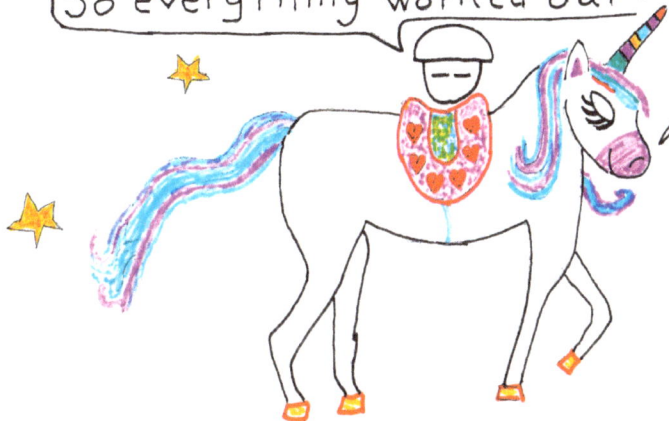

Turns out the toad and I both like ABBA songs so he barfed me up and we're going to a retro concert next week

☻ – If the only thing you've ever seen is a _drawing_ or _animation_ [GIF] of the ☼ coronavirus, well frankly, I don't blame you for not believing it is real. ☼ ← I mean, how convincing is that? Not at all.

– Seeing is believing. So go on a Google Images binge of:

'electron microscope coronavirus'
or
'electron microscope any pathogen named in this guide'

} Imagine if Dr. Snow could have seen Cholera! Pretend ♥ you're him.

☻ – Here is my suggestion if you are curious about ☼ coronavirus or any other medical topic.

⊙ Let's say it's Bubonic Plague, which is morbidly fascinating.

⊙ Search in this order:

1. 'Google Images bubonic plague' ➡ cool and/or gross images.
   ⊙ This is good if you're a visual learner. 👁

2. 'Wikipedia bubonic plague' 🌐 I♥ ↙ [I give $50/y to Wikipedia]
   ⊙ Wikipedia can be hit or miss on medical topics because the whole article can be a copy and paste from an uber-technical medical journal.
   ⊙ But the 1st paragraph is usually a nice summary.

3. 'Mayo Clinic bubonic plague' 🛡
   ⊙ Basic and short summary.
   ⊙ Always focuses on signs and symptoms.

4. 'CDC bubonic plague'
   ⊙ Crazy amounts of information ⟨ for everyone / for doctors

5. 'Medscape bubonic plague'
   ⊙ Unfortunately, this site is for doctors, cuz, you know, we're so SPECIAL
   ⊙ It is very technical medical language.
   ⊙ But the 'Overview' and 'Epidemiology' are superb and readable.
   ⊙ The 'Patho-physiology' explains _exactly_ why you are gonna croak.

6. uptodate.com
   ⊙ $559/year
   ⊙ Doctors only
   ⊙ Highly accurate

or like to think we are.

– That's just what I like. 'WHO bubonic plague' (very much the global perspective)
– You can also search ⟋ 'Medline bubonic plague' (it accesses the U.S. National Library of Medicine (NLM)).
– And if you wanna go mental on all the animals that ☼ coronavirus infects then Google this: 'NCBI taxonomy browser' ➡ Now enter 'coronaviridae' in the 'Search for' box at the top left.
   ↑
National Center for Biotechnology Information

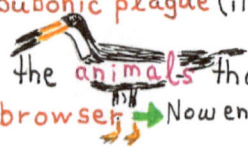

189

muco-ciliary escalator →

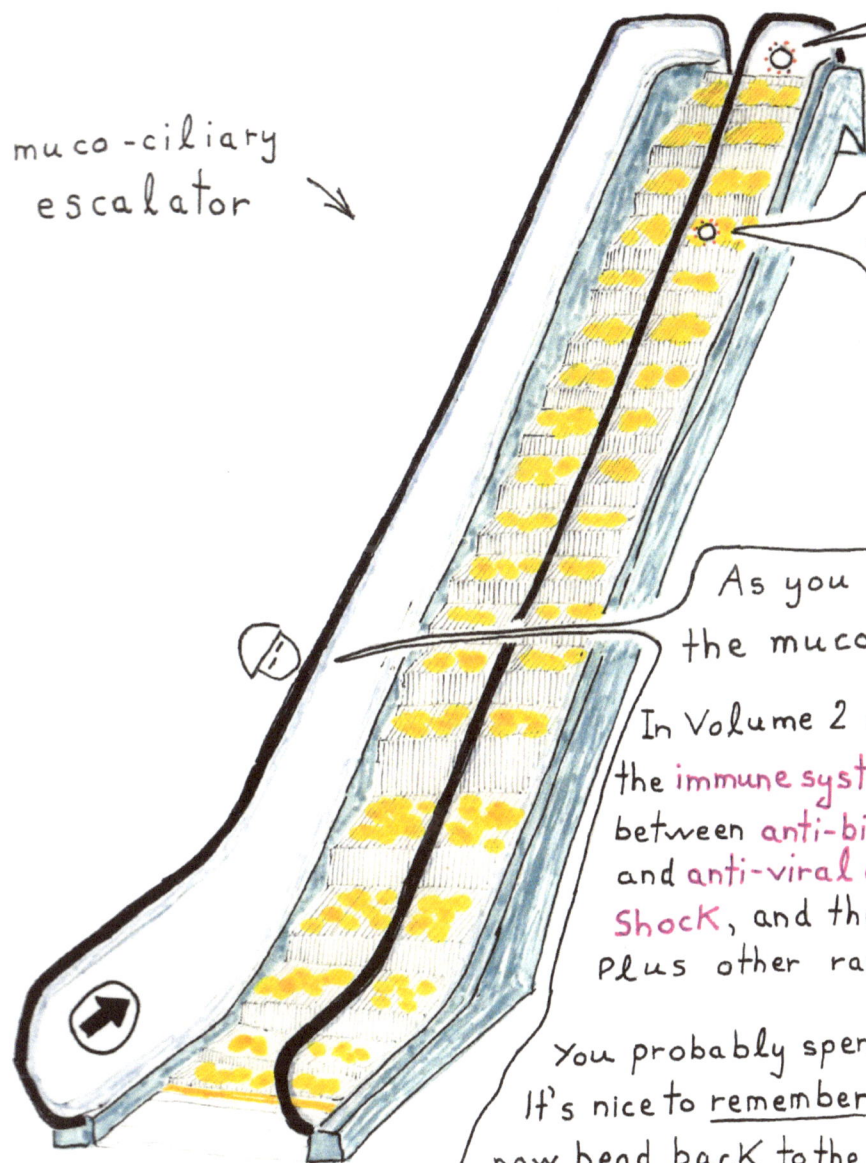

I just got here! I don't want to leave

See you in Volume 2

As you can see, I'm avoiding the mucous.

In Volume 2 we'll explore DNA/RNA, blood, the immune system, vaccines, the difference between anti-biotics (eg., penicillin for bacteria) and anti-viral drugs (for viruses), ventilators, Shock, and the Intensive Care Unit (ICU). Plus other random goodies.

You probably spent 12 hours reading this guide. It's nice to remember what you read. So if you now head back to the Table of Contents and rapidly scan it, you'll see what you've learned. That helps to cement it in your brain.

If you spend 60 minutes in a class (or making notes by yourself), take 2 minutes at the very end to summarize the lesson in 1 to 2 sentences (as in, write it/type it). Then 24 hours later do a quick 2 minute review of the notes plus your summary. This is a powerful tool for converting Short Term Memory (STM) to Long Term Memory (LTM). 4 minutes on top of 60 minutes. The 4 minutes creates cement.

Well, blah blah blah   Ciao for now, Sompoo

Acknowledgements

My great thanks to Jo Blackmore at Granville Island Publishing for your wisdom, oversight, kindness, and, above all, an uncanny sense of what is missing and what does not belong. To book designer Omar Gallegos, thank you for your precision and quest for perfection and for putting up with my incessant changes and multiple tiffs with the same file name. To proofreader Antoinette Mazumdar, thank you for your methodical and fine-grained approach. To publicist David Litvak, thank you for bright smiles, enthusiasm, and creative ideas.

My thanks to the following for suggestions to improve accuracy—some big, some small:
Dr. Anthony Chow, MD. Professor Emeritus of Infectious Disease, University of British Columbia, Vancouver, Canada;
Dr. Cam Goater, PhD. Professor Emeritus of Zoology, University of Victoria, Victoria, Canada;
Dr. Manish Sadarangani, MD. Associate Professor of Infectious Disease, University of British Columbia, Vancouver, Canada;
Dr. Tim Sly, PhD. Professor Emeritus of Epidemiology, Toronto Metropolitan University, Toronto, Canada; and
Dr. Ed Zegarra, PhD. Anthropology. Westwood Press, Portland, Oregon, USA.

My thanks to the following who answered specific questions:
Dr. William R. Gallaher, Ph.D. (Harvard '72) Professor of Microbiology, Immunology and Parasitology, Emeritus Louisiana State University School of Medicine, New Orleans;
Dr. B. L. (Bart) Haagmans, PhD. Associate Professor, Erasmus University Medical Center Department of Viroscience, Rotterdam, Netherlands;
Dr. Edward Holmes, PhD; Marie Bashir Institute for Infectious Diseases and Biosecurity, School of Life and Environmental Sciences and School of Medical Sciences, The University of Sydney, Sydney, Australia;
Dr. Marion Koopmans, DVM, PhD. Head of Erasmus University Medical Center Department of Viroscience, Rotterdam, Netherlands; and
Dr. Jeffery K. Taubenberger, M.D., Ph.D., Chief, Viral Pathogenesis and Evolution Section; Deputy Chief, Laboratory of Infectious Diseases; National Institute of Allergy and Infectious Diseases; National Institutes of Health, Bethesda, Maryland.
Any errors are entirely attributable to me.

My thanks also to Ritchie, Yukta, and the crew at Staples for their patience and care on a million scans of my drawings.
I am blessed with a massive circle of kith and kin, and I thank you all for the pixie dust you sprinkle into my life and for the encouragement during this journey. Some of these comments may appear cryptic, so I apologize dear reader, for the same.
My mother, Dr. Khorshed Karai-Jones, a tireless, devoted obstetrician who had the fortitude of a Viking mixed with the softness and warmth of a Golden Labrador (and would laugh gently at this sobriquet). My father, Richard Basil Jones, a librarian and aspiring writer, whose early morning staccato clacking on a manual typewriter was both inspirational and reveille. I wish both could have seen this funky guide.
Dr. George "Mafa" McMaster. You embody the quest for self-improvement. You taught me the *Attitude of Gratitude* ("Wake up in the morning and name three things to be grateful for"), *Suspend Judgement*, and *Keep Moving Forward*. But you are so not about platitudes. I am forever humbled by your words and wisdom. You are Hiawatha, Marcus Aurelius, and a fortune cookie all wrapped in one.
Sandi Wicks. I've never asked. You've never admitted. But I know you're from the clan of good witches.
Dale "D-Man Raygun Jack Fuenden" Evernden. Bro, it's been all highs since the Keg, that lost cell phone in NYC, the scorpion in Costa Rica, and David Gray's *White Ladder* in Amsterdam. Leah Maestri, from the day you stepped out of the Jetta, it's been hugs, laughs, and a whole lotta motivation. No better UX. Blake, it was you who dotted the eyes of the water mite on page 97. Good job, buddy!
Paul Franco. Always a taekwondo teammate, never a competitor—thank the lord—because you would've knocked me out. You are a true friend, and I treasure our shared moments, even when you elbowed me in the head at the hotel in Aruba at the Pan American Games. I will never forget the 5:30 a.m. gut laps and roundhouse kicks, painful as they were.
Jonny Jarvis. *People, Events, Ideas*—it was ever thus. Our conversations are consistently uplifting to the spirit. Your drive and passion are truly inspiring. You set the bar for no bars. It is always an honor.
Anthony "A-bomb" Volpe. Sci-fi, violence, graphic novels, popcorn. These are the things that make the world go round.
Iwona Szamra. Determination + astute + dark humor = very cool person = Don't go changin'.
Dr. Alan Frankland. "Pull for you, pull for you" (say with a thick Brazilian accent). Armbars, the stock market, tennis, psychiatry. Your breadth is wide, your friendship deep.
Dr. Fia Voutsilakos. Your smiles and kindness are ever-present and welcoming.

David Carstairs-Weir. Since our surprise meeting in the middle of nowhere in Uganda, I have come to know you as an inveterate traveler, canny lawyer, and quiet sage. Thank you for your candor—it's so on point and helpful.

Karl Toews. Too many memories to count, too many practical jokes to forget. I know you are creating a new society based on antimatter. Just send postcards is all I ask.

Roxy Toews. Unpasteurized milk, mashed potatoes, and ready to debate on absolutely any topic—you are the perfect person for a mission to Mars; except you'd refuse to fund such a mission. Oh, the bitter irony.

David Guigui. Tristar, sweat, Orange Julius, high-pitched laughter and friendship.

Reid Monk. Oh, my delightful comrade of etymology, when I say you are "meretricious trash," I know you will take no offense. Conversations with you sparkle like those kaleidoscope toys and are endless joy and laughter.

Dr. Robie Samanta Roy. No one smarter, no one humbler. You do MIT proud. I know you roll your eyes when I ask what angular momentum is and politely offer the Grade 2 explanation you know I will grasp: "Yes, Allen! You are correct. The Moon goes around the Earth. Excellent. Excellent."

Andrew Tang. Polite, fearless, measured. There is no such thing as quit in your DNA. Brutha, you routinely inspire me.

Kenny Yip. Thou most profane of the jet stream, please keep the jokes coming.

Habib Sadeed. You are the bright eyes that see the sky. Bouldering is extra-festive when you are present.

Audrey Farqaleet. Blindfold climbing—doesn't that just say it all? And 10^3 extra thanks for the perpetual support.

Raaf Sief. Here's to edamame and talk of empires, Ozymandias, and all else. You are the wise and humble pharaoh.

Sam Khalil. How did I become such a fan? I think it started with the fact we did more talking than belaying. And texts like this: *I don't think I'd be able to eat cat meat. (Life or death situation aside)*. You will always be my 5.10 Bruthaman.

Bo Trkulja. You are the only person I know who is famous in Japan AND the Czech Republic. Your sense of humor and insight are so refreshing.

Shy Kurtz. Wow, it goes far and wide, old friend. Bender Bay, Panache, drunk on the Brooklyn Bridge, jogging in Vienna, crazy cycling in Tel Aviv, and a wedding in Tanzania. I never tire of your fine mind or escapades.

Steen Sehnert. No greater philosopher hailed from Turks n Caicos. You think in poetry.

Will Jones. You are Ulysses reborn in slacks and a blazer. No one knows what to make of it, which is why you've never been defeated in court. You are unfathomably diligent and a beacon of good cheer.

Dr. Anthony Adili. What I never forget is that the (former) chief of surgery knows the name of every orderly. That's you, buddy. Wise, humble, full of great humor and warmth. Hi Elise. Keep the espresso ready.

Dr. Raj Gill. Your logic is so impressive, and I once opined that you are Spock in doctor greens. *Optics, remember optics*.

Dr. Victor Wong. You've been my second opinion on I don't know how many tough patients. Clinics are so fun with you.

Dr. Nimish Purohit. I marvel at your psychiatry expertise, precision, and adroitness of mind.

Lt. (Ret.) Mike Koren. CFB Gagetown infantryman meets Starbucks barista. What a strange combination, right up your alley: "Dr. Jones, Dr. Koren here. We're out of scalpels in the OR. Call me back."

Sayed Comte Najem. You are a glittering gem of unpredictability, philosophy, and energy. In other words, you either end up a multimillionaire or dead in a dumpster. And why is your Olympic silver medal in storage?

Ebrahim Sadaati. You are the indomitable spirit that wears a bright smile. You are the best of Iran and a true person.

Jack Witt. Gone But Not Forgotten. Our wrestling matches to the death—anywhere, anytime—are special memories.

Amy & Tim Cantor. The Amsterdam duo—you've added last-minute pizzazz, grace, and dreams to my life. I look forward to more mysterious synchronicity.

Robin Hamilton. It's been a long time since those lectures on genetics with Dr. Bush, stinky fruit flies, invertebrate zoology, and embryology. Your wonderful sense of humor, high bar, and calling a spade a spade are deeply valued.

Mike "My White Cousin" Templeton. Black Bond Books, ka-ra-tay, greasy spoon breakfasts, and a million cheesy jokes later. If there's a six-continent road trip, I call shotgun.

Tino "Did I tell you about my CrossFit workout?" Dossantos. Everything that people are supposed to do to live upright, to lead, to have integrity, to pour out joy and vigor—you have it all. I'm continually amazed by you. Such a bromance.

Jamilla Kitchell. I know the dishwasher is none of my business, I just can't help it. I know Tino is your man. You are a delight.

I.B., Julian, Camille, Nate—I send atomic hugs.

Mike Higgins. Boston Pizza. Pork buns. McDonald's on Boxing Day. Bird trivia. Japanese Joinery. You're a special one.

Ura Jones. Droplets, chamomile, hummingbirds, swirls, black ink, pitter patter on windowpanes, you are a beautiful haiku.

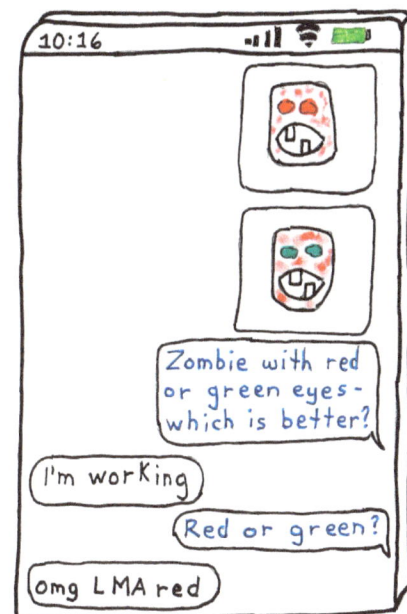

10:16

Zombie with red or green eyes—which is better?

I'm working

Red or green?

omg LMA red

Typical text

Index

Color coding
- Disease, Infection, or Medical Condition
- People

W

X

Y

Z

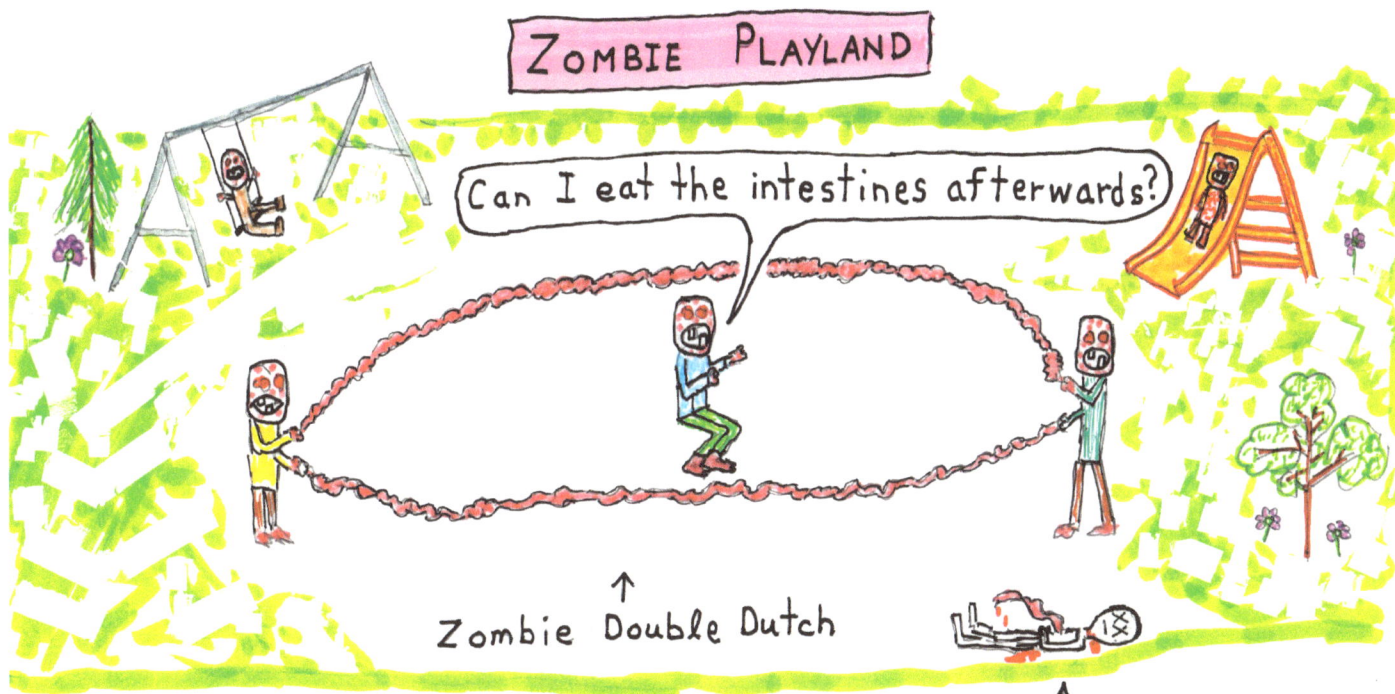

ZOMBIE PLAYLAND

"Can I eat the intestines afterwards?"

Zombie Double Dutch

Park warden (up until 15 minutes ago)

♀ - How many feet of intestines are required for Double Dutch?

♂ - That is an excellent question. The intestines are elastic and can be easily stretched after death. So it depends on how soon Double Dutch begins.

Pesky Organisms at Your Fingertips

Amoebas*	Infection
Amoeba proteus	Does not infect humans. Lives in ponds. 71
Entamoeba histolytica	Amoebic Dysentery, Alexander the Great 71
Plasmodium	Malaria 69, 70
Toxoplasma gondii	Toxoplasmosis (cat litter) 72, 84

*Technically, all these Amoebas are Protista (p. 85). Don't lose sleep over it.

Bacteria	Infection
Bacillus anthracis	Anthrax 58
Bartonella henselae	Cat Scratch Disease 72
Borrelia burgdorferi	Lyme disease 68
Brucella	Brucellosis 36
Clostridium botulinum	Botulism 63
Clostridium difficile	C. diff diarrhea 64
Clostridium perfringens	Gangrene 61, 62
Clostridium tetani	Tetanus 64
E. coli	Urinary Tract Infection (UTI) 59
E. coli O157:H7	Hemolytic Uremic Syndrome (Walkerton) 177, 178
Klebsiella pneumoniae	Pneumonia 110
Meningococcus	Meningitis 68
Mycobacterium tuberculosis	Tuberculosis (TB) 60, 74, 158–160
Pasteurella	Pasteurellosis (cat bite) 72
Propionibacterium acnes	Acne 59, 83
Pseudomonas aeruginosa	Cystic Fibrosis 110, 152
Rickettsia prowazekii	Typhus 8, 9, 17
Ruminococcus	Does not infect humans. Lives in cow stomach. 176
Salmonella	Food poisoning, Typhoid Fever, Typhoid Mary 58, 59
Shigella	Bloody diarrhea 177, 178
Staphylococcus aureus	Infection of bone, skin, lung, and heart valve 49, 65, 66, 165
Streptococcus	
Group A Strep (GAS)	Strep Throat, Flesh Eating Disease, Pneumonia 66
Group B Strep (GBS)	Chorioamnionitis during pregnancy 67
Strep pneumoniae	Pneumonia 65, 66
Vibrio cholera	Cholera 32, 60
Vibrio vulnificus	Necrotizing Soft Tissue Infection (NSTI) in SCUBA divers 60
Yersinia pestis	Plague 14, 17, 33, 51

Fungi	Infection
Aspergillus	Aspergillosis (lung infection) 74, 75, 94, 165, 167, 184
Sporothrix	Rose Handler's Disease 76
Trichophyton	Athlete's Foot, Ringworm 73, 83

Viruses

Human viruses   Infection

Human viruses	Infection
Chickenpox virus	Chickenpox 98
Cold virus (Rhinovirus)	Common Cold 98, 134
Coronavirus	COVID, MERS, SARS 111–152. See next page.
Cowpox virus	Cowpox 96, 98
Coxsackie virus	Myocarditis (Heart ♥ muscle inflammation) 98
Ebola virus	Ebola 18–20, 51
Epstein-Barr Virus	Mononucleosis (Kissing Disease) 98
Hepatitis (A, B, C, D, E) virus	Hepatitis 98
Herpes Simplex Virus	Oral Herpes 98
HIV / AIDS virus	AIDS 60, 84, 98
Influenza virus	Influenza 22–29
Measles virus	Measles 98
Mumps virus	Mumps 98
Polio virus	Polio 99
Rabies virus	Rabies 100–110
Rubella virus	Rubella, Congenital Rubella Syndrome 84, 98
Smallpox virus	Smallpox 21
Varicella Zoster Virus (VZV)	Shingles 98
Yellow Fever virus	Yellow Fever 15–17, 35, 98
Zika virus	Birth defects 84

Amoeba viruses
Matryoshka virus 94

Animal viruses
Chronic Bee Paralysis virus 96
Cowpox virus (humans also) 96, 98
Dragonfly Cyclovirus 97
Orsay virus 96
Rabies virus (humans also) 88, 90, 98

Bacteria viruses
Bacteriophage 93

Fungi viruses
Aspergillus fumigatus polymycovirus-1 94
Cryphonectria HypoVirus-1 (CHV-1) 94

Plant viruses
Rembrandt Tulip-Breaking virus 95
Tobacco Mosaic virus 122
Tulip-Breaking virus 95

TORCH infections of pregnancy 84
T: *Toxoplasma* 72, 84
O: Other: *Coronavirus, Zika virus, Syphilis corkscrew* 84
R: *Rubella virus* 84, 98
C: *Cytomegalovirus* 84
H: *Herpes simplex virus, HIV virus, Hepatitis C virus,* 84, 98

Vector

Think of the 'vector' as the courier from Hell delivering an awful package (the organism).

ABOUT THE AUTHOR

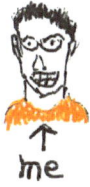

me

Allen Sohrab Jones
(but my mom always
called me Toto
which means 'little boy'
in Swahili)

Bachelor of Science (BSc) — MAJOR zoology
— MINOR chemistry

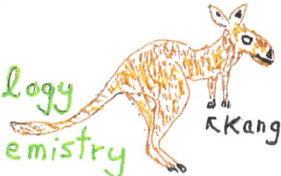

↖ Kangaroo

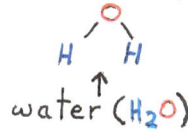

water (H_2O)

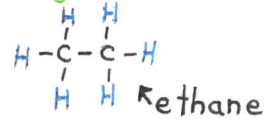

↖ ethane

Master of Science (MSc)
↳ neuro-science, specifically Spinal Cord Electro-physiology

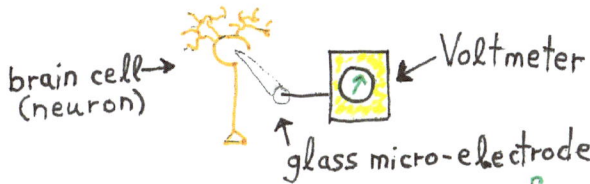

brain cell → (neuron)

Voltmeter

↑ glass micro-electrode

Medical Doctor (MD)

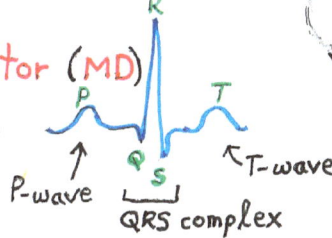

P-wave   QRS complex   ↖ T-wave

ECG

Electro Cardio Gram

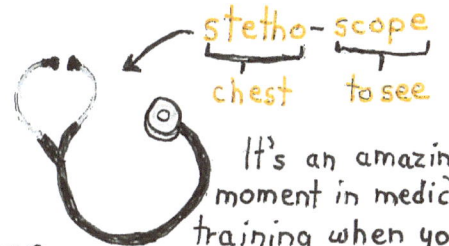

stetho- scope
chest   to see

It's an amazing
moment in medical
training when you
listen to the ♡ sounds
and understand how they
relate to the ECG.

Family Physician a.k.a. General Practitioner (GP)
officially, CCFP (AM)

Certification in the College of Family Physicians of Canada

That means added competence in
Addiction Medicine

So if I heard you
correctly, it burns
when you pee, and
you hate your mom?

Yes to
both

me   patient

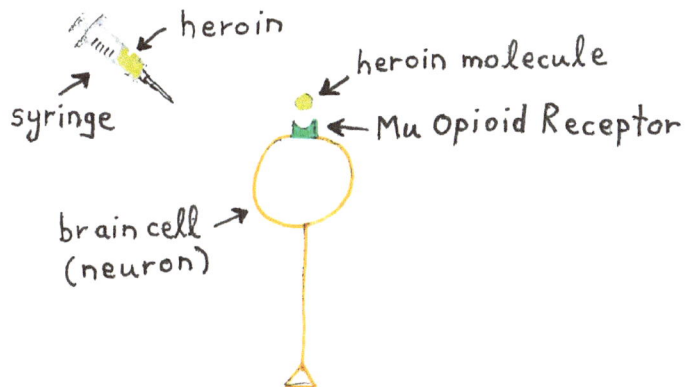

heroin

syringe

heroin molecule

← Mu Opioid Receptor

brain cell → (neuron)

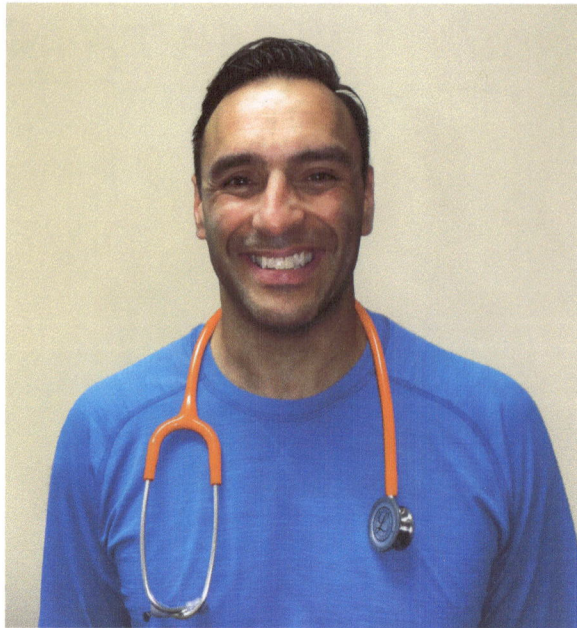

Allen Sohrab Jones was born in Nairobi, Kenya and is a dual citizen of the United States and Canada. Educated in Canada, he received a B.Sc. in zoology from Brandon University, Manitoba and an M.Sc. in neuroscience from the University of Manitoba, then an M.D. from the University of British Columbia, Vancouver. He completed his internship as a primary care physician at McMaster University in Hamilton. This was followed by ten months of emergency medicine training, including electives in toxicology at Bellevue Hospital in Manhattan, trauma at the R Adams Cowley Shock Trauma Center in Baltimore, and aerospace medicine at the Kennedy Space Center in Cape Canaveral. Subsequently, he became certified in addiction medicine, his current area of practice. Concurrently, he is a surgical assistant for procedures in orthopedic surgery, plastic surgery, and general surgery.

Dr. Jones started writing and drawing *The Hidden Zoo Inside You* during the pandemic after realizing the extent of misinformation regarding the coronavirus, and was further motivated by his passion for explaining and demystifying the language of medicine to his patients. When not working on his book or with his patients, he enjoys rock climbing and traveling. He currently lives in Vancouver.